HEALTH AND WELLNESS

ILLNESS AMONG AMERICANS

HEALTH AND WELLNESS

ILLNESS AMONG AMERICANS

Barbara Wexler

INFORMATION PLUS® REFERENCE SERIES
Formerly Published by Information Plus, Wylie, Texas

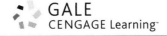

GALE
CENGAGE Learning™

Detroit • New York • San Francisco • New Haven, Conn • Waterville, Maine • London

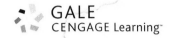

Health and Wellness: Illness among Americans

Barbara Wexler

Kepos Media, Inc.: Paula Kepos and Janice Jorgensen, Series Editors

Project Editors: Elizabeth Manar, Kathleen J. Edgar

Rights Acquisition and Management: Jhanay Williams

Composition: Evi Abou-El-Seoud, Mary Beth Trimper

Manufacturing: Cynde Lentz

For product information and technology assistance, contact us at
Gale Customer Support, 1-800-877-4253.
For permission to use material from this text or product,
submit all requests online at **www.cengage.com/permissions.**
Further permissions questions can be e-mailed to
permissionrequest@cengage.com

Cover photograph: Image copyright Vadim Ponomarenko, 2010. Used under license of Shutterstock.com.

While every effort has been made to ensure the reliability of the information presented in this publication, Gale, a part of Cengage Learning, does not guarantee the accuracy of the data contained herein. Gale accepts no payment for listing; and inclusion in the publication of any organization, agency, institution, publication, service, or individual does not imply endorsement of the editors or publisher. Errors brought to the attention of the publisher and verified to the satisfaction of the publisher will be corrected in future editions.

Gale
27500 Drake Rd.
Farmington Hills, MI 48331-3535

ISBN-13: 978-0-7876-5103-9 (set)   ISBN-10: 0-7876-5103-6 (set)
ISBN-13: 978-1-4144-4120-7   ISBN-10: 1-4144-4120-7

ISSN 1549-0971

This title is also available as an e-book.
ISBN-13: 978-1-4144-7003-0 (set)
ISBN-10: 1-4144-7003-7 (set)
Contact your Gale sales representative for ordering information.

Printed in the United States of America
1 2 3 4 5 6 7 14 13 12 11 10

TABLE OF CONTENTS

PREFACE vii

CHAPTER 1

Defining Health and Wellness 1

This chapter defines health and wellness and outlines measures of public health such as birthrates and fertility rates, the incidence of birth defects, and infant mortality. It also explores life expectancy, mortality, the leading causes of death, and Americans' assessments of their own health.

CHAPTER 2

Prevention of Disease 35

Americans have significantly improved their health through environmental and lifestyle changes. Many prevention measures, including programs to avert mental illness and suicide, are defined and described in this chapter.

CHAPTER 3

Diagnosing Disease: The Process of Detecting and Identifying Illness 53

An accurate diagnosis of disease can be made only when professionals understand a patient's medical history, conduct a physical examination, and use the appropriate diagnostic tests. This chapter surveys the procedures that physicians and other health professionals use, as well as technological advances that improve the speed and accuracy of diagnosis.

CHAPTER 4

Genetics and Health 63

Genetic disorders are conditions caused by mutations to genes, which are passed from one generation to the next. This chapter focuses on cystic fibrosis, Huntington's disease, muscular dystrophy, sickle-cell disease, and Tay-Sachs disease, which are all genetic disorders. The chapter also reports on the use, role, and ethical considerations of genetic testing.

CHAPTER 5

Chronic Diseases: Causes, Treatment, and Prevention 79

Chronic diseases are prolonged illnesses that do not resolve spontaneously and are rarely cured completely. The causes, treatment, prevalence, and prevention of cardiovascular diseases, cancer, respiratory diseases, and diabetes are investigated in this chapter.

CHAPTER 6

Degenerative Diseases 111

Degenerative diseases are noninfectious disorders that progressively disable otherwise healthy people. This chapter looks at the prevalence, causes, and treatment of arthritis, osteoporosis, multiple sclerosis, Parkinson's disease, and Alzheimer's disease.

CHAPTER 7

Infectious Diseases 125

Infectious diseases are caused by microorganisms transmitted from one person to another through casual contact or through bodily fluids. The focus of this chapter is on the most prevalent infectious diseases; the chapter also discusses how such diseases can be prevented through immunization. In-depth examinations of seasonal influenza, HIV/AIDS, tuberculosis, SARS, Lyme disease, and West Nile virus are included, as are emerging threats such as antibiotic-resistant bacteria and H1N1 pandemic influenza.

CHAPTER 8

Mental Health and Illness 151

Millions of American adults and children suffer from mental illnesses, including depression, schizophrenia, attention deficit hyperactivity disorder, autism spectrum disorders, anxiety disorders, and eating disorders. This chapter also examines the prevalence of suicide.

CHAPTER 9

Complementary and Alternative Medicine 175

Interest in complementary and alternative medicine has skyrocketed in the United States since the 1990s. This chapter details a variety of such treatments and considers the evidence about their effectiveness.

IMPORTANT NAMES AND ADDRESSES 193

RESOURCES 195

INDEX 197

PREFACE

Health and Wellness: Illness among Americans is part of the *Information Plus Reference Series*. The purpose of each volume of the series is to present the latest facts on a topic of pressing concern in modern American life. These topics include the most controversial and studied social issues in the 21st century: abortion, capital punishment, care for the elderly, crime, the environment, immigration, minorities, social welfare, women, world poverty, youth, and many more. Even though this series is written especially for high school and undergraduate students, it is an excellent resource for anyone in need of factual information on current affairs.

By presenting the facts, it is the intention of Gale, Cengage Learning to provide its readers with everything they need to reach an informed opinion on current issues. To that end, there is a particular emphasis in this series on the presentation of scientific studies, surveys, and statistics. These data are generally presented in the form of tables, charts, and other graphics placed within the text of each book. Every graphic is directly referred to and carefully explained in the text. The source of each graphic is presented within the graphic itself. The data used in these graphics are drawn from the most reputable and reliable sources, such as from the various branches of the U.S. government and from major organizations and associations. Every effort has been made to secure the most recent information available. Readers should bear in mind that many major studies take years to conduct and that additional years often pass before the data from these studies are made available to the public. Therefore, in many cases the most recent information available in 2010 is dated from 2007 or 2008. Older statistics are sometimes presented as well, if they are landmark studies or of particular interest and no more-recent information exists.

Even though statistics are a major focus of the *Information Plus Reference Series*, they are by no means its only content. Each book also presents the widely held positions and important ideas that shape how the book's subject is discussed in the United States. These positions are explained in detail and, where possible, in the words of their proponents. Some of the other material to be found in these books includes historical background, descriptions of major events related to the subject, relevant laws and court cases, and examples of how these issues play out in American life. Some books also feature primary documents or have pro and con debate sections that provide the words and opinions of prominent Americans on both sides of a controversial topic. All material is presented in an even-handed and unbiased manner; readers will never be encouraged to accept one view of an issue over another.

HOW TO USE THIS BOOK

"Health" describes the condition of being free from disease. "Wellness," however, is an important complement to health that represents a person's overarching efforts to live happily and successfully—emotionally, intellectually, occupationally, physically, socially, and spiritually. This book examines health and wellness among Americans, including the ways in which illness is currently prevented, identified, and treated. Many common types of chronic, degenerative, genetic, and infectious diseases are described, as are the concepts of mental health and illness. Both traditional and selected complementary and alternative medicine are covered.

Health and Wellness: Illness among Americans consists of nine chapters and three appendixes. Each chapter is devoted to a particular aspect of health and wellness in the United States. For a summary of the information covered in each chapter, please see the synopses provided in the Table of Contents. Chapters generally begin with an overview of the basic facts and background information on the chapter's topic, then proceed to examine subtopics of particular interest. For example, Chapter 7: Infectious Diseases describes illnesses caused by viruses, bacteria, parasites, and fungi.

Explored next are notifiable diseases, and the three most frequently reported infectious diseases in the United States in 2007. The chapter details resistant strains of bacteria, the appropriate use of antibiotics, and the prevention of infectious diseases via immunization. The remainder of the chapter describes influenza and the 2009–10 H1N1 influenza pandemic, as well as tuberculosis, HIV/AIDS, Lyme disease, West Nile virus, severe acute respiratory syndrome (SARS), and bioterrorism. Readers can find their way through a chapter by looking for the section and subsection headings, which are clearly set off from the text. Or, they can refer to the book's extensive index if they already know what they are looking for.

Statistical Information

The tables and figures featured throughout *Health and Wellness: Illness among Americans* will be of particular use to readers in learning about this issue. These tables and figures represent an extensive collection of the most recent and important statistics on health and wellness, as well as related issues—for example, graphics cover the prevalence of overweight and obesity, how Americans assess their own health, leading causes of death in the United States, recommended immunizations, the cases of H1N1 pandemic influenza, and the symptoms of depression. Gale, Cengage Learning believes that making this information available to readers is the most important way to fulfill the goal of this book: to help readers understand the issues and controversies surrounding health and wellness in the United States and reach their own conclusions.

Each table or figure has a unique identifier appearing above it, for ease of identification and reference. Titles for the tables and figures explain their purpose. At the end of each table or figure, the original source of the data is provided.

To help readers understand these often complicated statistics, all tables and figures are explained in the text. References in the text direct readers to the relevant statistics. Furthermore, the contents of all tables and figures are fully indexed. Please see the opening section of the index at the back of this volume for a description of how to find tables and figures within it.

Appendixes

Besides the main body text and images, *Health and Wellness: Illness among Americans* has three appendixes. The first is the Important Names and Addresses directory.

Here, readers will find contact information for a number of government and private organizations that can provide further information on aspects of health and wellness. The second appendix is the Resources section, which can also assist readers in conducting their own research. In this section, the author and editors of *Health and Wellness: Illness among Americans* describe some of the sources that were most useful during the compilation of this book. The final appendix is the index.

ADVISORY BOARD CONTRIBUTIONS

The staff of Information Plus would like to extend its heartfelt appreciation to the Information Plus Advisory Board. This dedicated group of media professionals provides feedback on the series on an ongoing basis. Their comments allow the editorial staff who work on the project to continually make the series better and more user-friendly. The staff's top priority is to produce the highest-quality and most useful books possible, and the Information Plus Advisory Board's contributions to this process are invaluable.

The members of the Information Plus Advisory Board are:

- Kathleen R. Bonn, Librarian, Newbury Park High School, Newbury Park, California

- Madelyn Garner, Librarian, San Jacinto College, North Campus, Houston, Texas

- Anne Oxenrider, Media Specialist, Dundee High School, Dundee, Michigan

- Charles R. Rodgers, Director of Libraries, Pasco-Hernando Community College, Dade City, Florida

- James N. Zitzelsberger, Library Media Department Chairman, Oshkosh West High School, Oshkosh, Wisconsin

COMMENTS AND SUGGESTIONS

The editors of the *Information Plus Reference Series* welcome your feedback on *Health and Wellness: Illness among Americans*. Please direct all correspondence to:

Editors
Information Plus Reference Series
27500 Drake Rd.
Farmington Hills, MI 48331-3535

CHAPTER 1
DEFINING HEALTH AND WELLNESS

The potential for us to help Americans live longer, healthier lives is almost unlimited.

—Thomas R. Frieden, director of the Centers for Disease Control and Prevention, quoted by Shelia M. Poole in "Science, Efficiency to Drive CDC Changes" (*Atlanta Journal-Constitution*, January 1, 2010)

Many definitions of health exist. Most definitions consider health as an outcome—the result of actions to produce it, such as good nutrition, immunization to prevent disease, or medical treatment to cure disease. The *American Heritage Dictionary* defines health as fixed and measurable: "The overall condition of an organism at a given time." However, health may also be viewed as the active process used by individuals and communities to adapt to ever-changing environments.

The 11th edition of *Merriam-Webster's Collegiate Dictionary* defines health as "the condition of being sound in body, mind, or spirit; *esp*: freedom from physical disease or pain." However, in 1948 the constitution of the World Health Organization (WHO; October 2006, http://www.who.int/gov ernance/eb/who_constitution_en.pdf) defined health as "a state of complete physical, mental and social well-being and not merely the absence of disease or infirmity." This still widely used definition is broader and more positive than simply defining health as the absence of illness or disability.

Expanding on the WHO definition of health and the commonly understood idea of well-being, the concept of wellness has been defined by the National Wellness Institute (2009, http://www.nationalwellness.org/index.php?id _tier= 2&id_c=26) as "an active process through which people become aware of, and make choices toward, a more successful existence." Wellness encompasses how people feel about various aspects of their life. Six interrelated aspects of human life are commonly known to make up wellness:

- Emotional wellness refers to awareness, sensitivity, and acceptance of feelings and the ability to successfully express and manage one's feelings. Emotional wellness enables people to cope with stress, maintain satisfying relationships with family and friends, and assume responsibility for their actions.

- Intellectual wellness emphasizes knowledge, learning, creativity, problem solving, and lifelong interest in learning and new ideas.

- Occupational wellness relates to preparing for and pursuing work that is meaningful, satisfying, and consistent with one's interests, aptitudes, and personal beliefs.

- Physical wellness is more than simply freedom from disease. The physical dimension of wellness concentrates on the prevention of illness and encourages exercise, healthy diet, and knowledgeable, appropriate use of the health care system. Physical wellness requires individuals to take personal responsibility for actions and choices that affect their health. Examples of healthy choices include wearing a seatbelt in automobiles, wearing a helmet when bicycling, and avoiding tobacco and illegal drugs.

- Social wellness is acting in harmony with nature, family, and others in the community. The pursuit of social wellness may involve actions to protect or preserve the environment or contribute to the health and well-being of the community by performing volunteer work.

- Spiritual wellness involves finding meaning in life and acting purposefully in a manner that is consistent with one's deeply held values and beliefs.

The concept of wellness is broader and includes more facets of human life than the traditional definition of health, and the two differ in an important way. When defined as the absence of disease, health may be measured and assessed objectively. For example, a physical examination and the results of laboratory testing enable a physician to determine that a patient is free of disease and thereby healthy.

In comparison, wellness is a more subjective quality and is more difficult to measure. The determination of wellness relies on self-assessment and self-report. Furthermore, it is not necessarily essential that individuals satisfy the traditional definition of good health to rate themselves high in terms of wellness. For instance, many people with chronic (ongoing or long-term) conditions—such as diabetes, heart disease, or asthma—or disabilities report high levels of satisfaction with each of the six dimensions of wellness. Similarly, people in apparently good health may not necessarily give themselves high scores in all six aspects of wellness.

THE HEALTH OF THE UNITED STATES

A primary indicator of the well-being of a nation is the health of its people. Many factors can affect a person's health: heredity, race or ethnicity, gender, income, education, geography, exposure to violent crime, exposure to environmental agents, exposure to infectious diseases, and access to and availability of health care.

Whereas physicians and other health practitioners observe the influences of these factors as they care for individual patients, epidemiologists (public health researchers who study the occurrence of disease) examine the distribution and rates of diseases and injuries in the population. Practitioners and epidemiologists each apply the scientific method to achieve their objectives, but they use it in varying ways. For instance, in the database step of the scientific method, practitioners use history and physical examination to determine a patient's health, and epidemiologists use surveillance and description. Practitioners seek to deliver appropriate treatment to individual patients, and epidemiologists recommend actions to prevent the spread of disease or otherwise improve the health of an entire community or population.

Epidemiologists and other public health professionals assess health by determining the incidence and prevalence rates of disease and disability in a given community. Incidence is a measure of the rate at which people without a disease develop the disease during a specific time period, and it describes the continuing occurrence of disease over time. For example, a researcher might report that men in a given community aged 65 and older have a 2% incidence of heart disease. Prevalence describes a group or population at a specific point in time. For example, the prevalence of high blood pressure found during screening at a health fair on a specific day might be 22%.

Other measures of the health of a population, such as natality (birth) and mortality (death) rates, are known as vital health statistics. This chapter provides an overview of vital health statistics and the health status of Americans.

BIRTHRATES AND FERTILITY RATES

The birthrate is the number of live births per 1,000 women. The fertility rate, however, is the number of live births per 1,000 women between 15 and 44 years of age,

which is generally considered a woman's prime childbearing years.

In "Births: Final Data for 2006" (*National Vital Statistics Reports*, vol. 57, no. 7, January 7, 2009), Joyce A. Martin et al. of the Centers for Disease Control and Prevention (CDC) report that there were 4.3 million live births in the United States in 2006, up 3% from 2005 and the largest number of births in more than four decades. This number translates to a birthrate of 14.2 births per 1,000 women in 2006, which was up slightly from 14 births per 1,000 women in 2005. (See Table 1.1.) Between the most recent high point, 16.7 in 1990, and the most recent low point, 13.9 in 2002, the crude birthrate declined 16.8%. Even though Martin et al. report that the number of live births has increased steadily since 1970, the birthrate and fertility rate have remained relatively stable since 2000.

Birthrates have continued to decline for teenagers aged 15 to 19. In 2006 the number of live births per 1,000 teens aged 15 to 17 was 22, down from the last most recent peak of 38.5 in 1991, a decrease of 43%. (See Table 1.1.) The number of live births per 1,000 young women aged 18 to 19 in 2006 was 73, down from a peak of 94 in 1991, a decrease of 22%.

In contrast, the birthrate for women aged 25 to 34 was relatively unchanged from 2005 to 2006. (See Table 1.1.) The birthrate for women aged 35 to 39, which has been increasing dramatically since 1980, increased in 2006—from 46.3 births per 1,000 women in 2005 to 47.3 births per 1,000 women. The birthrate for this age group increased from 31.7 births per 1,000 women in 1990 to 47.3 births per 1,000 women in 2006, an increase of 49%.

Women aged 20 to 29 continued to have the highest birthrates, although the proportion of births to these women has declined in recent years. (See Table 1.1.)

Fertility rates focus on live births to mothers in the primary childbearing age group: 15 to 44. In 2006 the fertility rate for American women was 68.5 births per 1,000 women, which is a slight increase from 2005 (66.7) but a decrease from 1990 (70.9). (See Table 1.1.) Total fertility rates, which offer an index of lifetime fertility among women, not only varied by age but also by race and ethnic origin. In 2006 the fertility rate for Hispanic women (101.5 births per 1,000 Hispanic women aged 15 to 44) was 41% higher than for non-Hispanic white women (59.5 births per 1,000).

Factors other than age, race, and ethnicity can have dramatic effects on fertility and birthrates. For example, even though women who are currently married and living with their husbands have much higher fertility rates than those women who have never married or are separated, widowed, or divorced, Martin et al. report that the birthrate for unmarried women has been increasing steadily over the years, from 24.5 births per 1,000 unmarried women aged 15

TABLE 1.1

Crude birth rates, fertility rates, and birth rates, by age of mother, according to race and Hispanic origin, selected years 1950–2006

[Data are based on birth certificates]

Race, Hispanic origin, and year	Crude birth rate[a]	Fertility rate[b]	10–14 years	15–19 years Total	15–17 years	18–19 years	20–24 years	25–29 years	30–34 years	35–39 years	40–44 years	45–54 years[c]
All races					Live births per 1,000 women							
1950	24.1	106.2	1.0	81.6	40.7	132.7	196.6	166.1	103.7	52.9	15.1	1.2
1960	23.7	118.0	0.8	89.1	43.9	166.7	258.1	197.4	112.7	56.2	15.5	0.9
1970	18.4	87.9	1.2	68.3	38.8	114.7	167.8	145.1	73.3	31.7	8.1	0.5
1980	15.9	68.4	1.1	53.0	32.5	82.1	115.1	112.9	61.9	19.8	3.9	0.2
1981	15.8	67.3	1.1	52.2	32.0	80.0	112.2	111.5	61.4	20.0	3.8	0.2
1982	15.9	67.3	1.1	52.4	32.3	79.4	111.6	111.0	64.1	21.2	3.9	0.2
1983	15.6	65.7	1.1	51.4	31.8	77.4	107.8	108.5	64.9	22.0	3.9	0.2
1984	15.6	65.5	1.2	50.6	31.0	77.4	106.8	108.7	67.0	22.9	3.9	0.2
1985	15.8	66.3	1.2	51.0	31.0	79.6	108.3	111.0	69.1	24.0	4.0	0.2
1986	15.6	65.4	1.3	50.2	30.5	79.6	107.4	109.8	70.1	24.4	4.1	0.2
1987	15.7	65.8	1.3	50.6	31.7	78.5	107.9	111.6	72.1	26.3	4.4	0.2
1988	16.0	67.3	1.3	53.0	33.6	79.9	110.2	114.4	74.8	28.1	4.8	0.2
1989	16.4	69.2	1.4	57.3	36.4	84.2	113.8	117.6	77.4	29.9	5.2	0.2
1990	16.7	70.9	1.4	59.9	37.5	88.6	116.5	120.2	80.8	31.7	5.5	0.2
1991	16.2	69.3	1.4	61.8	38.5	94.0	115.3	117.2	79.2	31.9	5.5	0.2
1992	15.8	68.4	1.4	60.3	37.5	93.7	113.7	115.7	79.6	32.3	5.9	0.3
1993	15.4	67.0	1.4	59.0	37.4	91.1	111.3	113.2	79.9	32.7	6.1	0.3
1994	15.0	65.9	1.4	58.2	37.2	90.3	109.2	111.0	80.4	33.4	6.4	0.3
1995	14.6	64.6	1.3	56.0	35.5	87.7	107.5	108.8	81.1	34.0	6.6	0.3
1996	14.4	64.1	1.2	53.5	33.3	84.7	107.8	108.6	82.1	34.9	6.8	0.3
1997	14.2	63.6	1.1	51.3	31.4	82.1	107.3	108.3	83.0	35.7	7.1	0.4
1998	14.3	64.3	1.0	50.3	29.9	80.9	108.4	110.2	85.2	36.9	7.4	0.4
1999	14.2	64.4	0.9	48.8	28.2	79.0	107.9	111.2	87.1	37.8	7.4	0.4
2000	14.4	65.9	0.9	47.7	26.9	78.1	109.7	113.5	91.2	39.7	8.0	0.5
2001	14.1	65.3	0.8	45.3	24.7	76.1	106.2	113.4	91.9	40.6	8.1	0.5
2002	13.9	64.8	0.7	43.0	23.2	72.8	103.6	113.6	91.5	41.4	8.3	0.5
2003	14.1	66.1	0.6	41.6	22.4	70.7	102.6	115.6	95.1	43.8	8.7	0.5
2004	14.0	66.3	0.7	41.1	22.1	70.0	101.7	115.5	95.3	45.4	8.9	0.5
2005	14.0	66.7	0.7	40.5	21.4	69.9	102.2	115.5	95.8	46.3	9.1	0.6
2006	14.2	68.5	0.6	41.9	22.0	73.0	105.9	116.7	97.7	47.3	9.4	0.6
Race of child:[d] white												
1950	23.0	102.3	0.4	70.0	31.3	120.5	190.4	165.1	102.6	51.4	14.5	1.0
1960	22.7	113.2	0.4	79.4	35.5	154.6	252.8	194.9	109.6	54.0	14.7	0.8
1970	17.4	84.1	0.5	57.4	29.2	101.5	163.4	145.9	71.9	30.0	7.5	0.4
1980	14.9	64.7	0.6	44.7	25.2	72.1	109.5	112.4	60.4	18.5	3.4	0.2
Race of mother:[e] white												
1980	15.1	65.6	0.6	45.4	25.5	73.2	111.1	113.8	61.2	18.8	3.5	0.2
1981	15.0	64.8	0.5	44.9	25.4	71.5	108.3	112.3	61.0	19.0	3.4	0.2
1982	15.1	64.8	0.6	45.0	25.5	70.8	107.7	111.9	64.0	20.4	3.6	0.2
1983	14.8	63.4	0.6	43.9	25.0	68.8	103.8	109.4	65.3	21.3	3.6	0.2
1984	14.8	63.2	0.6	42.9	24.3	68.4	102.7	109.8	67.7	22.2	3.6	0.2
1985	15.0	64.1	0.6	43.3	24.4	70.4	104.1	112.3	69.9	23.3	3.7	0.2
1986	14.8	63.1	0.6	42.3	23.8	70.1	102.7	110.8	70.9	23.9	3.8	0.2
1987	14.9	63.3	0.6	42.5	24.6	68.9	102.3	112.3	73.0	25.9	4.1	0.2
1988	15.0	64.5	0.6	44.4	26.0	69.6	103.7	114.8	75.4	27.7	4.5	0.2
1989	15.4	66.4	0.7	47.9	28.1	72.9	106.9	117.8	78.1	29.7	4.9	0.2
1990	15.8	68.3	0.7	50.8	29.5	78.0	109.8	120.7	81.7	31.5	5.2	0.2
1991	15.3	66.7	0.8	52.6	30.5	83.3	108.8	118.0	80.2	31.8	5.2	0.2
1992	15.0	66.1	0.8	51.4	29.9	83.2	107.7	116.9	80.8	32.1	5.7	0.2
1993	14.6	64.9	0.8	50.6	30.0	81.5	106.1	114.7	81.3	32.6	5.9	0.3
1994	14.3	64.2	0.8	50.5	30.4	81.2	105.0	113.0	82.2	33.5	6.2	0.3
1995	14.1	63.6	0.8	49.5	29.6	80.2	104.7	111.7	83.3	34.2	6.4	0.3
1996	13.9	63.3	0.7	47.5	28.0	77.6	105.3	111.7	84.6	35.3	6.7	0.3
1997	13.7	62.8	0.7	45.5	26.6	75.0	104.5	111.3	85.7	36.1	6.9	0.3
1998	13.8	63.6	0.6	44.9	25.6	74.1	105.4	113.6	88.5	37.5	7.3	0.4
1999	13.7	64.0	0.6	44.0	24.4	73.0	105.0	114.9	90.7	38.5	7.4	0.4
2000	13.9	65.3	0.6	43.2	23.3	72.3	106.6	116.7	94.6	40.2	7.9	0.4
2001	13.7	65.0	0.5	41.2	21.4	70.8	103.7	117.0	95.8	41.3	8.0	0.5
2002	13.5	64.8	0.5	39.4	20.5	68.0	101.6	117.4	95.5	42.4	8.2	0.5
2003	13.6	66.1	0.5	38.3	19.8	66.2	100.6	119.5	99.3	44.8	8.7	0.5
2004	13.5	66.1	0.5	37.7	19.5	65.0	99.2	118.6	99.1	46.4	8.9	0.5
2005	13.4	66.3	0.5	37.0	18.9	64.7	99.2	118.3	99.3	47.3	9.0	0.6
2006	13.7	68.0	0.5	38.2	19.4	67.5	102.5	119.1	100.9	48.2	9.2	0.6

TABLE 1.1

Crude birth rates, fertility rates, and birth rates, by age of mother, according to race and Hispanic origin, selected years 1950–2006

[CONTINUED]

[Data are based on birth certificates]

Race, Hispanic origin, and year	Crude birth rate[a]	Fertility rate[b]	10–14 years	15–19 years Total	15–17 years	18–19 years	20–24 years	25–29 years	30–34 years	35–39 years	40–44 years	45–54 years[c]
Race of child:[d] black or African American												
1960	31.9	153.5	4.3	156.1	—	—	295.4	218.6	137.1	73.9	21.9	1.1
1970	25.3	115.4	5.2	140.7	101.4	204.9	202.7	136.3	79.6	41.9	12.5	1.0
1980	22.1	88.1	4.3	100.0	73.6	138.8	146.3	109.1	62.9	24.5	5.8	0.3
Race of mother:[e] black or African American												
1980	21.3	84.7	4.3	97.8	72.5	135.1	140.0	103.9	59.9	23.5	5.6	0.3
1981	20.8	82.0	4.0	94.5	69.3	131.0	136.5	102.3	57.4	23.1	5.4	0.3
1982	20.7	80.9	4.0	94.3	69.7	128.9	135.4	101.3	57.5	23.3	5.1	0.4
1983	20.2	78.7	4.1	93.9	69.6	127.1	131.9	98.4	56.2	23.3	5.1	0.3
1984	20.1	78.1	4.4	94.1	69.2	128.1	132.2	98.4	56.7	23.3	4.8	0.2
1985	20.4	78.8	4.5	95.4	69.3	132.4	135.0	100.2	57.9	23.9	4.6	0.3
1986	20.5	78.9	4.7	95.8	69.3	135.1	137.3	101.1	59.3	23.8	4.8	0.3
1987	20.8	80.1	4.8	97.6	72.1	135.8	142.7	104.3	60.6	24.6	4.8	0.2
1988	21.5	82.6	4.9	102.7	75.7	142.7	149.7	108.2	63.1	25.6	5.1	0.3
1989	22.3	86.2	5.1	111.5	81.9	151.9	156.8	114.4	66.3	26.7	5.4	0.3
1990	22.4	86.8	4.9	112.8	82.3	152.9	160.2	115.5	68.7	28.1	5.5	0.3
1991	21.8	84.8	4.7	114.8	83.5	157.6	159.7	112.0	67.3	28.2	5.5	0.2
1992	21.1	82.4	4.6	111.3	80.5	156.3	156.2	109.7	67.0	28.6	5.6	0.2
1993	20.2	79.6	4.5	107.3	78.9	150.2	150.2	106.4	66.6	29.0	5.9	0.3
1994	19.1	75.9	4.5	102.9	75.1	146.2	142.9	101.5	65.0	28.7	5.9	0.3
1995	17.8	71.0	4.1	94.4	68.5	135.0	133.7	95.6	63.0	28.4	6.0	0.3
1996	17.3	69.2	3.5	89.6	63.3	130.5	133.2	94.3	62.0	28.7	6.1	0.3
1997	17.1	69.0	3.1	86.3	59.3	127.7	135.2	95.0	62.6	29.3	6.5	0.3
1998	17.1	69.4	2.8	83.5	55.4	124.8	138.4	97.5	63.2	30.0	6.6	0.3
1999	16.8	68.5	2.5	79.1	50.5	120.6	137.9	97.3	62.7	30.2	6.5	0.3
2000	17.0	70.0	2.3	77.4	49.0	118.8	141.3	100.3	65.4	31.5	7.2	0.4
2001	16.3	67.6	2.0	71.8	43.9	114.0	133.2	99.2	64.8	31.6	7.2	0.4
2002	15.7	65.8	1.8	66.6	40.0	107.6	127.1	99.0	64.4	31.5	7.4	0.4
2003	15.7	66.3	1.6	63.8	38.2	103.7	126.1	100.4	66.5	33.2	7.7	0.5
2004	16.0	67.6	1.6	63.3	37.2	104.4	127.7	103.6	67.9	34.0	7.9	0.5
2005	16.2	69.0	1.7	62.0	35.5	104.9	129.9	105.9	70.3	35.3	8.5	0.5
2006	16.8	72.1	1.5	64.6	36.6	110.2	135.8	109.4	74.0	36.6	8.5	0.5
American Indian or Alaska Native mothers[e]												
1980	20.7	82.7	1.9	82.2	51.5	129.5	143.7	106.6	61.8	28.1	8.2	*
1985	19.8	78.6	1.7	79.2	47.7	124.1	139.1	109.6	62.6	27.4	6.0	*
1990	18.9	76.2	1.6	81.1	48.5	129.3	148.7	110.3	61.5	27.5	5.9	*
1991	18.3	73.9	1.6	84.1	51.9	134.2	143.8	105.6	60.8	26.4	5.8	0.4
1992	17.9	73.1	1.6	82.4	52.3	130.5	142.3	107.0	61.0	26.7	5.9	*
1993	17.0	69.7	1.4	79.8	51.5	126.3	134.2	103.5	59.5	25.5	5.6	*
1994	16.0	65.8	1.8	76.4	48.4	123.7	126.5	98.2	56.6	24.8	5.4	0.3
1995	15.3	63.0	1.6	72.9	44.6	122.2	123.1	91.6	56.5	24.3	5.5	*
1996	14.9	61.8	1.6	68.2	42.7	113.3	123.5	91.1	56.5	24.4	5.5	*
1997	14.7	60.8	1.5	65.2	41.0	107.1	122.5	91.6	56.0	24.4	5.4	0.3
1998	14.8	61.3	1.5	64.7	39.7	106.9	125.1	92.0	56.8	24.6	5.3	*
1999	14.2	59.0	1.4	59.9	36.5	98.0	120.7	90.6	53.8	24.3	5.7	0.3
2000	14.0	58.7	1.1	58.3	34.1	97.1	117.2	91.8	55.5	24.6	5.7	0.3
2001	13.7	58.1	1.0	56.3	31.4	94.8	115.0	90.4	55.9	24.7	5.7	0.3
2002	13.8	58.0	0.9	53.8	30.7	89.2	112.6	91.8	56.4	25.4	5.8	0.3
2003	13.8	58.4	1.0	53.1	30.6	87.3	110.0	93.5	57.4	25.4	5.5	0.4
2004	14.0	58.9	0.9	52.5	30.0	87.0	109.7	92.8	58.0	26.8	6.0	0.2
2005	14.2	59.9	0.9	52.7	30.5	87.6	109.2	93.8	60.1	27.0	6.0	0.3
2006	14.9	63.1	0.9	55.0	30.7	93.0	115.4	97.8	61.8	28.4	6.1	0.4
Asian or Pacific Islander mothers[e]												
1980	19.9	73.2	0.3	26.2	12.0	46.2	93.3	127.4	96.0	38.3	8.5	0.7
1985	18.7	68.4	0.4	23.8	12.5	40.8	83.6	123.0	93.6	42.7	8.7	1.2
1990	19.0	69.6	0.7	26.4	16.0	40.2	79.2	126.3	106.5	49.6	10.7	1.1
1991	18.3	67.1	0.8	27.3	16.3	42.2	73.8	118.9	103.3	49.2	11.2	1.1
1992	17.9	66.1	0.7	26.5	15.4	41.9	71.7	114.6	102.7	50.7	11.1	0.9
1993	17.3	64.3	0.7	26.5	16.1	41.2	68.1	110.3	101.2	49.4	11.2	0.9
1994	17.1	63.9	0.7	26.6	16.3	41.3	66.4	108.0	102.2	50.4	11.5	1.0
1995	16.7	62.6	0.7	25.5	15.6	40.1	64.2	103.7	102.3	50.1	11.8	0.8
1996	16.5	62.3	0.6	23.5	14.7	36.8	63.5	102.8	104.1	50.2	11.9	0.8
1997	16.2	61.3	0.5	22.3	14.0	34.9	61.2	101.6	102.5	51.0	11.5	0.9

TABLE 1.1

Crude birth rates, fertility rates, and birth rates, by age of mother, according to race and Hispanic origin, selected years 1950–2006 [CONTINUED]

[Data are based on birth certificates]

Race, Hispanic origin, and year	Crude birth rate[a]	Fertility rate[b]	10–14 years	Age of mother 15–19 years Total	15–17 years	18–19 years	20–24 years	25–29 years	30–34 years	35–39 years	40–44 years	45–54 years[c]
Asian or Pacific Islander mothers[e]												
1998	15.9	60.1	0.5	22.2	13.8	34.5	59.2	98.7	101.6	51.4	11.8	0.9
1999	15.9	60.9	0.4	21.4	12.4	33.9	58.9	100.8	104.3	52.9	11.3	0.9
2000	17.1	65.8	0.3	20.5	11.6	32.6	60.3	108.4	116.5	59.0	12.6	0.8
2001	16.4	64.2	0.2	19.8	10.3	32.8	59.1	106.4	112.6	56.7	12.3	0.9
2002	16.5	64.1	0.3	18.3	9.0	31.5	60.4	105.4	109.6	56.5	12.5	0.9
2003	16.8	66.3	0.2	17.4	8.8	29.8	59.6	108.5	114.6	59.9	13.5	0.9
2004	16.8	67.1	0.2	17.3	8.9	29.6	59.8	108.6	116.9	62.1	13.6	1.0
2005	16.5	66.6	0.2	17.0	8.2	30.1	61.1	107.9	115.0	61.8	13.8	1.0
2006	16.6	67.5	0.2	17.0	8.8	29.5	63.2	108.4	116.9	63.0	14.1	1.0
Hispanic or Latina mothers[e,f]												
1980	23.5	95.4	1.7	82.2	52.1	126.9	156.4	132.1	83.2	39.9	10.6	0.7
1990	26.7	107.7	2.4	100.3	65.9	147.7	181.0	153.0	98.3	45.3	10.9	0.7
1991	26.5	106.9	2.4	104.6	69.2	155.5	184.6	150.0	95.1	44.7	10.7	0.6
1992	26.1	106.1	2.5	103.3	68.9	153.9	185.2	148.8	94.8	45.3	11.0	0.6
1993	25.4	103.3	2.6	101.8	68.5	151.1	180.0	146.0	93.2	44.1	10.6	0.6
1994	24.7	100.7	2.6	101.3	69.9	147.5	175.7	142.4	91.1	43.4	10.7	0.6
1995	24.1	98.8	2.6	99.3	68.3	145.4	171.9	140.4	90.5	43.7	10.7	0.6
1996	23.8	97.5	2.4	94.6	64.2	140.0	170.2	140.7	91.3	43.9	10.7	0.6
1997	23.0	94.2	2.1	89.6	61.1	132.4	162.6	137.5	89.6	43.4	10.7	0.6
1998	22.7	93.2	1.9	87.9	58.5	131.5	159.3	136.1	90.5	43.4	10.8	0.6
1999	22.5	93.0	1.9	86.8	56.9	129.5	157.3	135.8	92.3	44.5	10.6	0.6
2000	23.1	95.9	1.7	87.3	55.5	132.6	161.3	139.9	97.1	46.6	11.5	0.6
2001	23.0	96.0	1.6	86.4	52.8	135.5	163.5	140.4	97.6	47.9	11.6	0.7
2002	22.6	94.4	1.4	83.4	50.7	133.0	164.3	139.4	95.1	47.8	11.5	0.7
2003	22.9	96.9	1.3	82.3	49.7	132.0	163.4	144.4	102.0	50.8	12.2	0.7
2004	22.9	97.8	1.3	82.6	49.7	133.5	165.3	145.6	104.1	52.9	12.4	0.7
2005	23.1	99.4	1.3	81.7	48.5	134.6	170.0	149.2	106.8	54.2	13.0	0.8
2006	23.4	101.5	1.3	83.0	47.9	139.7	177.0	152.4	108.5	55.6	13.3	0.8
White, not Hispanic or Latina mothers[e,f]												
1980	14.2	62.4	0.4	41.2	22.4	67.7	105.5	110.6	59.9	17.7	3.0	0.1
1990	14.4	62.8	0.5	42.5	23.2	66.6	97.5	115.3	79.4	30.0	4.7	0.2
1991	13.9	60.9	0.5	43.4	23.6	70.6	95.7	112.1	77.7	30.2	4.7	0.2
1992	13.4	60.0	0.5	41.7	22.7	69.8	93.9	110.6	78.3	30.4	5.1	0.2
1993	13.1	58.9	0.5	40.7	22.7	67.7	92.2	108.2	79.0	31.0	5.4	0.2
1994	12.8	58.2	0.5	40.4	22.7	67.6	90.9	106.6	80.2	32.0	5.7	0.2
1995	12.5	57.5	0.4	39.3	22.0	66.2	90.2	105.1	81.5	32.8	5.9	0.3
1996	12.3	57.1	0.4	37.6	20.6	64.0	90.1	104.9	82.8	33.9	6.2	0.3
1997	12.2	56.8	0.4	36.0	19.3	62.1	90.0	104.8	84.3	34.8	6.5	0.3
1998	12.2	57.6	0.3	35.3	18.3	60.9	91.2	107.4	87.2	36.4	6.8	0.4
1999	12.1	57.7	0.3	34.1	17.1	59.4	90.6	108.6	89.5	37.3	6.9	0.4
2000	12.2	58.5	0.3	32.6	15.8	57.5	91.2	109.4	93.2	38.8	7.3	0.4
2001	11.8	57.7	0.3	30.3	14.0	54.8	87.1	108.9	94.3	39.8	7.5	0.4
2002	11.7	57.4	0.2	28.5	13.1	51.9	84.3	109.3	94.4	40.9	7.6	0.5
2003	11.8	58.5	0.2	27.4	12.4	50.0	83.5	110.8	97.6	43.2	8.1	0.5
2004	11.6	58.4	0.2	26.7	12.0	48.7	81.9	110.0	97.1	44.8	8.2	0.5
2005	11.5	58.3	0.2	25.9	11.5	48.0	81.4	109.1	96.9	45.6	8.3	0.5
2006	11.6	59.5	0.2	26.6	11.8	49.3	83.4	109.1	98.1	46.3	8.4	0.6
Black or African American, not Hispanic or Latina mothers[e,f]												
1980	22.9	90.7	4.6	105.1	77.2	146.5	152.2	111.7	65.2	25.8	5.8	0.3
1990	23.0	89.0	5.0	116.2	84.9	157.5	165.1	118.4	70.2	28.7	5.6	0.3
1991	22.4	87.0	4.9	118.2	86.1	162.2	164.8	115.1	68.9	28.7	5.6	0.2
1992	21.6	84.5	4.8	114.7	82.9	161.1	160.8	112.8	68.4	29.1	5.7	0.2
1993	20.7	81.5	4.6	110.5	81.1	154.6	154.5	109.2	68.1	29.4	5.9	0.3
1994	19.5	77.5	4.6	105.7	77.0	150.4	146.8	104.1	66.3	29.1	6.0	0.3
1995	18.2	72.8	4.2	97.2	70.4	139.2	137.8	98.5	64.4	28.8	6.1	0.3
1996	17.6	70.7	3.6	91.9	64.8	134.1	137.0	96.7	63.2	29.1	6.2	0.3
1997	17.4	70.3	3.2	88.3	60.7	131.0	138.8	97.2	63.6	29.6	6.5	0.3
1998	17.5	70.9	2.9	85.7	56.8	128.2	142.5	99.9	64.4	30.4	6.7	0.3
1999	17.1	69.9	2.6	81.0	51.7	123.9	142.1	99.8	63.9	30.6	6.5	0.3
2000	17.3	71.4	2.4	79.2	50.1	121.9	145.4	102.8	66.5	31.8	7.2	0.4
2001	16.6	69.1	2.1	73.5	44.9	116.7	137.2	102.1	66.2	32.1	7.3	0.4

TABLE 1.1

Crude birth rates, fertility rates, and birth rates, by age of mother, according to race and Hispanic origin, selected years 1950–2006

[CONTINUED]

[Data are based on birth certificates]

Race, Hispanic origin, and year	Crude birth rate[a]	Fertility rate[b]	10–14 years	Age of mother								
				15–19 years			20–24 years	25–29 years	30–34 years	35–39 years	40–44 years	45–54 years[c]
				Total	15–17 years	18–19 years						
Black or African American, not Hispanic or Latina mothers[e,f]												
2002	16.1	67.4	1.9	68.3	41.0	110.3	131.0	102.1	66.1	32.1	7.5	0.4
2003	15.9	67.1	1.6	64.7	38.7	105.3	128.1	102.1	67.4	33.4	7.7	0.5
2004	15.8	67.0	1.6	63.1	37.1	103.9	126.9	103.0	67.4	33.7	7.8	0.5
2005	15.7	67.2	1.7	60.9	34.9	103.0	126.8	103.0	68.4	34.3	8.2	0.5
2006	16.5	70.6	1.6	63.7	36.2	108.4	133.2	107.1	72.6	36.0	8.3	0.5

—Data not available.

*Rates based on fewer than 20 births are considered unreliable and are not shown.

[a]Live births per 1,000 population.

[b]Total number of live births regardless of age of mother per 1,000 women 15–44 years of age.

[c]Prior to 1997, data are for live births to mothers 45–49 years of age per 1,000 women 45–49 years of age. Starting with 1997 data, rates are for live births to mothers 45–54 years of age per 1,000 women 45–49 years of age.

[d]Live births are tabulated by race of child.

[e]Live births are tabulated by race and/or Hispanic origin of mother.

[f]Prior to 1993, data from states lacking an Hispanic-origin item on the birth certificate were excluded. Rates in 1985 were not calculated because estimates for the Hispanic and non-Hispanic populations were note available.

Notes: Data are based on births adjusted for under registration for 1950 and on registered births for all other years. Starting with 1970 data, births to persons who were not residents of the 50 states and the District of Columbia are excluded. Starting with *Health, United States,* 2003, rates for 1991–1999 were revised using intercensal population estimates based on the 2000 census. Rates for 2000 were computed using the 2000 census counts and starting in 2001 rates were computed using 2000-based postcensal estimates. The race groups, white, black, American Indian or Alaska Native, and Asian or Pacific Islander, include persons of Hispanic and non-Hispanic origin. Persons of Hispanic origin may be of any race. Starting with 2003 data, some states reported multiple-race data. The multiple-race data for these states were bridged to the single-race categories of the 1977 Office of Management and Budget standards for comparability with other states. Interpretation of trend data should take into consideration expansion of reporting areas and immigration.

SOURCE: "Table 4. Crude Birth Rates, Fertility Rates, and Birth Rates by Age, Race, and Hispanic Origin of Mother: United States, Selected Years 1950–2006," in *Health, United States, 2008. With Chartbook,* Centers for Disease Control and Prevention, National Center for Health Statistics, 2009, http://www.cdc.gov/nchs/data/hus/hus08.pdf (accessed December 12, 2009)

to 44 in 1975 to 50.6 births per 1,000 unmarried women in 2006. The proportion of all births to unmarried women grew to record levels—38.5% of all births in 2006, up from 36.9% in 2005. This increase has occurred in spite of the decrease in the birthrate among teenagers. The CDC cites successful health prevention programs that include education emphasizing prevention of pregnancy through abstinence (avoiding sexual contact) and contraception (measures to prevent pregnancy) as one factor that has contributed to the decline in teen birthrates along with a leveling-off of sexual activity among teens.

Prenatal Care, Prematurity, and Low Birth Weight

Early prenatal care, which is defined as pregnancy-related care started in the first trimester (one to three months), can detect and often correct many potential health problems early in pregnancy. Regular visits to a physician or clinic usually give the mother-to-be information and encouragement about eating properly, exercising regularly, taking prenatal vitamins, and avoiding harmful substances such as alcohol, drugs, and tobacco. The benefits of these preventive measures can literally make a lifetime of difference for a newborn.

Sophisticated diagnostic medical procedures, such as obstetric ultrasound scans and amniocentesis, can be performed to detect possible birth defects and other prenatal problems. Ultrasound uses high-frequency sound waves to compose a picture of the fetus and is used to detect and assess fetal development and malformations in the fetus. During amniocentesis, a physician inserts a needle through the abdominal wall into the uterus to obtain a small sample of the amniotic fluid surrounding the fetus. When tested in a laboratory, this fluid can reveal chromosomal abnormalities, metabolic disorders, and physical abnormalities.

Pregnant women older than age 35 are generally advised to undergo amniocentesis and other diagnostic testing, because they are at greater risk than younger women of giving birth to babies with chromosomal abnormalities such as Down syndrome (also called Down's syndrome). Instead of the normal 46 chromosomes, newborns with Down syndrome have an extra copy of chromosome 21, giving them a total of 47 chromosomes. These children have varying degrees of mental retardation, and, according to the Cincinnati Children's Hospital Medical Center, in "Heart-Related Syndromes: Down Syndrome (Trisomy 21)" (August 2009, http://www.cincinnatichildrens.org/health/heart-encyclopedia/disease/syndrome/down.htm), up to 50% have congenital heart diseases. Mikyong Shin et al. estimate in "Prevalence of Down Syndrome among Children and Adolescents in 10 Regions of the United States" (*Pediatrics*, vol. 124, no. 6, December 2009) that the average prevalence of children born with Down syndrome is 1 in 800 births, or 5,400 infants in the United States each year.

Ideally, every woman should receive prenatal care, and according to the National Center for Health Statistics (NCHS), the United States is capable of delivering prenatal care to nearly all pregnant women during the first trimester of pregnancy. However, not all mothers-to-be seek or receive early or adequate prenatal care. The Adequacy of Prenatal Care Utilization Index explains that adequate/adequate plus prenatal care is defined as pregnancy-related care beginning in the first four months of pregnancy with the appropriate number of visits for gestational age. The March of Dimes Foundation, a national voluntary organization that seeks to improve infant health by preventing birth defects, notes in "Quick Facts: Prenatal Care Overview" (2010, http://www.marchofdimes.com/peristats/tlanding.aspx?=&reg=99&lev=0&top=5&=&=&slev=1&=dv=qf) that 74.7% of expectant mothers received adequate/adequate plus prenatal care in 2002, whereas 14% received intermediate care (less than optimal but not inadequate) and 11.3% received inadequate care.

The percentage of expectant mothers receiving prenatal care beginning in the first trimester increased from 68% in 1970 to 83.9% in 2005. (See Table 1.2.) In *Health, United States, 2009* (2010, http://www.cdc.gov/nchs/data/hus/hus09.pdf), the NCHS indicates that this percentage decreased slightly to 83.2% in 2006. More Asian or Pacific Islander (84.8%) and white (84.7%) women received early prenatal care than did Hispanic or Latina (77.3%), African-American (76%), or Native American or Alaskan Native (69.5%) women in 2006. From 1970 to 2005 the percentage of expectant mothers who received inadequate prenatal care (care beginning during the third trimester or no prenatal care at all) declined by more than half, from 7.9% to 3.5%. (See Table 1.2.) The NCHS notes that by 2006 this percentage increased slightly to 3.6%. In 2006 more Native American or Alaskan Native (8.1%), African-American (5.7%), and Hispanic or Latina (5%) women failed to receive adequate prenatal care than did white (3.2%) or Asian or Pacific Islander (3.1%) women.

Overall, the percentage of women of all races and ethnicities who received early prenatal care increased slightly from the period of 1997–99 to the period of 2003–05. (See Table 1.3.) There was, however, a wide geographic variation in the percentage of women obtaining early prenatal care during the 2003–05 period, from a low of 69.8% of women in New Mexico to a high of 90.1% of women in Rhode Island. Within states, the percentage of women who received prenatal care varied widely. For example, in New Jersey 63.2% of African-American women received early prenatal care, compared with 88.6% of white women.

However, Martin et al. note that women were less likely to receive prenatal care in 2006 than in 2005. The percentage of mothers beginning prenatal care in the first trimester of pregnancy declined, whereas the percentage of mothers beginning late care (care beginning in the third trimester of pregnancy) or receiving no care increased. (See Table 1.4.)

The March of Dimes cites the lack of health insurance, transportation, and child care; inconvenient health care provider service hours; unplanned pregnancies; and cultural and personal factors as obstacles preventing expectant mothers from receiving prenatal care.

Early prenatal care can prevent or reduce the risk of low birth weight (LBW). Infants who weigh less than 5 pounds, 8 ounces (2,500 g) at birth are considered to be of LBW. Those born weighing less than 3 pounds, 4 ounces (1,500 g) are called very low birth weight (VLBW). LBW may result from premature birth (infants born before 37 weeks of pregnancy are considered premature), poor maternal nutrition, teen pregnancy, drug and alcohol use, smoking, or sexually transmitted diseases.

Infants who are premature or have LBWs are at greater risk of death and disability than infants of normal weight. About 80% of women at risk for delivering an LBW infant can be identified in the first prenatal visit, and interventions can be made to try to prevent problems. Between 1997–99 and 2003–05 the proportion of newborn babies weighing less than 2,500 grams increased from 7.6% to 8.1%. (See Table 1.5.) The NCHS notes in *Health, United States, 2009* that by 2004–06 this proportion increased slightly to 8.2%.

As with access to prenatal care, the percent of LBW live births varies by geography, race, and ethnicity. Among non-Hispanic African-Americans, 13.8% of live births in 2003–05 weighed less than 2,500 grams, compared with 7.9% of Asian or Pacific Islander births, 7.4% of Native American or Alaskan Native births, 7.2% of non-Hispanic white births, and 6.8% of Hispanic or Latina births. (See Table 1.5.) Over 15% of live births to non-Hispanic African-American mothers in Colorado and in South Carolina were LBW, compared with 5.3% of LBW live births to non-Hispanic white mothers in Alaska. In 2006 the percentage of LBW births increased to 7% of Hispanic births, 7.3% of white births, and 14% of African-American births. (See Table 1.6.)

The usual length of pregnancy is 40 weeks from the first day of the woman's last menstrual period. Infants born prematurely do not have fully formed organ systems. If, however, the premature infant is born with a birth weight comparable to a full-term baby and has organ systems only slightly undeveloped, the chances of survival are great. Premature infants of VLBW are susceptible to many risks and are less likely to survive than full-term infants. If they survive, they may suffer from mental retardation, developmental disabilities, and other abnormalities of the nervous system.

TABLE 1.2

Crude birth rates, fertility rates, and birth rates, by age of mother, according to race and Hispanic origin, selected years 1970–2005

[Data are based on birth certificates]

Prenatal care, race, and Hispanic origin of mother	1970	1980	1990	2000	37 states, DC, and NYC		7 states	
					2004[a]	2005[a]	2004[b]	2005[b]
					Percent of live births[c]			
Prenatal care began during 1st trimester								
All races	68.0	76.3	75.8	83.2	84.2	83.9	72.9	72.8
White	72.3	79.2	79.2	85.0	85.9	85.5	75.9	75.6
Black or African American	44.2	62.4	60.6	74.3	76.2	76.3	57.8	58.1
American Indian or Alaska Native	38.2	55.8	57.9	69.3	69.5	69.6	58.7	59.5
Asian or Pacific Islander[d]	—	73.7	75.1	84.0	85.3	85.3	69.1	70.0
Hispanic or Latina[e]	—	60.2	60.2	74.4	77.7	77.6	56.5	57.0
Mexican	—	59.6	57.8	72.9	77.5	77.6	53.2	53.3
Puerto Rican	—	55.1	63.5	78.5	79.7	80.1	62.6	63.3
Cuban	—	82.7	84.8	91.7	86.4	86.2	71.2	72.5
Central and South American	—	58.8	61.5	77.6	77.5	76.6	56.6	58.2
Other and unknown Hispanic or Latina	—	66.4	66.4	75.8	76.7	76.9	58.8	59.0
Not Hispanic or Latina:[e]								
White	—	81.2	83.3	88.5	89.0	88.7	78.0	77.8
Black or African American	—	60.8	60.7	74.3	76.3	76.5	58.9	59.3
Prenatal care began during 3rd trimester or no prenatal care								
All races	7.9	5.1	6.1	3.9	3.5	3.5	6.2	6.0
White	6.3	4.3	4.9	3.3	3.0	3.0	5.1	5.0
Black or African American	16.6	8.9	11.3	6.7	5.7	5.7	11.9	11.3
American Indian or Alaska Native	28.9	15.2	12.9	8.6	8.1	8.2	11.2	11.8
Asian or Pacific Islander[d]	—	6.5	5.8	3.3	3.0	3.0	6.8	6.8
Hispanic or Latina[e]	—	12.0	12.0	6.3	5.2	5.1	11.0	10.8
Mexican	—	11.8	13.2	6.9	5.3	5.0	12.7	12.4
Puerto Rican	—	16.2	10.6	4.5	4.0	4.1	8.5	7.8
Cuban	—	3.9	2.8	1.4	2.8	2.5	*6.5	*5.2
Central and South American	—	13.1	10.9	5.4	5.1	5.6	9.4	9.7
Other and unknown Hispanic or Latina	—	9.2	8.5	5.9	6.0	5.6	11.4	11.3
Not Hispanic or Latina:[e]								
White	—	3.5	3.4	2.3	2.1	2.2	4.5	4.4
Black or African American	—	9.7	11.2	6.7	5.7	5.6	11.4	10.8

— Data not available.

[a]Data for 2004 and 2005 include the 39 reporting areas (37 states, DC, and NYC) that used the 1989 revision of the U.S. Standard Certificate of Live Birth in 2005. Reporting areas that have adopted the 2003 revision of the U.S. Standard Certificate of Live Birth are excluded because prenatal care data based on the 2003 revision are not comparable with data based on the 1989 and earlier revisions of the U.S. Standard Certificate of Live Birth.

[b]Data for 2004 and 2005 include the 7 reporting areas that adopted the 2003 revision of the U.S. Standard Certificate of Live Birth in 2004. Reporting areas that used the 1989 revision of the U.S. Standard Certificate of Live Birth are excluded because prenatal care data based on the 2003 revision are not comparable with data based on the 1989 or earlier revisions.

[c]Excludes live births where trimester when prenatal care began is unknown.

[d]Starting with 2003 data, estimates are not available for Asian or Pacific Islander subgroups during the transition from single-race to multiple-race reporting.

[e]Prior to 1993, data from states lacking an Hispanic-origin item on the birth certificate were excluded. Data for non-Hispanic white and non-Hispanic black women for years prior to 1989 are not nationally representative and are provided for comparison with Hispanic data.

Notes: Prior to 2003, all data are based on the 1989 and earlier revisions of the U.S. Standard Certificate of Live Birth. Data for 1970 and 1975 exclude births that occurred in states not reporting prenatal care. Starting with 2004 data, data for states adopting the 2003 revision of the U.S. Standard Certificate of Live Birth are shown separately. The race groups, white, black, American Indian or Alaska Native, and Asian or Pacific Islander, include persons of Hispanic and non-Hispanic origin. Persons of Hispanic origin may be of any race. Starting with 2003 data, some states reported multiple-race data. The multiple-race data for these states were bridged to the single-race categories of the 1977 Office of Management and Budget standards for comparability with other states. Interpretation of trend data should take into consideration changes in reporting areas and immigration. Data for additional years are available.

SOURCE: "Table 7. Prenatal Care for Live Births, by Detailed Race and Hispanic Origin of Mother: United States, Selected Years 1970–2000, and Selected States, 2004–2005," in *Health, United States, 2008. With Chartbook*, Centers for Disease Control and Prevention, National Center for Health Statistics, 2009, http://www.cdc.gov/nchs/data/hus/hus08.pdf (accessed December 12, 2009)

A severe medical condition called hyaline membrane disease (or respiratory distress syndrome) commonly affects premature infants. It is caused by the inability of immature lungs to function properly. Occurring immediately after birth, the disease may cause infant death within hours. Intensive care of affected infants includes the use of a mechanical ventilator to facilitate breathing. Also, premature infants' immature gastrointestinal systems preclude them from taking in nourishment properly. Unable to suck and swallow, they must be fed through a nasogastric feeding tube (nutrient-rich formula enters through a tube inserted into the stomach via the nose).

LBW and VLBW are major predictors of infant morbidity (illness or disease) and mortality. Martin et al. explain that for LBW infants, the risk of dying during the first year of life is more than five times that of normal-weight infants; the risk for VLBW infants is nearly 100 times higher. The risk of

TABLE 1.3

Early prenatal care, 1997–99, 2000–02, and 2003–05

[Data are based on birth certificates]

Percent of live births with early prenatal care (beginning in the 1st trimester)

Geographic division and state	All races 1997–1999	All races 2000–2002	All races 2003–2005	Not Hispanic or Latina — White 1997–1999	White 2000–2002	White 2003–2005	Not Hispanic or Latina — Black or African American 1997–1999	Black 2000–2002	Black 2003–2005	Hispanic or Latina[c] 1997–1999	Hispanic 2000–2002	Hispanic 2003–2005	American Indian or Alaska Native[d] 1997–1999	AIAN 2000–2002	AIAN 2003–2005	Asian or Pacific Islander[d] 1997–1999	API 2000–2002	API 2003–2005
United States	82.9	83.4	84.1	88.1	88.6	88.9	73.2	74.6	76.3	74.1	75.7	77.7	68.8	69.5	69.8	83.0	84.3	85.2
New England:										79.1	80.9	80.8	78.4	82.9	83.8	84.2	85.6	86.3
Connecticut	88.8	88.8	87.6	92.4	92.5	92.4	80.6	82.3	78.1	78.5	78.3	76.6	78.5	83.8	85.1	86.3	88.0	87.7
Maine	89.0	88.3	88.0	89.5	88.6	88.4	82.7	76.8	78.5	82.0	80.4	81.1	71.0	81.3	77.3	82.2	85.2	84.9
Massachusetts	89.3	89.6	89.6	92.1	92.5	92.2	79.4	78.9	80.4	78.7	81.4	82.9	78.1	84.5	88.5	83.9	84.8	86.3
New Hampshire[a]	90.0	91.1	—	90.5	91.9	—	75.8	78.4	—	79.2	81.9	—	84.5	85.2	—	84.5	86.7	—
Rhode Island	90.1	90.6	90.1	92.6	93.1	92.8	81.2	83.2	82.6	83.4	86.7	86.6	82.7	80.9	81.1	81.9	84.0	80.6
Vermont[a]	87.8	88.9	—	87.9	89.2	—	78.1	73.2	—	79.1	82.5	—	*82.8	*80.0	—	77.5	85.9	—
Middle Atlantic:[b]										71.5	72.1	73.4	76.0	77.4	71.7	78.6	79.0	80.8
New Jersey	81.4	80.2	79.3	89.5	89.1	88.6	64.2	63.6	63.2	70.7	68.2	67.2	71.9	72.9	66.9	83.6	83.6	84.9
New York[a]	85.7	84.7	—	89.3	88.7	—	71.1	70.2	—	74.6	73.7	—	74.9	75.0	—	83.6	82.6	—
New York City	80.4	76.6	79.9	87.2	86.0	88.4	70.3	71.5	74.4	70.9	74.0	77.7	79.4	78.7	85.1	74.7	74.2	77.8
East North Central:										72.6	74.1	77.8	73.5	75.5	76.6	82.9	84.2	86.4
Illinois	82.6	83.7	85.6	89.7	90.2	90.9	69.9	72.8	74.7	73.0	76.0	80.9	72.8	80.9	83.1	85.9	85.6	88.8
Indiana	80.2	80.9	80.7	82.8	84.0	84.3	66.2	69.0	67.9	65.2	63.5	64.0	70.7	72.6	71.1	81.7	81.3	83.8
Michigan	84.1	84.8	85.9	88.4	89.1	89.7	70.5	70.1	72.1	72.8	73.5	78.4	74.7	77.4	79.6	85.9	88.0	88.4
Ohio	85.7	87.2	87.6	88.1	89.4	89.6	74.0	77.1	78.6	77.3	76.9	78.7	80.2	80.7	80.7	86.5	89.5	90.4
Wisconsin	84.3	84.1	85.2	88.0	88.0	88.7	68.5	70.3	75.8	71.6	69.3	71.8	70.9	71.8	72.8	63.6	67.2	71.4
West North Central:										68.5	70.8	74.3	67.2	65.4	64.4	75.0	79.3	80.7
Iowa	87.5	88.5	88.3	88.9	90.0	90.1	74.4	78.2	76.3	71.7	74.4	75.2	73.0	73.6	76.4	82.7	85.5	86.8
Kansas	85.7	86.8	—	89.2	90.3	—	76.3	79.4	—	67.0	70.7	—	77.0	80.9	—	83.3	85.6	—
Minnesota	84.4	84.9	86.4	87.8	89.2	90.3	65.6	68.1	73.9	62.4	65.2	70.6	61.6	62.3	64.6	64.2	71.2	75.7
Missouri	86.4	87.8	88.1	88.9	89.8	90.1	74.8	79.1	80.5	76.8	78.4	79.4	77.1	78.4	81.0	85.3	87.9	88.7
Nebraska	84.1	83.3	—	87.1	86.9	—	72.3	68.8	—	68.3	68.3	—	67.1	67.1	—	82.9	81.4	—
North Dakota	85.6	86.1	86.3	87.8	89.0	89.2	75.0	79.8	83.1	76.7	78.4	79.1	69.9	65.3	67.6	81.9	87.9	87.9
South Dakota	82.7	78.2	78.6	86.6	82.6	84.0	73.4	63.6	62.2	71.1	67.0	63.2	65.0	59.7	57.6	77.3	78.0	73.3
South Atlantic:										78.3	77.1	69.6	73.6	74.9	81.0	86.4	86.2	85.8
Delaware	83.2	86.5	83.8	88.0	90.9	89.0	73.9	80.5	79.7	70.3	73.6	67.7	73.1	84.9	86.1	85.5	91.0	88.8
District of Columbia	70.1	75.4	77.2	90.4	90.7	91.2	65.0	69.8	72.5	65.6	73.4	66.7	73.1	84.9	*	75.1	81.1	78.1
Florida[a]	83.8	84.4	—	88.8	89.4	—	73.0	75.1	—	81.6	82.2	—	67.0	66.0	—	87.8	88.3	—
Georgia	86.5	85.9	83.8	91.4	91.2	90.1	79.6	80.1	79.2	78.1	75.8	71.0	83.6	79.8	84.4	88.8	89.9	88.6
Maryland	87.8	84.7	82.5	92.7	90.8	90.2	79.5	76.9	75.0	81.5	73.8	65.6	81.8	82.5	78.1	89.8	84.8	84.6
North Carolina	84.5	84.4	84.0	90.5	90.9	90.5	74.8	75.7	76.6	68.8	69.6	69.4	73.6	77.9	80.7	82.4	83.8	85.5
South Carolina[a]	80.9	79.0	—	87.6	85.6	—	70.3	70.2	—	64.3	61.3	—	77.8	77.9	—	77.7	77.4	—
Virginia	85.2	85.2	85.3	90.2	90.4	90.5	74.1	76.4	78.7	73.3	70.5	70.4	79.4	84.1	80.4	85.1	85.3	85.0
West Virginia	83.6	86.1	85.4	84.2	86.7	85.9	68.7	74.0	73.7	74.9	69.7	74.5	*82.9	*66.7	*71.4	81.6	83.3	83.0

TABLE 1.3

Early prenatal care, 1997–99, 2000–02, and 2003–05 [CONTINUED]

[Data are based on birth certificates]

Percent of live births with early prenatal care (beginning in the 1st trimester)

Geographic division and state	All races 1997–1999	All races 2000–2002	All races 2003–2005	White[d] (Not Hispanic or Latina) 1997–1999	White[d] 2000–2002	White[d] 2003–2005	Black or African American (Not Hispanic or Latina) 1997–1999	Black 2000–2002	Black 2003–2005	Hispanic or Latina[c] 1997–1999	Hispanic 2000–2002	Hispanic 2003–2005	American Indian or Alaska Native[d] 1997–1999	Am. Indian 2000–2002	Am. Indian 2003–2005	Asian or Pacific Islander[d] 1997–1999	Asian 2000–2002	Asian 2003–2005
East South Central:										65.9	60.0	56.8	77.7	77.9	77.3	84.4	84.5	87.4
Alabama	82.6	82.8	83.6	89.3	89.7	89.8	70.6	72.4	76.7	61.8	53.9	52.3	78.6	80.4	82.7	84.3	87.6	87.5
Kentucky[a]	86.3	86.8	—	87.4	88.0	—	77.3	79.5	—	72.5	69.6	—	81.1	85.5	—	86.3	86.0	—
Mississippi	80.7	82.6	84.5	89.4	89.9	90.7	70.8	74.4	77.7	75.4	73.7	76.4	76.3	74.6	74.2	80.9	84.5	87.1
Tennessee[a]	84.0	82.9	—	88.0	87.7	—	73.0	72.2	—	64.0	57.4	—	76.8	76.4	—	84.6	82.6	—
West South Central:										72.0	73.3	70.0	70.7	70.9	71.1	86.3	87.4	84.2
Arkansas	77.5	79.7	81.4	81.8	83.8	84.8	66.5	69.8	74.7	61.9	67.6	70.3	69.8	74.3	73.5	74.6	79.0	83.1
Louisiana	82.1	83.5	85.5	89.4	90.7	91.5	72.1	73.9	77.3	85.0	84.2	84.4	77.9	82.0	85.9	84.4	86.0	89.5
Oklahoma	79.2	77.7	77.7	82.6	81.7	81.9	70.0	69.8	71.3	68.2	65.1	65.2	69.5	69.1	69.9	81.8	80.3	79.7
Texas	79.0	79.9	—	87.0	87.8	—	75.7	76.7	—	72.0	73.6	—	74.8	75.3	—	87.3	88.4	—
Mountain:										65.4	65.4	67.5	62.1	63.8	65.5	78.7	78.9	79.4
Arizona	75.5	76.6	76.9	85.3	87.2	87.6	73.1	75.7	78.2	64.9	66.3	67.8	62.9	65.8	68.9	83.3	85.0	84.3
Colorado	82.2	79.8	79.9	88.1	87.1	86.0	76.2	72.9	72.8	67.9	65.5	68.9	72.2	66.4	68.0	81.5	82.0	81.3
Idaho[a]	79.3	81.6	—	82.0	83.9	—	70.8	78.8	—	62.8	68.6	—	61.6	69.1	—	80.0	80.6	—
Montana	82.9	83.2	83.9	85.3	86.2	87.0	79.5	80.8	87.0	77.5	80.2	79.3	66.2	65.1	65.7	84.1	79.3	85.0
Nevada	75.3	75.4	74.9	83.0	85.2	83.6	67.7	68.0	69.4	62.8	62.3	64.2	68.3	68.6	67.9	78.9	79.4	79.8
New Mexico	68.2	68.9	69.8	76.0	76.7	77.5	62.3	66.8	69.0	65.6	66.2	67.7	56.7	59.2	59.4	75.7	75.5	77.3
Utah	82.1	79.4	80.2	85.4	83.5	83.9	65.2	58.9	58.8	63.9	61.2	65.0	57.8	56.1	58.3	68.1	64.4	66.1
Wyoming	82.3	83.5	85.5	83.9	85.0	87.3	74.0	79.1	89.8	72.9	75.2	78.8	68.0	71.7	69.3	83.6	83.8	79.8
Pacific:[b]										77.9	81.7	84.4	72.9	72.8	72.7	84.1	86.1	87.2
Alaska	80.4	80.3	80.2	82.9	84.1	84.7	82.7	83.3	82.8	79.5	79.7	78.7	74.9	70.6	70.6	74.6	77.2	72.6
California	82.6	85.4	87.0	88.4	90.1	90.5	79.7	82.5	83.5	78.4	82.4	84.9	72.5	75.0	75.2	84.9	87.2	88.8
Hawaii	84.8	84.5	81.9	90.8	89.4	85.6	90.7	92.5	86.5	83.1	83.2	80.8	83.2	82.5	83.5	82.8	82.9	80.4
Oregon	80.7	81.5	80.9	83.5	84.5	84.3	78.4	76.3	74.2	67.5	70.1	69.8	67.6	70.0	68.9	81.2	82.0	81.8
Middle Atlantic:																		
Pennsylvania[b]	—	—	74.0	—	—	79.0	—	—	56.6	—	—	57.6	—	—	64.2	—	—	67.0
Pacific:																		
Washington[b]	—	—	72.1	—	—	75.8	—	—	66.6	—	—	61.6	—	—	57.9	—	—	69.7

—Data not available.

*Percents preceded by an asterisk are based on fewer than 50 births in the numerator. Percents not shown are based on fewer than 20 births in the numerator. Percents not shown are based on fewer than 20 births.

[a]Reporting areas that adopted the 2003 revision of the U.S. Standard Certificate of Live Birth in 2004 and 2005 are excluded for 2003–2005 because prenatal care data based on the 2003 revision are not comparable with data based on the 1989 revision of the U.S. Standard Certificate of Live Birth.

[b]In 2003, Pennsylvania and Washington adopted the 2003 revision; data are shown separately for 2003–2005 for these two states and are based on the 2003 revision of the U.S. Standard Certificate of Live Birth, and are not comparable with data in this table based on the 1989 revision.

[c]Persons of Hispanic origin may be of any race.

[d]Includes persons of Hispanic and non-Hispanic origin.

Notes: Data are based on the 1989 revision of the U.S. Standard Certificate of Live Birth (except for 2003–2005 data for Pennsylvania and Washington). Starting with 2003 data, some states reported multiple-race data. The multiple-race data for these states were bridged to the single-race categories of the 1977 Office of Management and Budget standards for comparability with other states. Some data have changed from previous editions of *Health, United States*.

SOURCE: "Table 8. Early Prenatal Care by Race and Hispanic Origin of Mother, Geographic Division, and State: United States, Average Annual 1997–1999, 2000–2002, and 2003–2005," in *Health, United States, 2008. With Chartbook*, Centers for Disease Control and Prevention, National Center for Health Statistics, 2009, http://www.cdc.gov/nchs/data/hus/hus08.pdf (accessed December 12, 2009)

TABLE 1.4

Women receiving timely, late, or no prenatal care in selected states, 2005 and 2006

	Timing of prenatal care (PNC)							
Race and Hispanic origin of mother	Revised (12 reporting areas)[a, b]				Unrevised (34 reporting areas)[c]			
	First trimester PNC		Late or no PNC		First trimester PNC		Late or no PNC	
	2006	2005	2006	2005	2006	2005	2006	2005
All races and origins[d]	68.3	70.2	8.2	7.7	83.2	83.8	3.6	3.5
Non-Hispanic white	76.0	77.2	5.3	4.9	88.1	88.7	2.3	2.2
Non-Hispanic black	58.2	60.1	11.9	11.3	76.1	76.3	5.7	5.6
Hispanic[e]	57.6	60.0	12.2	11.9	77.3	77.6	5.0	5.0

[a]Data are based on the 2003 Revision of the U.S. Certificate of Live Birth; these data are not comparable with those based on the 1989 Revision of the U.S. Certificate of Live Birth.
[b]Data are for all reporting areas that had implemented the 2003 Revision of the U.S. Certificate of Live Birth as of January 2005; Florida, Idaho, Kansas, Kentucky, Nebraska, New Hampshire, New York State (excluding New York City), Pennsylvania, South Carolina, Tennessee, Texas, and Washington.
[c]Data are for all reporting areas that had not implemented the 2003 Revision of the U.S. Certificate of Live Birth as of January 2006. Also includes data for California, which implemented a partial revision of the 2003 Revision of the U.S. Certificate of Live Birth in 2006. Data are based on the 1989 Revision of the U.S. Certificate of Live Birth; these data are not comparable with those based on the 2003 Revision of the U.S. Certificate of Live Birth. Excludes data from Delaware, Florida, Idaho, Kansas, Kentucky, Nebraska, New Hampshire, New York State (excluding New York City), North Dakota, Ohio, Pennsylvania, South Carolina, South Dakota, Tennessee, Texas, Vermont, Washington, and Wyoming.
[d]Includes races other than white and black and origina not stated.
[e]Includes all persons of Hispanic origin of any race.
[f]Excludes data for California.
Notes: Race and Hispanic origin are reported separately on birth certificates. Persons of Hispanic origin may be of any race. Race categories are consistent with the 1977 Office of Management and Budget (OMB) standards. Twenty-three states reported multiple-race data. The multiple-race data for these states were bridged to the single-race categories of the 1977 OMB standards for comparability with other states.

SOURCE: Adapted from Joyce A. Martin et al., "Table II. Timing of Prenatal Care and Primary Cesarean and Vaginal Birth (VBAC) after Previous Cesarean, by Race and Hispanic Origin of Mother: 12 States (revised) and 34 States (unrevised), District of Columbia, and New York City, 2005 and 2006," in "Births: Final Data for 2006," *National Vital Statistics Reports*, vol. 57, no. 7, January 7, 2009, http://www.cdc.gov/nchs/data/nvsr/nvsr57/nvsr57_07.pdf (accessed December 15, 2009)

delivering an LBW infant is greatest among the youngest and oldest mothers; however, many of the LBW births among older mothers are attributable to their higher rates of multiple births. Even though older mothers and multiples account for many LBW infants, between 1990 and 2006 there was an increase in LBW singletons. (See Figure 1.1.) The increase in LBW singletons may also be attributable to shorter gestational age—intervention during pregnancy to deliver babies earlier, before gestation is complete, to safeguard the health of the mother or the child.

Birth Weight Influences the Risk of Disease

Even though the precise mechanisms of the relationship between birth weight and the development of disease in adulthood have not yet been completely described, and researchers do not yet know exactly how or why birth weight can predict health and illness in adulthood, there is ample evidence that lower- and higher-than-average birth weight are associated with health in later life. LBW infants are more likely than normal-weight infants to develop disease as they age and male LBW infants—who gain weight rapidly before their first birthday—are disproportionately affected and seem to be at the highest risk for future health problems. Researchers conjecture that LBW infants have fewer muscle cells at birth and that rapid weight gain during the first year of life may lead to different ratios of fat to muscle and above-average body mass. People with LBW who later develop above-average body mass are at higher risk of developing diseases such as Type 2 diabetes, hypertension (high blood pressure), and cardiovascular disease (heart disease and

stroke) than those with average birth weights who do not gain weight rapidly in the first year of life.

Magnus Kaijser et al. find in "Perinatal Risk Factors for Ischemic Heart Disease" (*Circulation*, vol. 117, no. 3, January 22, 2008) that LBW is associated with an increased risk of developing heart disease. Based on a review of 6,425 subjects born with LBW, Kaijser et al. determine that this association reflects the length of pregnancy and problems in pregnancy such as maternal malnutrition that might limit the growth of the unborn child.

In "Low Birth Weight and Increased Cardiovascular Risk: Fetal Programming" (*International Journal of Cardiology*, January 25, 2009), Mustafa Mucahit Balci, Sadik Acikel, and Ramazan Akdemir posit that LBW infants may have hyper-responsive immune systems that predispose them to inflammatory conditions such as certain forms of heart disease, diabetes, arthritis, and asthma.

Evidence also indicates that birth weight is related to a risk of developing breast cancer. Xiaohui Xu et al. review relevant medical literature to determine whether studies conducted between 1996 and 2008 confirm that birth weight influences the risk of developing breast cancer in adulthood. The results of this meta-analysis were published in "Birth Weight as a Risk Factor for Breast Cancer: A Meta-analysis of 18 Epidemiological Studies" (*Journal of Women's Health*, vol. 18, no. 8, August 2009). By examining 18 studies and 16,424 cases of breast cancer, the researchers determine that size at birth was associated with breast

TABLE 1.5

Low birthweight live births, 1997–99, 2000–02, and 2003–05

[Data are based on birth certificates]

Percent of live births weighing less than 2,500 grams[a]

Geographic division and state	All races			Not Hispanic or Latina — White			Not Hispanic or Latina — Black or African American			Hispanic or Latina[b]			American Indian or Alaska Native[c]			Asian or Pacific Islander[d]		
	1997–1999	2000–2002	2003–2005	1997–1999	2000–2002	2003–2005	1997–1999	2000–2002	2003–2005	1997–1999	2000–2002	2003–2005	1997–1999	2000–2002	2003–2005	1997–1999	2000–2002	2003–2005
United States	7.57	7.69	8.07	6.56	6.75	7.18	13.17	13.19	13.77	6.41	6.48	6.79	6.90	7.11	7.39	7.37	7.54	7.89
New England	6.96	7.14	7.55	6.25	6.46	6.89	11.92	11.83	12.08	8.33	8.08	8.37	8.59	7.93	8.28	7.39	7.64	7.87
Connecticut	7.56	7.52	7.74	6.31	6.48	6.60	12.94	12.28	12.88	9.05	8.25	8.49	*9.63	10.06	7.45	7.59	8.07	7.83
Maine	5.93	6.12	6.58	6.00	6.13	6.57	*12.07	*9.47	8.47	*	*6.03	*4.74	*	*	*	*4.79	*5.46	8.69
Massachusetts	6.99	7.26	7.77	6.35	6.56	7.15	11.31	11.54	11.82	8.11	8.37	8.41	*7.74	*7.11	*7.62	7.26	7.57	7.63
New Hampshire	5.91	6.40	6.65	5.75	6.24	6.59	*7.81	10.58	10.85	6.80	4.84	6.55	*	*	*	*7.27	5.95	5.75
Rhode Island	7.43	7.47	8.12	6.65	6.75	7.39	11.23	12.32	11.22	7.57	7.20	8.61	11.76	*10.32	13.66	9.19	9.31	10.11
Vermont	6.15	6.15	6.57	6.08	6.12	6.55	*	*	*	*	*	*	*	*	*	*	*	*8.08
Middle Atlantic	7.83	7.84	8.16	6.42	6.62	6.97	13.03	12.69	13.15	7.71	7.47	7.67	8.34	8.66	8.74	7.52	7.42	7.97
New Jersey	8.01	7.89	8.19	6.44	6.59	7.11	14.02	13.20	13.48	7.33	7.15	7.27	9.87	11.09	9.83	7.71	7.57	8.10
New York	7.83	7.76	8.11	6.34	6.48	6.82	12.26	12.02	12.78	7.66	7.38	7.59	7.56	7.81	7.31	7.43	7.33	7.89
Pennsylvania	7.69	7.93	8.20	6.49	6.78	7.06	13.93	13.79	13.67	9.23	8.97	9.00	9.03	9.15	10.95	7.54	7.48	7.99
East North Central	7.72	7.79	8.19	6.54	6.71	7.18	13.80	13.78	14.21	6.46	6.33	6.58	6.87	7.17	7.40	7.75	7.92	8.17
Illinois	7.96	8.04	8.40	6.47	6.74	7.22	14.12	14.04	14.70	6.29	6.31	6.60	8.08	8.60	9.46	8.02	8.49	8.28
Indiana	7.84	7.54	8.10	7.20	6.95	7.54	13.33	12.89	13.46	6.77	6.09	6.33	*10.65	*7.74	*10.00	7.06	7.41	7.87
Michigan	7.84	7.94	8.28	6.34	6.55	7.00	13.89	14.24	14.43	6.67	6.26	6.46	6.75	7.26	6.98	7.94	7.46	8.33
Ohio	7.78	8.07	8.51	6.75	7.08	7.53	13.47	13.45	13.83	7.57	7.20	7.13	7.23	8.86	10.22	7.44	7.86	8.27
Wisconsin	6.53	6.58	6.93	5.71	5.83	6.18	13.43	13.25	13.59	6.42	6.13	6.34	6.08	6.12	6.04	7.21	6.97	7.50
West North Central	6.75	6.87	7.17	6.24	6.36	6.68	12.94	12.44	12.79	6.07	6.10	6.06	6.33	6.99	7.07	7.32	7.29	7.53
Iowa	6.31	6.39	6.92	6.05	6.19	6.72	11.99	11.77	12.22	6.10	6.01	6.12	8.53	7.23	9.15	7.64	7.13	7.71
Kansas	7.01	6.96	7.28	6.58	6.66	6.97	12.80	12.37	13.42	6.01	5.93	6.09	6.42	6.20	7.09	7.87	6.69	7.34
Minnesota	5.92	6.23	6.43	5.62	5.80	5.93	11.08	10.54	10.71	6.15	6.02	5.70	6.57	7.10	6.87	7.23	7.28	7.43
Missouri	7.75	7.74	8.12	6.70	6.79	7.18	13.77	13.27	13.90	6.07	6.18	6.33	8.58	8.67	7.63	6.83	7.34	7.61
Nebraska	6.75	6.88	6.97	6.42	6.52	6.76	12.33	13.07	12.16	6.19	6.30	6.20	6.89	7.27	6.78	8.03	8.05	7.61
North Dakota	6.31	6.28	6.49	6.36	6.13	6.37	*9.35	*9.02	*9.43	*4.98	*8.10	*5.84	6.03	6.62	6.78	*	*	*8.39
South Dakota	5.75	6.58	6.71	5.75	6.37	6.62	*10.81	*11.51	*7.27	*5.29	6.89	5.94	5.47	6.84	7.04	*6.86	*11.39	*9.50
South Atlantic	8.53	8.63	8.97	6.87	7.09	7.49	13.13	13.15	13.70	6.35	6.39	6.65	9.24	9.17	9.91	7.53	7.95	8.17
Delaware	8.57	9.29	9.31	6.53	7.80	7.62	14.32	14.08	14.32	7.52	6.81	7.03	*	*	*	7.89	9.89	9.33
District of Columbia	13.21	11.85	11.06	6.05	6.35	6.28	16.05	14.60	13.96	6.06	8.04	7.46	*	*	*	*8.67	*7.00	8.97
Florida	8.09	8.18	8.59	6.93	6.98	7.38	12.31	12.58	13.28	6.55	6.61	6.98	7.52	7.11	7.38	8.29	8.35	8.73
Georgia	8.68	8.79	9.27	6.69	6.92	7.44	12.84	12.98	13.81	5.51	5.77	5.96	8.43	9.29	9.00	7.54	8.18	8.35
Maryland	8.82	8.88	9.17	6.50	6.79	7.19	13.41	13.00	13.13	6.65	6.73	7.18	9.48	9.74	10.87	7.19	7.42	7.93
North Carolina	8.84	8.90	9.07	7.22	7.49	7.73	13.77	13.83	14.33	6.24	6.13	6.27	10.35	10.30	11.01	7.26	8.20	7.77
South Carolina	9.52	9.74	10.15	7.09	7.40	7.82	14.11	14.29	15.19	5.71	6.87	6.66	*8.88	10.22	10.75	7.66	8.02	8.13
Virginia	7.80	7.90	8.23	6.39	6.54	7.01	12.44	12.56	12.83	6.23	6.07	6.28	*7.58	*10.73	*9.20	7.08	7.50	7.71
West Virginia	8.12	8.60	9.16	7.97	8.39	9.03	12.88	13.81	13.15	*	*	*6.06	*	*	*	*7.16	*9.16	*9.51
East South Central	9.07	9.45	9.89	7.52	7.88	8.43	13.61	14.24	14.94	6.47	6.74	6.45	7.73	7.84	7.64	7.92	7.95	7.80
Alabama	9.28	9.75	10.35	7.37	7.77	8.46	13.34	14.10	15.02	6.57	6.95	6.92	*7.03	9.68	10.53	8.24	7.38	8.02
Kentucky	8.06	8.38	8.86	7.58	7.84	8.50	13.15	13.84	13.52	6.76	7.73	6.85	*9.51	*7.17	*8.54	7.37	7.75	7.56
Mississippi	10.18	10.82	11.62	7.35	7.97	8.67	13.63	14.48	15.60	5.41	6.61	6.42	*6.44	7.30	6.24	7.70	6.83	8.06
Tennessee	9.01	9.20	9.35	7.65	7.95	8.26	14.06	14.23	14.51	6.49	6.28	6.04	*9.37	*7.11	*6.63	8.13	8.60	7.76

TABLE 1.5

Low birthweight live births, 1997–99, 2000–02, and 2003–05 [CONTINUED]

[Data are based on birth certificates]

Geographic division and state	All races			Not Hispanic or Latina						Hispanic or Latina[b]			American Indian or Alaska Native[c]			Asian or Pacific Islander[c]		
				White			Black or African American											
	1997–1999	2000–2002	2003–2005	1997–1999	2000–2002	2003–2005	1997–1999	2000–2002	2003–2005	1997–1999	2000–2002	2003–2005	1997–1999	2000–2002	2003–2005	1997–1999	2000–2002	2003–2005
						Percent of live births weighing less than 2,500 grams[a]												
West South Central	7.81	8.00	8.48	6.81	7.07	7.61	13.30	13.51	14.44	6.62	6.85	7.20	6.33	6.71	7.04	7.80	7.80	8.17
Arkansas	8.62	8.64	9.04	7.45	7.48	7.83	13.21	13.81	14.86	6.28	5.79	6.54	*5.60	8.11	8.86	8.55	7.73	6.74
Louisiana	10.09	10.40	11.02	7.00	7.56	8.12	14.57	14.44	15.33	6.37	6.56	7.62	8.00	9.06	10.11	8.39	7.89	8.46
Oklahoma	7.28	7.75	7.92	6.91	7.35	7.63	12.22	13.57	13.62	5.86	6.41	6.46	6.19	6.48	6.69	6.52	7.87	6.82
Texas	7.35	7.54	8.07	6.61	6.81	7.43	12.58	12.82	13.91	6.65	6.88	7.23	6.68	6.67	7.33	7.82	7.78	8.33
Mountain	7.36	7.36	7.67	7.11	7.09	7.44	13.45	13.65	13.77	7.18	7.23	7.40	6.97	7.01	7.43	8.70	8.27	9.14
Arizona	6.86	6.91	7.05	6.60	6.78	7.01	12.83	13.16	12.38	6.64	6.56	6.69	6.83	6.85	7.11	7.67	7.95	7.92
Colorado	8.60	8.60	9.04	8.18	8.24	8.81	14.12	14.59	15.20	8.54	8.33	8.53	8.85	9.05	9.45	10.05	10.17	10.26
Idaho	6.15	6.41	6.65	6.01	6.29	6.60	*9.68	*	*7.03	6.71	6.95	6.67	7.18	6.15	8.31	*6.47	7.38	6.67
Montana	6.71	6.65	7.02	6.56	6.60	6.81	*	*	*15.58	6.69	7.44	8.63	7.37	7.14	7.80	*7.38	*5.95	*8.70
Nevada	7.59	7.44	8.11	7.42	7.19	7.78	13.32	13.40	13.98	6.23	6.34	6.74	6.87	6.80	7.58	9.11	7.56	10.35
New Mexico	7.68	7.99	8.38	7.83	7.89	8.33	13.30	13.88	15.01	7.66	8.13	8.45	6.55	6.88	7.32	8.83	7.67	8.60
Utah	6.72	6.48	6.68	6.55	6.28	6.45	14.76	13.09	12.05	7.08	7.20	7.26	7.54	6.37	7.46	7.95	7.23	8.20
Wyoming	8.75	8.35	8.71	8.77	8.12	8.74	*16.76	*13.29	*	7.09	8.81	8.43	7.39	9.55	8.39	*16.31	*12.04	*
Pacific	6.09	6.22	6.63	5.50	5.70	6.11	11.69	11.50	12.25	5.58	5.66	6.09	6.28	6.36	6.59	6.99	7.27	7.55
Alaska	5.90	5.71	6.02	5.36	4.84	5.34	11.24	10.70	11.74	6.69	6.07	5.31	5.89	5.81	5.86	6.88	7.33	6.57
California	6.17	6.29	6.71	5.61	5.86	6.30	11.87	11.66	12.46	5.57	5.66	6.10	6.06	6.21	6.49	6.86	7.15	7.42
Hawaii	7.44	7.98	8.23	5.48	6.17	6.42	10.34	11.01	11.44	7.71	8.00	8.34	*7.65	*4.99	*	7.96	8.45	8.84
Oregon	5.41	5.65	6.09	5.21	5.44	6.02	10.51	10.32	11.16	5.47	5.54	5.43	6.13	7.23	7.34	6.07	6.78	7.00
Washington	5.72	5.75	6.13	5.33	5.43	5.63	10.10	10.34	10.63	5.46	5.31	5.93	7.13	7.08	7.31	6.61	6.37	6.90

*Percents preceded by an asterisk are based on fewer than 50 births. Percents not shown are based on fewer than 20 births.

[a]Excludes live births with unknown birthweight.

[b]Persons of Hispanic origin may be of any race.

[c]Includes persons of Hispanic and non-Hispanic origin.

Notes: Starting with 2003 data, some states reported multiple-race data. The multiple-race data for these states were bridged to the single-race categories of the 1977 Office of Management and Budget standards for comparability with other states.

SOURCE: "Table 14. Low Birthweight Live Births, by Race and Hispanic Origin of Mother, Geographic Division, and State: United States, Average Annual 1997–1999, 2000–2002, and 2003–2005," in *Health, United States, 2008. With Chartbook*, Centers for Disease Control and Prevention, National Center for Health Statistics, 2009, http://www.cdc.gcv/nchs/data/hus/hus08.pdf (accessed December 12, 2009)

TABLE 1.6

Low-birthweight births by race, ethnicity, and state, 2006

[By place of residence. Low birthweight is birthweight of less than 2,500 grams (5 lb. 8 oz.)]

State	Number All races[a]	Number Non-Hispanic White[b]	Number Non-Hispanic Black[b]	Number Hispanic[c]	Percent All races[a]	Percent Non-Hispanic White[b]	Percent Non-Hispanic Black[b]	Percent Hispanic[c]
United States[d]	351,974	168,871	86,122	72,538	8.3	7.3	14.0	7.0
Alabama	6,624	3,251	3,001	287	10.5	8.5	15.5	6.1
Alaska	654	377	38	37	6.0	6.0	9.6	4.9
Arizona	7,289	2,930	459	3,128	7.1	6.8	12.8	6.9
Arkansas	3,749	2,192	1,172	303	9.2	7.9	15.0	6.9
California	38,411	10,056	3,850	18,332	6.8	6.4	12.0	6.3
Colorado	6,317	3,654	467	1,914	8.9	8.7	15.7	8.4
Connecticut	3,395	1,782	646	747	8.1	6.9	12.5	8.8
Delaware	1,108	506	442	117	9.3	7.7	14.8	6.2
District of Columbia	980	156	703	102	11.5	7.3	14.5	7.7
Florida	20,614	8,134	6,862	4,936	8.7	7.6	13.4	7.0
Georgia	14,232	5,234	7,021	1,452	9.6	7.5	14.4	6.1
Hawaii	1,531	269	51	238	8.1	5.9	10.2	7.8
Idaho	1,671	1,368	17	232	6.9	7.0	*	6.1
Illinois	15,577	7,033	4,474	3,180	8.6	7.4	14.3	7.2
Indiana	7,268	5,114	1,459	564	8.2	7.6	14.1	6.7
Iowa	2,809	2,339	168	205	6.9	6.8	10.6	6.4
Kansas	2,933	2,047	371	371	7.2	6.9	12.4	5.6
Kentucky	5,327	4,275	769	201	9.1	8.7	14.6	7.2
Louisiana	7,231	2,994	3,934	169	11.4	8.5	16.2	7.2
Maine	967	901	22	21	6.8	6.8	7.5	9.6
Maryland	7,269	2,807	3,393	681	9.4	7.6	13.4	6.8
Massachusetts	6,138	3,855	859	906	7.9	7.2	12.1	8.4
Michigan	10,637	6,144	3,224	605	8.4	7.1	14.2	7.0
Minnesota	4,807	3,264	651	357	6.5	6.0	10.3	5.9
Mississippi	5,698	2,006	3,514	111	12.4	8.9	16.7	7.1
Missouri	6,555	4,439	1,673	266	8.1	7.1	13.6	5.8
Montana	912	716	3	27	7.3	7.3	*	6.8
Nebraska	1,900	1,313	239	266	7.1	6.6	14.0	6.7
Nevada	3,335	1,400	470	1,037	8.3	8.3	14.1	6.6
New Hampshire	994	875	23	54	6.9	6.8	10.8	9.3
New Jersey	9,882	4,241	2,464	2,197	8.6	7.4	14.1	7.5
New Mexico	2,668	744	76	1,499	8.9	8.7	15.0	9.1
New York	20,790	8,853	5,343	4,738	8.3	7.1	12.6	8.0
North Carolina	11,585	5,547	4,218	1,315	9.1	7.8	14.2	6.2
North Dakota	576	478	9	22	6.7	6.7	*	8.8
Ohio	13,180	8,860	3,432	481	8.8	7.7	14.5	7.2
Oklahoma	4,503	2,757	753	465	8.3	7.9	15.4	6.6
Oregon	2,963	2,016	93	583	6.1	6.0	8.5	5.9
Pennsylvania	12,562	7,875	2,877	1,148	8.5	7.4	14.0	8.7
Rhode Island	988	473	115	204	8.0	7.7	11.6	8.0
South Carolina	6,292	2,674	3,099	373	10.1	7.8	15.2	6.4
South Dakota	836	617	24	33	7.0	6.7	11.2	8.3
Tennessee	8,108	4,823	2,578	526	9.6	8.4	14.8	6.6
Texas	33,727	10,681	6,518	15,139	8.4	7.6	14.2	7.6
Utah	3,700	2,805	51	618	6.9	6.6	11.0	7.5
Vermont	447	413	10	4	6.9	6.7	*	*
Virginia	8,914	4,446	3,031	862	8.3	7.1	13.0	6.0
Washington	5,641	3,340	399	987	6.5	6.0	10.7	6.3
West Virginia	2,024	1,877	112	10	9.7	9.5	16.3	*
Wisconsin	4,974	3,356	938	427	6.9	6.2	13.4	6.2
Wyoming	682	564	7	61	8.9	9.1	*	6.8

cancer risk. Risk was higher among women who weighed 8.5 pounds (3.9 kg) or more.

In "Birth Weight and the Risk of Testicular Cancer: A Meta-Analysis" (*International Journal of Cancer*, vol. 121, no. 5, September 1, 2007), Athanasios Michos, Fei Xue, and Karin B. Michels indicate that both high and low birth weights increase the risk of testicular cancer in men. Men with LBW were 18% more likely to develop testicular cancer, and men with a high birth weight were 12% more likely to develop the cancer than men of average birth weight.

Marilyn Rogers et al. report in "Aerobic Capacity, Strength, Flexibility, and Activity Level in Unimpaired Extremely Low Birth Weight (≤800 g) Survivors at 17 Years of Age Compared with Term-Born Control Subjects" (*Pediatrics*, vol. 116, no. 1, July 2005) that infants born either prematurely or with a VLBW were significantly more likely to suffer lower levels of fitness later in life—including less strength, endurance, and flexibility—and had a greater risk of health problems as adults. When compared with normal-birth-weight teens, the VLBW teens had lower aerobic

TABLE 1.6

Low-birthweight births by race, ethnicity, and state, 2006 [CONTINUED]

[By place of residence. Low birthweight is birthweight of less than 2,500 grams (5 lb. 8 oz.)]

	Number				Percent			
		Non-Hispanic				Non-Hispanic		
State	All races[a]	White[b]	Black[b]	Hispanic[c]	All races[a]	White[b]	Black[b]	Hispanic[c]
Puerto Rico	6,316	195	14	6,099	13.0	12.2	*	13.0
Virgin Islands	175	8	123	35	10.4	*	11.3	9.3
Guam	268	7	4	1	7.9	*	*	*
American Samoa	41	—	—	—	2.8	—	—	—
Northern Marianas	120	—	—	—	8.5	—	—	—

*Figure does not meet standards of reliability or precision based on fewer than 20 births in the numerator.
—Data not available.
[a]Includes races other than white and black and origin not stated.
[b]Race and Hispanic origina are reported separately on birth certificates. Persons of Hispanic origin may be of any race. Race categories are consistent with the 1977 Office of Management and Budget (OMB) standards. In 2006, 23 states reported multiple-race data. Multiple-race data for these states were bridged to the single-race categories of the 1977 OMB standards for comparability with other states.
[c]Includes all persons of Hispanic origin of any race.
[d]Excludes data for the territories.

SOURCE: Joyce A. Martin et al., "Table 36. Number and Percentage of Births of Low Birthweight, by Race and Hispanic Origin of Mother: United States, Each State and Territory, 2006," in "Births: Final Data for 2006," *National Vital Statistics Reports*, vol. 57, no. 7, January 7, 2009, http://www.cdc.gov/nchs/data/nvsr/nvsr57/nvsr57_07.pdf (accessed December 15, 2009)

capacity, grip strength, leg power, and vertical jump. They were unable to perform as many pushups, had less abdominal strength as measured by curl-ups, had less lower-back flexibility, and had tighter hamstrings. The VLBW teens reported less previous and current sports participation, lower physical activity levels, and poorer coordination compared with full-term-born control subjects. VLBW teens also had more trouble maintaining rhythm and tempo than their normal-birth-weight peers.

The only action able to alter the birth weight of an infant is to modify weight gain by the mother during pregnancy. In 2010 health professionals concurred that for normal-weight women the ideal weight gain during pregnancy ranges from 25 to 35 pounds (11.3 to 15.9 kg) of fat and lean mass. Furthermore, research published in 2003 revealed that a newborn's birth weight and mother's post-pregnancy weight are influenced not only by how much weight is gained during pregnancy but also by the source of the excess weight. In "Composition of Gestational Weight Gain Impacts Maternal Fat Retention and Infant Birth Weight" (*American Journal of Obstetrics and Gynecology*, vol. 189, no. 5, November 2003), Nancy F. Butte et al. of the Children's Nutrition Research Center in Houston, Texas, conducted body scans of 63 women before, during, and after their pregnancies and recorded changes in the women's weight from water, protein, fat, and potassium—a marker for changes in muscle tissue, which is one component of lean mass. The researchers find that only increases in lean mass, and not fat mass, appeared to influence infant size. Independent of how much fat was gained by women during pregnancy, only lean body mass increased the birth weight of the infant, with women who gained more lean body mass giving birth to larger infants.

Kathleen M. Rasmussen et al. report in *Weight Gain during Pregnancy: Reexamining the Guidelines* (May 28, 2009, http://www.iom.edu/) that in 2009 the Institute of Medicine and the National Research Council issued new recommendations for pregnancy weight gain. (See Table 1.7.) The guidelines caution that obese expectant mothers (with a body mass index [BMI; a measure of body fat based on weight and height] of 30 or higher) should limit weight gain to between 11 and 20 pounds (5 and 9.1 kg). This recommendation replaces the 1990 guideline, which advised obese expectant mothers to gain no less than 15 pounds (6.8 kg). The updated guidelines are based on the findings that the offspring of overweight or obese moms face increased risk for preterm birth or being larger than normal at delivery, with extra fat. Large babies may suffer stuck shoulders and broken collar bones during birth and are at greater risk of becoming overweight, obese, and diabetic in adulthood.

Birth Defects

In "Birth Defects" (October 28, 2009, http://www.cdc.gov/ncbddd/bd/default.htm), the CDC states that birth defects affect one out of 33 babies and that birth defects account for more than 20% of all infant deaths. A birth defect may be a structural defect, a deficiency of function, or a disease that an infant has at birth (congenital). Some common birth defects are genetic—inherited abnormalities such as Tay-Sachs disease (a fatal disease that generally affects children of east European Jewish ancestry) or chromosomal irregularities such as Down syndrome. Other birth defects result from environmental factors—infections during pregnancy, such as rubella (German measles), or drugs used by the pregnant woman. Even though the specific causes of some birth defects are unknown, scientists

FIGURE 1.1

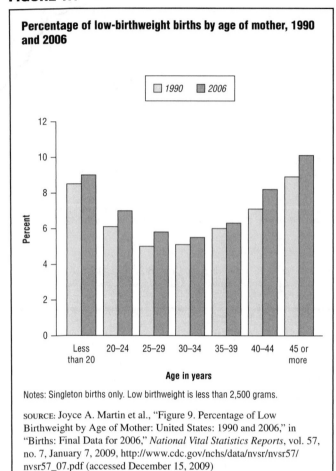

Percentage of low-birthweight births by age of mother, 1990 and 2006

Notes: Singleton births only. Low birthweight is less than 2,500 grams.

SOURCE: Joyce A. Martin et al., "Figure 9. Percentage of Low Birthweight by Age of Mother: United States: 1990 and 2006," in "Births: Final Data for 2006," *National Vital Statistics Reports*, vol. 57, no. 7, January 7, 2009, http://www.cdc.gov/nchs/data/nvsr/nvsr57/nvsr57_07.pdf (accessed December 15, 2009)

TABLE 1.7

New recommendations for weight gain during pregnancy by prepregnancy body mass index (BMI), 2009

Prepregnancy BMI	BMI (kg/m²)	Total weight gain (lbs)	Rates of weight gain 2nd and 3rd trimester (lbs/week)
Underweight	<18.5	28–40	1 (1–1.3)
Normal weight	18.5–24.9	25–35	1 (0.8–1)
Overweight	25.0–29.9	15–25	0.6 (0.5–0.7)
Obese (includes all classes)	≥30.0	11–20	0.5 (0.4–0.6)

Notes: To calculate BMI go to www.nhlbisupport.com/bmi. Calculations assume a 0.5 = 2 kg (1.1–4.4 lbs) weight gain in the first trimester (based on Siega-Riz et al., 1994; Abrams et al., 1995; Carmichael et al., 1997)

SOURCE: Kathleen M. Rasmussen et al., "Table 1. New Recommendations for Total and Rate of Weight Gain during Pregnancy, by Prepregnancy BMI," in *Weight Gain during Pregnancy: Reexamining the Guidelines*, Institute of Medicine of the National Academies, May 28, 2009, http://www.iom.edu/~/media/Files/Report%o20Files/2009/Weight-Gain-During-Pregnancy-Reexamining-the-Guidelines/Resource%20Page%20-%20Weight%20Gain%20During%20Pregnancy.ashx (accessed December 16, 2009)

believe that many result from a combination of genetic and environmental factors.

NEURAL TUBE DEFECTS. Neural tube defects (NTDs) are abnormalities of the brain and spinal cord resulting from the failure of the neural tube to develop properly during early pregnancy. The neural tube is the embryonic nerve tissue that eventually develops into the brain and the spinal cord. The two most common NTDs are anencephaly and spina bifida.

ANENCEPHALY. According to the National Institutes of Health, in "Anencephaly" (February 23, 2010, http://www.nlm.nih.gov/medlineplus/ency/article/001580.htm), anencephaly (the absence of a major part of the brain, skull, and scalp) occurs in about one out of 10,000 births. The exact number is unknown because many of these pregnancies end in miscarriage. Infants with anencephaly either die before birth (in utero or stillborn) or shortly thereafter.

T. J. Matthews of the CDC notes in *Trends in Spina Bifida and Anencephalus in the United States, 1991–2006* (April 2009, http://www.cdc.gov/nchs/data/hestat/spine_anen.pdf) that the incidence of anencephaly decreased significantly from 1991 to 2001. In 1991, 18.4 infants per 100,000 live births were reported with the condition; this number dropped to 9.4 infants per 100,000 live births in 2001. However, the rate for the period 2003 to 2006 rose to around 11 infants per 100,000 live births, which was higher than the rate of 10 infants per 100,000 live births reported for the period 1998 to 2002.

SPINA BIFIDA. Spina bifida, which literally means "divided spine," is caused by the failure of the vertebrae (backbone) to completely cover the spinal cord early in fetal development, leaving the spinal cord exposed. Depending on the amount of nerve tissue exposed, spina bifida defects range from minor developmental disabilities to paralysis. The March of Dimes reports in "Spina Bifida" (2010, http://www.marchofdimes.com/professionals/14332_1224.asp) that spina bifida occurs in about 1,500 infants per year.

Matthews indicates that after an increase in the spina bifida rates from 1992 to 1995, there was a significant decline from 1995 to 1999. From 1999 to 2002 the rates did not change much, but from 1999 to 2002 the rates were much lower than in 1997. The rate of spina bifida decreased from 20.1 infants per 100,000 live births in 2002 to 18 infants per 100,000 live births in 2006. The 2006 rate was nearly identical to the rate for 2005, which was the lowest ever reported, at 17.9 infants per 100,000 live births. (See Figure 1.2.)

PREVENTION. Scientists now know that daily consumption of 0.4 milligrams (400 micrograms) of the B vitamin folic acid by women before and during the first trimester of pregnancy greatly reduces the risk of spina bifida and other birth defects. Because half of all pregnancies in the United States are unplanned or incorrectly timed and because NTDs occur during the first month of pregnancy—before most

FIGURE 1.2

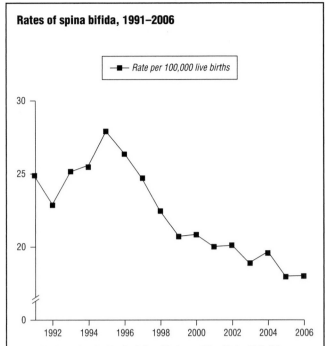

Rates of spina bifida, 1991–2006

■ Rate per 100,000 live births

Notes: Excludes data for Maryland, New Mexico, and New York, which did not require reporting for spina bifida for some years.

SOURCE: T. J. Mathews, "Figure 1. Spina Bifida Rates, 1991–2006," in *Trends in Spina Bifida and Anencephalus in the United States, 1991–2006*, Health E-Stats, National Center for Health Statistics, April 2009, http://www.cdc.gov/nchs/data/hestat/spine_anen.pdf (accessed December 16, 2009)

women know they are pregnant—the U.S. Public Health Service began recommending in 1992 that all women of childbearing age consume 0.4 milligrams of folic acid daily. To comply with a mandate from the U.S. Food and Drug Administration, as of January 1998 all enriched cereal grain products must be fortified with folic acid. According to the March of Dimes, in "Folic Acid" (2010, http://www.march ofdimes.com/professionals/690_1151.asp), the occurrence of NTDs can be reduced by up to 70% if women consume the recommended amount of folic acid before conception and throughout the first month of pregnancy.

In "Blood Folate Levels: The Latest NHANES Results" (May 2008, http://www.cdc.gov/nchs/data/data briefs/db06 .pdf), Margaret A. McDowell et al. of the CDC find that the prevalence of low folate levels among U.S. women of childbearing age declined from 37.6% in 1988–94 to 5.1% in 1999–2000. By 2005–06 the prevalence dropped even further, to 4.5%. This decline is an indicator of the successful efforts to prevent birth defects by increasing folic acid consumption and folate levels among women of childbearing age.

LEGISLATION TO PREVENT BIRTH DEFECTS. In April 1998 President Bill Clinton (1946–) signed into law the Birth Defects Prevention Act, which authorized a nationwide network of birth defects research and prevention programs and called for a nationwide information clearinghouse on birth defects.

In December 2003 the Birth Defects and Development Disabilities Prevention Act was passed into law. This bill revises and extends the Birth Defects Prevention Act to expand and adjust research and reporting requirements. According to the U.S. Department of Health and Human Services (June 4, 2009, http://www.hhs.gov/asrt/ob/docbud get/2010budgetinbriefg.html), the budget for activities related to the Birth Defects and Developmental Disabilities Program included $142 million for fiscal year 2010.

INFANT MORTALITY

Since 1958 infant mortality has declined or remained unchanged, except for a slight increase in 2002. In 2006 there were 6.7 deaths per 1,000 live births. (See Figure 1.3.)

Advances in neonatology (the medical subspecialty concerned with the care of newborns, especially those at risk) have contributed to the huge decline in infant death rates. Infants born prematurely or with LBWs, who were once likely to die, can survive life-threatening conditions due to the development of neonatal intensive care units. Improved access to health care has also contributed to the decline, as have public health initiatives such as education

FIGURE 1.3

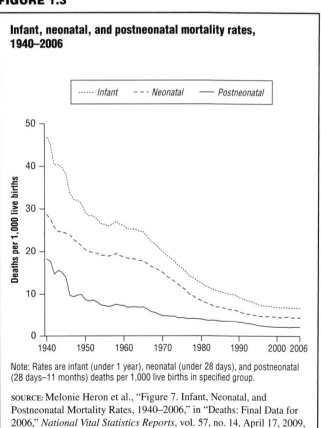

Infant, neonatal, and postneonatal mortality rates, 1940–2006

······ Infant   - - - Neonatal   —— Postneonatal

Note: Rates are infant (under 1 year), neonatal (under 28 days), and postneonatal (28 days–11 months) deaths per 1,000 live births in specified group.

SOURCE: Melonie Heron et al., "Figure 7. Infant, Neonatal, and Postneonatal Mortality Rates, 1940–2006," in "Deaths: Final Data for 2006," *National Vital Statistics Reports*, vol. 57, no. 14, April 17, 2009, http://www.cdc.gov/nchs/data/nvsr/nvsr57/nvsr57_14.pdf (accessed December 16, 2009)

about how to prevent sudden infant death syndrome—specifically the Back to Sleep campaign, which teaches caregivers to place sleeping infants on their back.

Table 1.8 shows the U.S. infant mortality rate compared with those of other industrialized nations. In 2006 the United States had a higher infant mortality rate than 27 other countries and at least twice the rate of infant deaths as Singapore, Hong Kong, Japan, Sweden, Norway, and Finland.

LIFE EXPECTANCY

Along with infant mortality, life expectancy rates are an important measure of the health of the population. Life expectancy at birth is strongly influenced by infant and child mortality. Life expectancy in adulthood reflects death rates at or beyond specified ages and is independent of the effect of mortality at younger ages.

Figure 1.4 shows the upward trend from 1970 to 2005 in U.S. life expectancy for males and females at birth and

TABLE 1.8

Infant mortality rates and international rankings by selected countries, selected years 1960–2006

[Data are based on reporting by countries]

Country[b]	1960	1970	1980	1990	2000	2001	2002	2003	2004	2005	2006	International rankings[a] 1960	2005	2006
					Infant[c] deaths per 1,000 live births									
Australia	20.2	17.9	10.7	8.2	5.2	5.3	5.0	4.8	4.7	5.0	4.7	5	21	20
Austria	37.5	25.9	14.3	7.8	4.8	4.8	4.1	4.5	4.5	4.2	3.6	24	15	9
Belgium	23.9	21.1	12.1	6.5	4.8	4.5	4.4	4.3	4.3	3.7	—	11	9	—
Bulgaria	45.1	27.3	20.2	14.8	13.3	14.4	13.3	12.0	11.7	—	—	30	—	—
Canada	27.3	18.8	10.4	6.8	5.3	5.2	5.4	5.3	5.3	5.4	—	15	25	—
Chile	120.3	82.2	33.0	16.0	8.9	8.3	7.8	7.8	8.4	7.9	7.6	36	32	29
Costa Rica	77.9	68.4	19.9	15.0	10.3	10.8	10.5	10.1	9.3	9.8	9.6	35	34	30
Cuba	37.3	38.7	19.6	10.7	7.2	6.2	6.5	6.3	5.8	6.2	5.3	23	27	24
Czech Republic	20.0	20.2	16.9	10.8	4.1	4.0	4.1	3.9	3.7	3.4	3.3	4	7	7
Denmark	21.5	14.2	8.4	7.5	5.3	4.9	4.4	4.4	4.4	4.4	3.8	8	17	12
England and Wales	22.4	18.5	12.0	7.9	5.6	5.4	5.2	5.3	5.0	5.0	5.0	9	21	21
Finland	21.0	13.2	7.6	5.6	3.8	3.2	3.0	3.1	3.3	3.0	2.8	6	5	4
France	27.7	18.2	10.0	7.3	4.5	4.5	4.1	4.0	4.0	3.8	3.8	16	10	12
Germany[d]	35.0	22.5	12.4	7.0	4.4	4.3	4.2	4.2	4.1	3.9	3.8	22	13	12
Greece	40.1	29.6	17.9	9.7	5.4	5.1	5.1	4.0	4.1	3.8	3.7	25	10	10
Hong Kong	41.5	19.2	11.2	5.9	2.9	2.7	2.4	2.3	2.5	2.4	1.8	26	2	1
Hungary	47.6	35.9	23.2	14.8	9.2	8.1	7.2	7.3	6.6	6.2	5.7	31	27	25
Ireland	29.3	19.5	11.1	8.2	6.2	5.7	5.0	5.3	4.6	4.0	3.7	18	14	10
Israel[e]	31.0	18.9	15.6	9.9	5.4	5.1	5.4	4.9	4.5	4.6	4.3	20	18	16
Italy	43.3	29.0	14.6	8.2	4.5	4.7	4.3	3.9	4.1	4.7	—	27	19	—
Japan	30.7	13.1	7.5	4.6	3.2	3.1	3.0	3.0	2.8	2.8	2.6	19	4	2
Netherlands	17.9	12.7	8.6	7.1	5.1	5.4	5.0	4.8	4.4	4.9	4.4	2	20	17
New Zealand	22.6	16.7	13.0	8.4	6.3	5.6	5.6	4.9	5.9	5.0	5.2	10	21	23
Northern Ireland	27.2	22.9	13.4	7.5	5.0	6.1	4.7	5.3	5.5	6.1	5.1	14	26	22
Norway	18.9	12.7	8.1	6.9	3.8	3.9	3.5	3.4	3.2	3.1	3.2	3	6	6
Poland	54.8	36.7	25.5	19.3	8.1	7.7	7.5	7.0	6.8	6.4	6.0	32	29	26
Portugal	77.5	55.5	24.2	11.0	5.5	5.0	5.0	4.1	3.8	3.5	3.3	34	8	7
Puerto Rico	43.3	28.6	19.0	13.4	9.9	9.2	9.8	9.8	8.1	9.2	—	27	33	—
Romania	75.7	49.4	29.3	26.9	18.6	18.4	17.3	16.7	16.8	15.0	13.9	33	36	32
Russian Federation[f]	—	—	22.0	17.6	15.2	14.6	13.2	12.4	11.5	11.0	10.2	—	35	31
Scotland	26.4	19.6	12.1	7.7	5.7	5.5	5.3	5.1	4.9	5.2	4.5	13	24	19
Singapore	34.8	21.4	11.7	6.7	2.5	2.2	2.9	2.5	2.0	2.1	2.6	21	1	2
Slovakia	28.6	25.7	20.9	12.0	8.6	6.2	7.6	7.9	6.8	7.2	6.6	17	31	27
Spain	43.7	28.1	12.3	7.6	4.4	3.4	4.1	3.9	4.0	3.8	3.8	29	10	12
Sweden	16.6	11.0	6.9	6.0	3.4	3.7	3.3	3.1	3.1	2.4	2.8	1	2	4
Switzerland	21.1	15.1	9.1	6.8	4.9	5.0	5.0	4.3	4.2	4.2	4.4	7	15	17
United States	26.0	20.0	12.6	9.2	6.9	6.8	7.0	6.9	6.8	6.9	6.7	12	30	28

—Data not available.

[a]Rankings are from lowest to highest infant mortality rates (IMR). Countries with the same IMR receive the same rank. The country with the next highest IMR is assigned the rank it would have received had the lower-ranked countries not been tied, i.e., skip a rank. Some of the variation in IMRs is due to differences among countries in distinguishing between fetal and infant deaths.
[b]Refers to countries, territories, cities, or geographic areas with at least 1 million population and with complete counts of live births and infant deaths according to the United Nations Demographic Yearbook.
[c]Under 1 year of age.
[d]Rates for 1990 and earlier years were calculated by combining information from the Federal Republic of Germany and the German Democratic Republic.
[e]Includes data for East Jerusalem and Israeli residents in certain other territories under occupation by Israeli military forces since June 1967.
[f]Excludes infants born alive after less than 28 weeks gestation, of less than 1,000 grams in weight and 35 centimeters in length, who die within 7 days of birth.
Note: Some rates for selected countries and selected years were revised and differ from previous editions of *Health, United States*.

SOURCE: Table 24. Infant Mortality Rates and International Rankings: Selected Countries and Territories, Selected Years 1960–2006, in *Health, United States, 2008. With Chartbook*, Centers for Disease Control and Prevention, National Center for Health Statistics, 2009, http://www.cdc.gov/nchs/data/hus/hus08.pdf (accessed December 12, 2009)

FIGURE 1.4

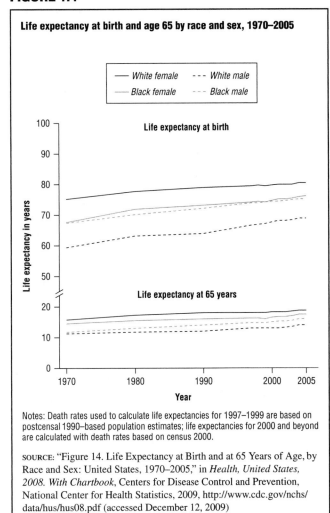

Life expectancy at birth and age 65 by race and sex, 1970–2005

— White female - - - White male
— Black female - - - Black male

Life expectancy at birth

Life expectancy at 65 years

Year

Notes: Death rates used to calculate life expectancies for 1997–1999 are based on postcensal 1990–based population estimates; life expectancies for 2000 and beyond are calculated with death rates based on census 2000.

SOURCE: "Figure 14. Life Expectancy at Birth and at 65 Years of Age, by Race and Sex: United States, 1970–2005," in *Health, United States, 2008. With Chartbook*, Centers for Disease Control and Prevention, National Center for Health Statistics, 2009, http://www.cdc.gov/nchs/data/hus/hus08.pdf (accessed December 12, 2009)

Many factors contribute to the significantly lower life expectancy for African-American men. Besides issues of access to health care, some observers suggest that African-American males must deal with greater social, economic, and psychological stress than other men, leaving African-American men more susceptible to various diseases. Among African-American males in 2006, the observed number of deaths resulting from homicides, the human immunodeficiency virus (HIV; the virus that produces the acquired immunodeficiency syndrome), and cardiovascular disease was much higher than would be expected based on their proportion in the overall population. (See Table 1.9.)

As deaths from infectious diseases declined, mortality from chronic diseases, such as heart disease, cancer, and diabetes, increased. Table 1.9 displays the 10 leading causes of death in the United States in 1980 and 2006. Being overweight or obese is considered to be a contributing factor to at least four of the 10 leading causes of death in 2006: diseases of the heart, malignant neoplasms (cancer), cerebrovascular diseases (diseases affecting the supply of blood to the brain), and diabetes mellitus. Obesity may also be implicated in another leading cause of death: nephritis, nephrotic syndrome, and nephrosis (kidney disease or chronic renal failure). Table 1.9 also reveals the rise of diabetes as a cause of death. In 1980 it was the seventh-leading cause of death, claiming 34,851 lives. By 2006 it was the sixth-leading cause of death, claiming 72,449 lives. Epidemiologists and medical researchers believe the increasing prevalence of diabetes in the U.S. population and the resultant rise in deaths attributable to diabetes are direct consequences of the obesity epidemic in the United States.

at age 65. In *Health, United States, 2009*, the NCHS indicates that life expectancy increased throughout the latter part of the 20th century, from 67.1 years in 1970 to 75.1 years in 2006 for males and from 74.7 years in 1970 to 80.2 in 2006 for females. Similarly, life expectancy at age 65 also increased during the 20th century. Unlike life expectancy at birth, which rose early in the 20th century, much of the rise in life expectancy at age 65 occurred after 1950, in response to improved access to health care, advances in medicine, healthier current lifestyles, and better health throughout the lifespan.

The CDC estimates in the press release "Life Expectancy at All Time High; Death Rates Reach New Low, New Report Shows" (August 19, 2009, http://www.cdc.gov/media/pressrel/2009/r090819.htm) that a child born in 2007 could expect to live 77.9 years. In *Health, United States, 2009*, the NCHS states that white females in 2006 had the longest life expectancy, at 80.6 years, compared with 76.5 years for African-American females, 75.7 years for white males, and 69.7 years for African-American males.

Recent research suggests that the steady increase in life expectancy that the U.S. population has experienced over the past two centuries is likely to end in the coming years and that U.S. life expectancy may actually decline. In "Forecasting the Effects of Obesity and Smoking on U.S. Life Expectancy" (*New England Journal of Medicine*, vol. 361, no. 23, December 3, 2009), Susan T. Stewart, David M. Cutler, and Allison B. Rosen of the National Bureau of Economic Research in Cambridge, Massachusetts, use obesity prevalence data to predict that nearly half the U.S. population will be obese by 2020. When the researchers combine these data with past trends in smoking to project life expectancy, they find that the negative effects of obesity, as measured by BMI, far outweighed the positive effects of declines in smoking in terms of life expectancy. Stewart, Cutler, and Rosen conclude that "if past obesity trends continue unchecked, the negative effects on the health of the U.S. population will increasingly outweigh the positive effects gained from declining smoking rates. Failure to address continued increases in obesity could result in an erosion of the pattern of steady gains in health observed since early in the 20th century."

TABLE 1.9

Leading causes of death and numbers of deaths, by sex, race, and Hispanic origin, 1980 and 2006

[Data are based on death certificates]

Sex, race, Hispanic origin, and rank order	1980 Cause of death	Deaths	2006 Cause of death	Deaths
All persons				
...	All causes	1,989,841	All causes	2,426,264
1	Diseases of heart	761,085	Diseases of heart	631,636
2	Malignant neoplasms	416,509	Malignant neoplasms	559,888
3	Cerebrovascular diseases	170,225	Cerebrovascular diseases	137,119
4	Unintentional injuries	105,718	Chronic lower respiratory diseases	124,583
5	Chronic obstructive pulmonary diseases	56,050	Unintentional injuries	121,599
6	Pneumonia and influenza	54,619	Diabetes mellitus	72,449
7	Diabetes mellitus	34,851	Alzheimer's disease	72,432
8	Chronic liver disease and cirrhosis	30,583	Influenza and pneumonia	56,326
9	Atherosclerosis	29,449	Nephritis, nephrotic syndrome and nephrosis	45,344
10	Suicide	26,869	Septicemia	34,234
Male				
...	All causes	1,075,078	All causes	1,201,942
1	Diseases of heart	405,661	Diseases of heart	315,706
2	Malignant neoplasms	225,948	Malignant neoplasms	290,069
3	Unintentional injuries	74,180	Unintentional injuries	78,941
4	Cerebrovascular diseases	69,973	Chronic lower respiratory diseases	59,260
5	Chronic obstructive pulmonary diseases	38,625	Cerebrovascular diseases	54,524
6	Pneumonia and influenza	27,574	Diabetes mellitus	36,006
7	Suicide	20,505	Suicide	26,308
8	Chronic liver disease and cirrhosis	19,768	Influenza and pneumonia	25,650
9	Homicide	18,779	Nephritis, nephrotic syndrome and nephrosis	22,094
10	Diabetes mellitus	14,325	Alzheimer's disease	21,151
Female				
...	All causes	914,763	All causes	1,224,322
1	Diseases of heart	355,424	Diseases of heart	315,930
2	Malignant neoplasms	190,561	Malignant neoplasms	269,819
3	Cerebrovascular diseases	100,252	Cerebrovascular diseases	82,595
4	Unintentional injuries	31,538	Chronic lower respiratory diseases	65,323
5	Pneumonia and influenza	27,045	Alzheimer's disease	51,281
6	Diabetes mellitus	20,526	Unintentional injuries	42,658
7	Atherosclerosis	17,848	Diabetes mellitus	36,443
8	Chronic obstructive pulmonary diseases	17,425	Influenza and pneumonia	30,676
9	Chronic liver disease and cirrhosis	10,815	Nephritis, nephrotic syndrome and nephrosis	23,250
10	Certain conditions originating in the perinatal period	9,815	Septicemia	18,712
White				
...	All causes	1,738,607	All causes	2,077,549
1	Diseases of heart	683,347	Diseases of heart	545,974
2	Malignant neoplasms	368,162	Malignant neoplasms	482,575
3	Cerebrovascular diseases	148,734	Cerebrovascular diseases	115,864
4	Unintentional injuries	90,122	Chronic lower respiratory diseases	114,993
5	Chronic obstructive pulmonary diseases	52,375	Unintentional injuries	103,853
6	Pneumonia and influenza	48,369	Alzheimer's disease	67,088
7	Diabetes mellitus	28,868	Diabetes mellitus	57,204
8	Atherosclerosis	27,069	Influenza and pneumonia	49,401
9	Chronic liver disease and cirrhosis	25,240	Nephritis, nephrotic syndrome and nephrosis	35,793
10	Suicide	24,829	Suicide	30,138
Black or African American				
...	All causes	233,135	All causes	289,971
1	Diseases of heart	72,956	Diseases of heart	72,253
2	Malignant neoplasms	45,037	Malignant neoplasms	63,082
3	Cerebrovascular diseases	20,135	Cerebrovascular diseases	17,045
4	Unintentional injuries	13,480	Unintentional injuries	13,917
5	Homicide	10,172	Diabetes mellitus	12,813
6	Certain conditions originating in the perinatal period	6,961	Homicide	9,032
7	Pneumonia and influenza	5,648	Nephritis, nephrotic syndrome and nephrosis	8,397
8	Diabetes mellitus	5,544	Chronic lower respiratory diseases	7,730
9	Chronic liver disease and cirrhosis	4,790	Human immunodeficiency virus (HIV) disease	6,854
10	Nephritis, nephrotic syndrome, and nephrosis	3,416	Septicemia	6,108

MORTALITY

Years of Potential Life Lost

Years of potential life lost (YPLL) is a term used by medical and public health professionals to describe the number of years deceased people might have lived if they had not died prematurely (before their life expectancy). In 2006 most YPLL resulted from malignant neoplasms, unintentional injuries (accidents), and heart disease. (See Table 1.10.)

TABLE 1.9

Leading causes of death and numbers of deaths, by sex, race, and Hispanic origin, 1980 and 2006 [CONTINUED]

[Data are based on death certificates]

Sex, race, Hispanic origin, and rank order	1980		2006	
	Cause of death	Deaths	Cause of death	Deaths
American Indian or Alaska Native				
...	All causes	6,923	All causes	14,037
1	Diseases of heart	1,494	Diseases of heart	2,736
2	Unintentional injuries	1,290	Malignant neoplasms	2,447
3	Malignant neoplasms	770	Unintentional injuries	1,704
4	Chronic liver disease and cirrhosis	410	Diabetes mellitus	811
5	Cerebrovascular diseases	322	Chronic liver disease and cirrhosis	596
6	Pneumonia and influenza	257	Cerebrovascular diseases	548
7	Homicide	217	Chronic lower respiratory diseases	508
8	Diabetes mellitus	210	Suicide	395
9	Certain conditions originating in the perinatal period	199	Nephritis, nephrotic syndrome and nephrosis	288
10	Suicide	181	Influenza and pneumonia	267
Asian or Pacific Islander				
...	All causes	11,071	All causes	44,707
1	Diseases of heart	3,265	Malignant neoplasms	11,784
2	Malignant neoplasms	2,522	Diseases of heart	10,673
3	Cerebrovascular diseases	1,028	Cerebrovascular diseases	3,662
4	Unintentional injuries	810	Unintentional injuries	2,125
5	Pneumonia and influenza	342	Diabetes mellitus	1,621
6	Suicide	249	Chronic lower respiratory diseases	1,352
7	Certain conditions originating in the perinatal period	246	Influenza and pneumonia	1,347
8	Diabetes mellitus	227	Nephritis, nephrotic syndrome and nephrosis	866
9	Homicide	211	Suicide	813
10	Chronic obstructive pulmonary diseases	207	Alzheimer's disease	720
Hispanic or Latino				
...	—	—	All causes	133,004
1	—	—	Diseases of heart	28,921
2	—	—	Malignant neoplasms	26,633
3	—	—	Unintentional injuries	12,052
4	—	—	Cerebrovascular diseases	7,005
5	—	—	Diabetes mellitus	6,287
6	—	—	Chronic liver disease and cirrhosis	3,592
7	—	—	Homicide	3,524
8	—	—	Chronic lower respiratory diseases	3,310
9	—	—	Influenza and pneumonia	2,966
10	—	—	Certain conditions originating in the perinatal period	2,804
White male				
...	All causes	933,878	All causes	1,022,328
1	Diseases of heart	364,679	Diseases of heart	272,117
2	Malignant neoplasms	198,188	Malignant neoplasms	250,322
3	Unintentional injuries	62,963	Unintentional injuries	66,843
4	Cerebrovascular diseases	60,095	Chronic lower respiratory diseases	54,043
5	Chronic obstructive pulmonary diseases	35,977	Cerebrovascular diseases	45,198
6	Pneumonia and influenza	23,810	Diabetes mellitus	29,060
7	Suicide	18,901	Suicide	23,767
8	Chronic liver disease and cirrhosis	16,407	Influenza and pneumonia	22,310
9	Diabetes mellitus	12,125	Alzheimer's disease	19,654
10	Atherosclerosis	10,543	Nephritis, nephrotic syndrome and nephrosis	17,715
Black or African American male				
...	All causes	130,138	All causes	148,602
1	Diseases of heart	37,877	Diseases of heart	36,230
2	Malignant neoplasms	25,861	Malignant neoplasms	32,556
3	Unintentional injuries	9,701	Unintentional injuries	9,605
4	Cerebrovascular diseases	9,194	Homicide	7,677
5	Homicide	8,274	Cerebrovascular diseases	7,424
6	Certain conditions originating in the perinatal period	3,869	Diabetes mellitus	5,772
7	Pneumonia and influenza	3,386	Human immunodeficiency virus (HIV) disease	4,443
8	Chronic liver disease and cirrhosis	3,020	Chronic lower respiratory diseases	4,136
9	Chronic obstructive pulmonary diseases	2,429	Nephritis, nephrotic syndrome and nephrosis	3,812
10	Diabetes mellitus	2,010	Certain conditions originating in the perinatal period	2,811

The increase in life expectancy during the 20th and 21st centuries has meant a decrease in the YPLL rate. In 1980 a total of 10,448.4 years per 100,000 population were lost to people younger than age 75; by 2006 this number had declined to 7,214.3 total years lost. (See Table 1.10.) Even though heart disease remains the number-one killer in the United States (see Table 1.9), it has been responsible for a smaller proportion of YPLL since 1980 (2,238.7 in 1980

TABLE 1.9

[Data are based on death certificates]

Sex, race, Hispanic origin, and rank order	1980 Cause of death	Deaths	2006 Cause of death	Deaths
American Indian or Alaska Native male				
...	All causes	4,193	All causes	7,630
1	Unintentional injuries	946	Diseases of heart	1,532
2	Diseases of heart	917	Malignant neoplasms	1,217
3	Malignant neoplasms	408	Unintentional injuries	1,184
4	Chronic liver disease and cirrhosis	239	Diabetes mellitus	362
5	Cerebrovascular diseases	163	Chronic liver disease and cirrhosis	330
6	Homicide	162	Suicide	309
7	Pneumonia and influenza	148	Chronic lower respiratory diseases	234
8	Suicide	147	Cerebrovascular diseases	231
9	Certain conditions originating in the perinatal period	107	Homicide	206
10	Diabetes mellitus	86	Influenza and pneumonia	137
Asian or Pacific Islander male				
...	All causes	6,809	All causes	23,382
1	Diseases of heart	2,174	Malignant neoplasms	5,974
2	Malignant neoplasms	1,485	Diseases of heart	5,827
3	Unintentional injuries	556	Cerebrovascular diseases	1,671
4	Cerebrovascular diseases	521	Unintentional injuries	1,309
5	Pneumonia and influenza	227	Chronic lower respiratory diseases	847
6	Suicide	159	Diabetes mellitus	812
7	Chronic obstructive pulmonary diseases	158	Influenza and pneumonia	717
8	Homicide	151	Suicide	563
9	Certain conditions originating in the perinatal period	128	Nephritis, nephrotic syndrome and nephrosis	432
10	Diabetes mellitus	103	Homicide	320
Hispanic or Latino male				
...	—	—	All causes	74,250
1	—	—	Diseases of heart	15,518
2	—	—	Malignant neoplasms	13,856
3	—	—	Unintentional injuries	9,102
4	—	—	Cerebrovascular diseases	3,269
5	—	—	Diabetes mellitus	3,140
6	—	—	Homicide	3,004
7	—	—	Chronic liver disease and cirrhosis	2,527
8	—	—	Suicide	1,813
9	—	—	Chronic lower respiratory diseases	1,708
10	—	—	Certain conditions originating in the perinatal period	1,565
White female				
...	All causes	804,729	All causes	1,055,221
1	Diseases of heart	318,668	Diseases of heart	273,857
2	Malignant neoplasms	169,974	Malignant neoplasms	232,253
3	Cerebrovascular diseases	88,639	Cerebrovascular diseases	70,666
4	Unintentional injuries	27,159	Chronic lower respiratory diseases	60,950
5	Pneumonia and influenza	24,559	Alzheimer's disease	47,434
6	Diabetes mellitus	16,743	Unintentional injuries	37,010
7	Atherosclerosis	16,526	Diabetes mellitus	28,144
8	Chronic obstructive pulmonary diseases	16,398	Influenza and pneumonia	27,091
9	Chronic liver disease and cirrhosis	8,833	Nephritis, nephrotic syndrome and nephrosis	18,078
10	Certain conditions originating in the perinatal period	6,512	Septicemia	14,923
Black or African American female				
...	All causes	102,997	All causes	141,369
1	Diseases of heart	35,079	Diseases of heart	36,023
2	Malignant neoplasms	19,176	Malignant neoplasms	30,526
3	Cerebrovascular diseases	10,941	Cerebrovascular diseases	9,621
4	Unintentional injuries	3,779	Diabetes mellitus	7,041
5	Diabetes mellitus	3,534	Nephritis, nephrotic syndrome and nephrosis	4,585
6	Certain conditions originating in the perinatal period	3,092	Unintentional injuries	4,312
7	Pneumonia and influenza	2,262	Chronic lower respiratory diseases	3,594
8	Homicide	1,898	Septicemia	3,391
9	Chronic liver disease and cirrhosis	1,770	Alzheimer's disease	3,265
10	Nephritis, nephrotic syndrome, and nephrosis	1,722	Influenza and pneumonia	2,825

and 1,077.8 in 2006). Similarly, the years lost to cerebrovascular diseases (e.g., strokes), liver diseases, pneumonia, and motor vehicle accidents have also declined since 1980. After increasing dramatically between 1980 and 1995, the years lost to HIV infection steadily decreased between 1996 and 2006. However, YPLL rates for diabetes increased over this same period (dropping slightly from 2005 to 2006) and chronic lower respiratory diseases remained roughly the same with substantial decreases in 2004 and 2006.

TABLE 1.9

Leading causes of death and numbers of deaths, by sex, race, and Hispanic origin, 1980 and 2006 [CONTINUED]

[Data are based on death certificates]

Sex, race, Hispanic origin, and rank order	1980		2006	
	Cause of death	Deaths	Cause of death	Deaths
American Indian or Alaska Native female				
...	All causes	2,730	All causes	6,407
1	Diseases of heart	577	Malignant neoplasms	1,230
2	Malignant neoplasms	362	Diseases of heart	1,204
3	Unintentional injuries	344	Unintentional injuries	520
4	Chronic liver disease and cirrhosis	171	Diabetes mellitus	449
5	Cerebrovascular diseases	159	Cerebrovascular diseases	317
6	Diabetes mellitus	124	Chronic lower respiratory diseases	274
7	Pneumonia and influenza	109	Chronic liver disease and cirrhosis	266
8	Certain conditions originating in the perinatal period	92	Nephritis, nephrotic syndrome and nephrosis	153
9	Nephritis, nephrotic syndrome, and nephrosis	56	Influenza and pneumonia	130
10	Homicide	55	Septicemia	108
Asian or Pacific Islander female				
...	All causes	4,262	All causes	21,325
1	Diseases of heart	1,091	Malignant neoplasms	5,810
2	Malignant neoplasms	1,037	Diseases of heart	4,846
3	Cerebrovascular diseases	507	Cerebrovascular diseases	1,991
4	Unintentional injuries	254	Unintentional injuries	816
5	Diabetes mellitus	124	Diabetes mellitus	809
6	Certain conditions originating in the perinatal period	118	Influenza and pneumonia	630
7	Pneumonia and influenza	115	Chronic lower respiratory diseases	505
8	Congenital anomalies	104	Alzheimer's disease	475
9	Suicide	90	Nephritis, nephrotic syndrome and nephrosis	434
10	Homicide	60	Essential hypertension and hypertensive renal disease	338
Hispanic or Latina female				
...	—	—	All causes	58,754
1	—	—	Diseases of heart	13,403
2	—	—	Malignant neoplasms	12,777
3	—	—	Cerebrovascular diseases	3,736
4	—	—	Diabetes mellitus	3,147
5	—	—	Unintentional injuries	2,950
6	—	—	Chronic lower respiratory diseases	1,602
7	—	—	Alzheimer's disease	1,587
8	—	—	Influenza and pneumonia	1,527
9	—	—	Nephritis, nephrotic syndrome and nephrosis	1,297
10	—	—	Certain conditions originating in the perinatal period	1,239

...Category not applicable.
—Data not available.
Notes: For cause of death codes based on the International Classification of Diseases, 9th Revision (ICD-9) in 1980 and icd-10 IN 2006.

SOURCE: "Table 28. Leading Causes of Death and Numbers of Deaths, by Sex, Race, and Hispanic Origin: United States, 1980 and 2006," in *Health, United States, 2009. With Special Feature on Medical Technology*, Centers for Disease Control and Prevention, National Center for Health Statistics, 2010, http://www.cdc.gov/nchs/data/hus/hus09.pdf (accessed March 12, 2010)

Except for suicide, the YPLL due to all causes for African-Americans was significantly higher than for whites. In 2006, for all causes, African-Americans lost 11,646.3 years per 100,000 population, compared with 6,713.1 years for whites. (See Table 1.10.) African-Americans lost considerably more years of life to heart disease, cerebrovascular diseases, cancers, HIV, and homicide than did whites.

RACIAL AND GENDER DIFFERENCES. Significant racial and ethnic variations exist in the 10 leading causes of death. (See Table 1.9.) In 2006 chronic liver disease and cirrhosis were not listed as leading causes of death for all Americans; they were, however, listed as leading causes of death among Native Americans or Alaskan Natives and Hispanics. Homicide was a leading cause of death for African-American and Hispanic men; however, it ranked ninth for Native American or Alaskan Native men and was the tenth-leading cause of death for Asian or Pacific Islander men. In 2006 homicide did not rank as a leading cause of death for women of any race or ethnicity.

AGE DIFFERENCES. The NCHS indicates in *Health, United States, 2009* that, as would be expected, death rates were highest for people aged 85 and older (13,253.1 per 100,000 population) in 2006. From age 25 on, death rates doubled with each additional decade.

The 10 leading causes of death vary by age. In 2006 accidents (unintentional injuries) were the leading cause of death for children one to four years of age, followed by congenital malformations and malignant neoplasms. (See Table 1.11.) Among children five to 14 years old, accidents

TABLE 1.10

Years of potential life lost before age 75 for selected causes of death, by sex and race, selected years 1980–2006

[Data are based on death certificates]

Sex, race, Hispanic origin, and cause of death[b]	Age-adjusted[a]			1992	1993	1994	1995	1996	1997	1998	1999[c]	2000[c]	2001[c]	2002[c]	2003[c]	2004[c]	2005[c]	2006[c]
	1980	1990	1991															
	Years lost before age 75 per 100,000 population under 75 years of age																	
All persons																		
All causes	10,448.4	9,085.5	8,965.7	8,752.2	8,858.1	8,765.7	8,626.2	8,229.2	7,852.5	7,667.0	7,599.4	7,578.1	7,531.2	7,499.6	7,466.9	7,270.6	7,299.8	7,214.3
Diseases of heart	2,238.7	1,617.7	1,584.4	1,546.2	1,542.7	1,501.5	1,475.4	1,430.6	1,387.5	1,345.4	1,294.7	1,253.0	1,221.1	1,212.7	1,187.9	1,128.9	1,110.4	1,077.8
Ischemic heart disease	1,729.3	1,153.6	1,122.3	1,085.7	1,073.1	1,038.6	1,013.2	981.5	934.1	892.5	874.6	841.8	809.7	792.0	765.1	720.6	701.8	675.5
Cerebrovascular diseases	357.5	259.6	252.2	246.2	246.2	247.4	246.5	244.5	240.1	232.4	218.9	223.3	211.9	208.1	203.6	198.1	193.3	190.2
Malignant neoplasms	2,108.8	2,003.8	1,980.2	1,939.8	1,910.5	1,881.5	1,841.6	1,800.5	1,760.5	1,720.4	1,694.4	1,674.1	1,651.7	1,622.7	1,586.9	1,543.4	1,525.2	1,490.5
Trachea, bronchus, and lung	548.5	561.4	546.5	535.2	525.7	509.1	497.3	486.4	471.0	461.2	441.4	443.1	431.2	423.4	412.2	402.8	392.9	378.7
Colorectal	190.0	164.7	162.1	157.7	156.2	156.1	152.0	146.2	145.4	143.5	142.6	141.9	142.4	141.0	133.8	127.3	124.7	126.1
Prostate[d]	84.9	96.8	94.4	93.4	89.2	87.3	83.5	81.2	74.7	71.6	67.4	63.6	61.8	60.1	58.6	55.8	55.1	54.8
Breast[e]	463.2	451.6	441.3	421.5	407.6	402.5	398.6	379.1	366.6	352.2	328.9	332.6	328.1	316.8	313.7	302.1	296.2	286.7
Chronic lower respiratory diseases	169.1	187.4	191.6	184.4	196.0	193.5	190.4	189.6	187.7	186.5	195.9	188.1	185.8	184.5	183.9	173.7	181.2	171.0
Influenza and pneumonia	160.2	141.5	137.9	127.4	135.1	130.4	126.9	125.7	123.5	121.7	86.0	87.1	82.3	82.7	90.8	79.1	83.6	76.4
Chronic liver disease and cirrhosis	300.3	196.9	188.2	182.2	180.1	178.6	173.7	169.3	164.5	159.9	162.1	164.1	164.7	160.5	159.6	153.9	152.6	149.9
Diabetes mellitus	134.4	155.9	158.4	159.1	164.3	170.4	174.7	178.4	174.0	174.1	178.3	178.4	180.5	184.3	184.6	178.4	179.9	176.5
Human immunodeficiency virus (HIV) disease	—	383.8	437.7	487.9	534.9	593.6	595.3	420.4	217.6	171.8	183.3	174.6	167.8	161.8	153.3	143.4	133.6	126.0
Unintentional injuries	1,543.5	1,162.1	1,106.0	1,033.5	1,066.6	1,060.3	1,057.2	1,039.0	1,018.6	1,008.8	1,021.3	1,026.5	1,036.8	1,079.2	1,084.6	1,098.0	1,132.7	1,167.5
Motor vehicle-related injuries	912.9	716.4	658.7	603.7	610.7	613.0	616.3	610.9	592.0	579.6	561.6	574.3	572.5	585.8	569.6	567.6	564.4	561.2
Suicide[f]	392.0	393.1	388.2	381.7	387.4	389.1	384.7	371.3	361.1	355.0	334.0	334.5	342.6	346.7	343.3	353.0	347.3	348.7
Homicide[f]	425.5	417.4	445.0	427.8	437.6	416.8	378.6	343.1	318.9	290.8	271.0	266.5	311.0	274.4	274.3	264.8	276.8	281.8
Male																		
All causes	13,777.2	11,973.5	11,804.0	11,523.9	11,648.2	11,519.5	11,289.2	10,632.7	10,021.1	9,728.2	9,606.8	9,572.2	9,507.1	9,470.0	9,416.4	9,143.1	9,206.1	9,092.6
Diseases of heart	3,352.1	2,356.0	2,299.0	2,236.3	2,220.2	2,155.7	2,117.4	2,037.7	1,975.9	1,903.0	1,823.0	1,766.0	1,708.3	1,706.9	1,664.2	1,583.4	1,561.6	1,517.5
Ischemic heart disease	2,715.1	1,766.3	1,710.9	1,651.8	1,627.5	1,570.8	1,531.5	1,473.5	1,405.1	1,337.4	1,302.5	1,255.4	1,201.8	1,179.6	1,138.8	1,070.5	1,044.3	1,009.2
Cerebrovascular diseases	396.7	286.6	281.1	275.3	275.3	277.4	276.9	272.5	267.4	258.0	241.0	244.6	233.5	227.6	225.9	219.6	213.7	212.0
Malignant neoplasms	2,360.8	2,214.6	2,185.6	2,133.6	2,106.8	2,065.9	2,008.5	1,964.6	1,911.5	1,872.8	1,844.4	1,810.8	1,782.4	1,754.2	1,711.4	1,663.3	1,639.7	1,595.2
Trachea, bronchus, and lung	821.1	764.8	738.7	713.0	699.2	671.0	645.6	629.2	601.6	584.5	557.2	554.9	535.9	520.5	504.6	490.3	476.3	454.5
Colorectal	214.9	194.3	189.9	186.2	183.7	184.7	179.4	172.8	171.7	168.9	165.9	167.3	166.6	168.2	157.7	149.7	146.2	145.4
Prostate	84.9	96.8	94.4	93.4	89.2	87.3	83.5	81.2	74.7	71.6	67.4	63.6	61.8	60.1	58.6	55.8	55.1	54.8
Chronic lower respiratory diseases	235.1	224.8	223.6	216.7	225.9	221.5	213.1	210.0	210.1	207.3	216.8	206.0	200.7	200.7	199.5	188.4	195.8	182.4
Influenza and pneumonia	202.5	180.0	172.6	160.4	167.2	162.4	155.7	154.1	150.0	144.0	100.1	102.8	96.9	97.3	106.4	93.6	97.8	88.9
Chronic liver disease and cirrhosis	415.0	283.9	269.6	266.8	261.1	259.0	254.8	246.5	238.2	232.1	236.9	236.9	233.6	226.6	229.4	219.0	216.1	210.9
Diabetes mellitus	140.4	170.4	173.2	176.7	181.5	189.4	194.6	200.8	194.1	197.8	202.7	203.8	209.6	217.2	218.2	212.6	216.5	213.2
Human immunodeficiency virus (HIV) disease	—	686.2	774.8	855.0	921.5	1,004.1	991.2	680.3	337.7	261.0	275.5	258.9	247.7	237.0	223.7	205.1	192.0	178.3

TABLE 1.10

Years of potential life lost before age 75 for selected causes of death, by sex and race, selected years 1980–2006 [CONTINUED]

[Data are based on death certificates]

Sex, race, Hispanic origin, and cause of death[b]	1980	Age-adjusted[a]		1992	1993	1994	1995	1996	1997	1998	1999[c]	2000[c]	2001[c]	2002[c]	2003[c]	2004[c]	2005[c]	2006[c]
		1990	1991															
Unintentional injuries	2,342.7	1,715.1	1,622.5	1,516.8	1,560.9	1,542.7	1,531.6	1,490.9	1,458.2	1,447.1	1,463.9	1,475.6	1,490.1	1,542.2	1,537.7	1,547.4	1,608.5	1,659.2
Motor vehicle-related injuries	1,359.7	1,018.4	928.2	846.3	855.0	848.6	851.1	835.5	803.3	792.9	771.1	796.4	803.5	817.2	795.0	789.1	795.9	790.9
Suicide[f]	605.6	634.8	628.8	618.3	626.8	633.8	628.4	602.4	581.2	570.9	537.5	539.1	552.3	555.7	548.2	553.0	548.0	549.0
Homicide[f]	675.0	658.0	700.6	676.7	685.5	660.5	589.6	533.3	499.1	445.6	411.1	410.5	480.5	425.0	430.5	414.3	439.0	447.1
Female																		
All causes	7,350.3	6,333.1	6,251.3	6,094.7	6,176.0	6,113.1	6,057.5	5,912.8	5,763.1	5,678.7	5,659.2	5,644.6	5,609.2	5,580.0	5,560.5	5,435.8	5,425.7	5,364.7
Diseases of heart	1,246.0	948.5	934.2	915.9	922.4	901.1	883.9	870.5	842.8	827.9	803.4	774.6	765.4	748.8	739.5	699.9	682.6	660.6
Ischemic heart disease	852.1	600.3	588.9	570.7	567.5	552.2	537.8	529.4	500.1	481.5	478.3	457.6	444.3	430.2	415.0	391.8	379.0	360.6
Cerebrovascular diseases	324.0	235.9	226.7	219.9	220.1	220.3	218.7	219.0	215.2	208.7	198.8	203.9	192.1	190.3	183.0	178.1	174.4	169.8
Malignant neoplasms	1,896.8	1,826.6	1,806.2	1,775.4	1,742.6	1,723.5	1,698.9	1,659.9	1,631.1	1,588.6	1,564.0	1,555.3	1,538.4	1,507.7	1,477.3	1,437.6	1,424.3	1,398.6
Trachea, bronchus, and lung	310.4	382.2	376.6	377.6	371.3	364.9	365.2	358.5	354.0	350.6	337.2	342.1	336.6	335.4	328.1	323.2	316.9	309.7
Colorectal	168.7	138.7	137.6	132.4	131.8	130.6	127.5	122.4	121.8	120.6	121.5	118.7	120.4	115.9	111.9	106.8	104.9	108.4
Breast	463.2	451.6	441.3	421.5	407.6	402.5	398.6	379.1	366.6	352.2	328.9	332.6	328.1	316.8	313.7	302.1	296.2	286.7
Chronic lower respiratory diseases	114.0	155.9	164.6	156.9	170.3	169.4	171.0	172.1	168.2	168.4	177.9	172.3	172.8	170.0	169.9	160.4	168.2	160.5
Influenza and pneumonia	122.0	106.2	105.8	96.8	105.6	100.5	100.2	99.4	99.0	101.3	73.0	72.3	68.7	69.1	76.0	65.3	70.0	64.7
Chronic liver disease and cirrhosis	194.5	115.1	111.6	102.2	103.3	102.4	96.6	95.8	94.3	91.1	90.9	94.5	98.8	97.4	92.6	91.3	91.6	91.3
Diabetes mellitus	128.5	142.3	144.4	142.2	148.2	152.4	155.9	157.3	155.1	152.0	155.3	154.4	153.0	153.1	152.9	146.0	145.1	141.7
Human immunodeficiency virus (HIV) disease	—	87.8	107.0	127.1	154.7	189.7	205.7	164.7	99.4	84.2	92.8	92.0	89.4	88.1	84.1	82.7	76.2	74.5
Unintentional injuries	755.3	607.4	587.4	548.0	569.7	575.1	580.1	584.2	576.6	567.5	575.4	573.2	578.3	610.3	624.6	641.1	648.0	666.1
Motor vehicle-related injuries	470.4	411.6	386.4	358.3	363.3	374.2	378.4	383.1	377.9	363.3	349.0	348.5	337.2	349.8	339.2	341.1	327.1	325.4
Suicide[f]	184.2	153.3	149.0	145.9	148.5	144.2	140.8	140.3	141.0	138.9	130.0	129.1	131.9	136.6	136.6	150.9	144.1	145.7
Homicide[f]	181.3	174.3	185.9	174.5	184.9	168.3	163.2	148.7	134.7	132.5	127.6	118.9	137.4	119.6	112.9	110.2	108.7	110.4
White[g]																		
All causes	9,554.1	8,159.5	8,038.1	7,836.0	7,909.5	7,833.2	7,744.9	7,412.3	7,127.2	6,980.5	6,937.2	6,949.5	6,941.6	6,936.6	6,910.6	6,743.7	6,775.6	6,713.1
Diseases of heart	2,100.8	1,490.3	1,457.0	1,418.6	1,413.4	1,378.0	1,353.0	1,313.5	1,275.8	1,231.1	1,186.1	1,149.4	1,115.0	1,111.8	1,081.3	1,031.0	1,011.7	985.9
Ischemic heart disease	1,682.7	1,113.4	1,079.3	1,044.9	1,029.7	999.0	975.2	946.2	898.3	858.3	836.4	805.3	773.0	759.5	731.5	690.4	672.0	648.2
Cerebrovascular diseases	300.7	213.1	207.4	203.7	205.4	204.1	205.2	204.1	198.8	193.6	183.1	187.1	175.6	173.5	166.7	165.4	160.4	158.1
Malignant neoplasms	2,035.9	1,929.3	1,912.3	1,870.9	1,844.8	1,819.9	1,780.5	1,745.2	1,703.4	1,664.2	1,644.6	1,627.8	1,610.2	1,582.8	1,546.5	1,502.0	1,485.9	1,456.6
Trachea, bronchus, and lung	529.9	544.2	531.4	520.1	513.0	498.3	487.1	477.6	461.7	452.5	434.0	436.3	427.5	418.5	407.9	398.3	389.4	374.8
Colorectal	186.8	157.8	156.4	151.3	149.6	148.4	145.0	138.8	138.1	135.9	135.5	134.1	135.0	134.0	125.5	120.5	117.3	118.9
Prostate[d]	74.8	86.6	84.0	81.9	78.2	76.6	73.0	71.0	64.6	61.8	57.9	54.3	53.1	51.3	50.5	48.4	47.0	47.3
Breast[e]	460.2	441.7	428.7	408.3	393.9	388.5	381.5	361.9	349.9	334.5	309.8	315.6	309.6	297.5	295.0	282.1	275.1	269.0
Chronic lower respiratory diseases	165.4	182.3	185.9	180.5	191.7	189.0	185.7	184.1	184.2	181.7	193.6	185.3	184.7	183.5	184.2	174.3	182.2	172.0
Influenza and pneumonia	130.8	116.9	115.2	106.8	115.3	111.1	108.3	107.3	107.5	105.2	74.2	77.7	72.7	75.1	82.2	71.5	76.3	70.4
Chronic liver disease and cirrhosis	257.3	175.8	172.0	168.7	167.6	167.6	164.6	163.2	160.4	156.8	159.5	162.7	164.4	162.9	162.3	157.2	156.7	155.3

TABLE 1.10

Years of potential life lost before age 75 for selected causes of death, by sex and race, selected years 1980–2006 [CONTINUED]

[Data are based on death certificates]

Sex, race, Hispanic origin, and cause of death[b]	1980	Age-adjusted[a] 1990	1991	1992	1993	1994	1995	1996	1997	1998	1999[c]	2000[c]	2001[c]	2002[c]	2003[c]	2004[c]	2005[c]	2006[c]
Diabetes mellitus	115.7	133.7	135.8	136.8	140.9	146.9	149.4	153.2	147.9	148.8	153.3	155.6	156.2	160.3	160.3	155.2	156.3	152.8
Human immunodeficiency virus (HIV) disease	—	309.0	347.0	377.8	402.5	431.5	422.6	273.8	125.4	94.4	101.5	94.7	88.4	84.7	82.1	74.5	69.8	64.6
Unintentional injuries	1,520.4	1,139.7	1,080.8	1,011.9	1,039.6	1,034.8	1,040.9	1,025.1	1,006.2	1,002.4	1,020.2	1,031.8	1,049.0	1,101.6	1,117.7	1,134.9	1,170.9	1,209.8
Motor vehicle-related injuries	939.9	726.7	670.0	609.9	617.6	620.4	623.6	618.1	597.2	586.0	571.0	586.1	585.1	604.0	588.5	587.6	585.7	580.5
Suicide[f]	414.5	417.7	415.1	406.2	411.1	412.9	411.6	397.6	387.9	383.1	359.8	362.0	373.5	380.1	375.0	386.0	381.2	383.5
Homicide[f]	271.7	234.9	248.1	241.6	238.6	231.8	220.2	195.8	184.5	172.1	163.2	156.6	204.0	159.7	159.3	157.0	159.7	160.1
Black or African American[g]																		
All causes	17,873.4	16,593.0	16,506.2	16,136.3	16,453.7	16,212.2	15,809.7	14,917.8	13,812.7	13,339.8	13,112.4	12,897.1	12,579.7	12,401.0	12,304.0	11,922.4	11,890.7	11,646.3
Diseases of heart	3,619.9	2,891.8	2,862.1	2,806.0	2,822.5	2,704.5	2,681.8	2,582.3	2,489.3	2,456.9	2,360.8	2,275.2	2,248.9	2,212.8	2,205.7	2,090.5	2,046.0	1,969.3
Ischemic heart disease	2,305.1	1,676.1	1,662.0	1,597.7	1,615.9	1,534.8	1,510.2	1,448.3	1,390.9	1,336.6	1,345.7	1,300.1	1,260.6	1,218.7	1,182.6	1,119.0	1,080.2	1,034.5
Cerebrovascular diseases	883.2	656.4	628.8	603.6	590.0	607.3	583.6	575.0	568.3	542.5	500.3	507.0	491.3	474.1	479.6	452.0	441.7	431.8
Malignant neoplasms	2,946.1	2,894.8	2,808.4	2,778.0	2,724.4	2,652.1	2,597.1	2,512.5	2,471.6	2,418.6	2,344.9	2,294.7	2,228.4	2,196.6	2,163.9	2,107.3	2,069.7	2,003.1
Trachea, bronchus, and lung	776.0	811.3	769.7	762.3	731.8	699.9	683.0	662.0	641.4	627.1	595.1	593.0	557.5	561.9	542.1	529.3	511.8	496.4
Colorectal	232.3	241.8	230.4	225.9	230.1	236.9	226.9	223.4	220.4	219.8	220.2	222.4	219.6	213.7	214.4	196.6	199.6	198.9
Prostate[d]	200.3	223.5	221.9	232.7	220.8	218.4	210.0	202.0	194.1	186.3	179.4	171.0	164.1	160.3	154.3	143.0	144.8	140.0
Breast[e]	524.2	592.9	594.1	586.1	572.6	564.5	577.4	562.6	550.0	529.9	516.5	500.0	501.7	495.9	490.6	477.7	485.7	450.1
Chronic lower respiratory diseases	203.7	240.6	252.0	230.8	245.8	246.0	244.0	246.0	231.5	240.6	239.4	232.7	220.5	222.8	212.3	201.8	211.0	197.6
Influenza and pneumonia	384.9	330.8	314.1	280.9	288.6	276.0	269.8	266.8	247.4	242.6	172.9	161.2	152.1	146.7	157.5	141.2	145.3	127.6
Chronic liver disease and cirrhosis	644.0	371.8	326.9	295.6	284.3	273.7	250.3	231.0	209.8	195.1	193.2	185.6	181.5	161.3	158.9	148.4	138.4	127.0
Diabetes mellitus	305.3	361.5	370.5	366.1	382.1	385.3	400.8	399.9	402.0	393.7	396.5	383.4	392.6	396.7	396.0	378.8	379.9	375.4
Human immunodeficiency virus (HIV) disease	—	1,014.7	1,195.6	1,394.4	1,597.9	1,873.5	1,945.4	1,540.3	906.6	741.7	786.1	763.3	743.5	720.6	670.1	637.8	594.4	566.8
Unintentional injuries	1,751.5	1,392.7	1,378.2	1,258.8	1,343.0	1,324.0	1,272.1	1,239.1	1,209.3	1,188.4	1,185.0	1,152.8	1,133.4	1,129.3	1,082.1	1,095.5	1,134.6	1,170.7
Motor vehicle-related injuries	750.2	699.5	644.5	613.3	620.8	622.2	621.8	623.6	623.3	608.7	580.0	580.6	571.7	558.5	536.2	543.8	532.3	541.6
Suicide[f]	238.0	261.4	250.5	257.6	269.6	265.8	254.2	242.6	231.1	215.6	207.7	208.7	201.5	196.5	199.5	200.6	194.0	187.3
Homicide[f]	1,580.8	1,612.9	1,704.6	1,608.0	1,674.1	1,560.4	1,352.8	1,243.5	1,134.5	1,016.4	924.9	941.6	963.6	962.2	965.0	918.7	967.8	998.6
American Indian or Alaska Native[g]																		
All causes	13,390.9	9,506.2	9,274.0	9,393.9	9,493.8	9,405.2	9,332.5	8,799.1	8,716.0	8,496.1	8,277.2	7,758.2	7,991.8	8,278.0	8,541.6	8,405.4	8,624.4	8,517.6
Diseases of heart	1,819.9	1,391.0	1,244.3	1,358.4	1,376.8	1,317.2	1,296.3	1,232.1	1,240.2	1,182.1	1,076.0	1,030.1	1,027.7	959.9	1,099.3	975.8	1,010.2	1,008.6
Ischemic heart disease	1,208.2	901.8	906.8	952.4	949.5	891.0	877.3	820.1	829.0	752.8	729.2	709.3	695.2	648.4	708.1	628.3	625.2	614.2
Cerebrovascular diseases	269.3	223.3	200.6	200.3	222.5	216.4	255.3	230.6	216.4	201.5	210.3	198.1	193.5	201.7	190.7	171.4	209.4	178.2
Malignant neoplasms	1,101.3	1,141.1	1,181.9	1,190.7	1,124.9	1,085.8	1,099.5	1,148.3	1,197.6	1,104.9	1,020.7	995.7	1,099.5	1,066.0	997.2	1,068.4	1,084.3	983.9
Trachea, bronchus, and lung	181.1	268.1	300.6	290.5	261.3	284.5	267.7	286.0	283.4	285.1	254.8	227.8	238.7	226.3	223.9	264.1	268.2	225.3
Colorectal	78.8	82.4	106.9	93.6	96.9	94.6	103.5	102.8	120.2	103.6	84.4	93.8	87.9	115.7	85.5	92.1	109.7	88.1
Prostate[d]	66.7	42.0	66.3	62.9	75.2	57.1	51.1	68.6	44.5	46.6	*	44.5	35.2	36.3	34.7	37.1	37.6	38.8
Breast[e]	205.5	213.4	177.3	225.2	185.4	184.4	195.9	227.3	162.7	183.3	167.3	174.1	175.2	187.1	146.8	186.0	149.2	172.9

TABLE 1.10

Years of potential life lost before age 75 for selected causes of death, by sex and race, selected years 1980–2006 [CONTINUED]

[Data are based on death certificates]

Sex, race, Hispanic origin, and cause of death[b]	1980	Age-adjusted[a]																
		1990	1991	1992	1993	1994	1995	1996	1997	1998	1999[c]	2000[c]	2001[c]	2002[c]	2003[c]	2004[c]	2005[c]	2006[c]
Chronic lower respiratory diseases	89.3	129.0	111.0	117.3	144.7	123.3	145.3	114.0	166.2	151.8	146.6	151.8	139.3	137.0	163.6	148.6	155.3	144.6
Influenza and pneumonia	307.9	206.3	192.5	214.5	205.9	203.6	199.7	205.4	185.9	200.1	144.5	124.0	141.3	100.9	171.8	116.1	113.6	101.6
Chronic liver disease and cirrhosis	1,190.3	535.1	524.6	576.9	562.4	553.3	604.8	504.2	501.2	520.8	532.8	519.4	506.0	495.8	504.6	480.5	498.9	479.2
Diabetes mellitus	305.5	292.3	276.4	314.3	324.3	350.8	360.6	372.9	365.0	377.7	385.2	305.6	297.3	344.7	355.2	323.5	347.3	324.8
Human immunodeficiency virus (HIV) disease	—	70.1	140.3	101.9	173.2	201.1	246.9	148.9	81.7	70.5	90.5	68.4	88.1	79.9	80.7	93.8	89.9	76.1
Unintentional injuries	3,541.0	2,183.9	2,094.4	2,034.7	1,965.3	1,999.9	1,980.9	1,898.0	1,854.6	1,723.2	1,708.0	1,700.1	1,632.0	1,764.6	1,818.4	1,732.9	1,875.6	1,885.1
Motor vehicle-related injuries	2,102.4	1,301.5	1,255.2	1,180.7	1,187.1	1,136.2	1,210.3	1,193.6	1,085.2	1,057.4	995.4	1,032.2	989.4	1,089.3	1,081.8	968.3	1,004.9	1,021.7
Suicide[f]	515.0	495.9	442.2	429.0	459.5	526.8	445.2	465.1	444.1	466.0	415.6	403.1	420.6	420.8	418.2	511.6	498.6	487.8
Homicide[f]	628.9	434.2	484.4	417.9	415.9	467.9	432.7	363.5	391.4	334.2	359.9	278.5	287.0	366.5	323.1	304.7	337.5	328.3
Asian or Pacific Islander[g]																		
All causes	5,378.4	4,705.2	4,418.2	4,451.6	4,436.0	4,487.3	4,333.2	4,153.6	4,077.3	3,906.1	3,828.8	3,811.1	3,798.7	3,635.5	3,657.5	3,452.1	3,533.2	3,450.6
Diseases of heart	952.8	702.2	701.7	705.7	679.4	718.2	664.9	659.6	641.8	614.7	587.9	567.9	547.1	539.4	534.3	474.9	513.8	471.8
Ischemic heart disease	697.7	486.6	495.0	496.2	457.7	490.2	440.6	440.4	430.7	403.8	405.8	381.1	369.4	352.0	354.7	303.4	326.5	305.7
Cerebrovascular diseases	266.9	233.5	241.6	227.1	220.6	217.3	220.0	217.2	221.0	200.8	203.9	199.4	198.8	186.5	192.9	167.5	162.8	163.9
Malignant neoplasms	1,218.6	1,166.4	1,172.9	1,165.3	1,146.3	1,150.5	1,122.1	1,071.4	1,059.5	1,061.3	1,042.2	1,033.8	1,029.6	990.3	959.1	949.9	945.3	912.7
Trachea, bronchus, and lung	238.2	204.7	218.5	211.1	217.5	200.2	197.0	180.1	180.8	189.8	181.7	185.8	180.8	173.8	173.9	176.0	169.2	171.3
Colorectal	115.9	105.1	97.7	113.0	101.6	102.4	99.5	94.3	96.5	99.7	87.2	91.6	97.2	92.8	94.4	87.7	78.7	81.2
Prostate[d]	17.0	32.4	23.9	24.1	23.1	21.9	25.3	27.2	20.5	20.3	18.8	18.8	13.3	20.8	14.6	15.1	20.4	18.3
Breast[e]	222.2	216.5	247.3	196.9	203.0	221.5	237.8	187.9	193.4	206.6	183.5	200.8	205.0	188.4	192.3	193.4	178.4	173.3
Chronic lower respiratory diseases	56.4	72.8	69.7	63.4	66.7	67.2	65.8	75.9	64.2	59.2	57.5	56.5	52.1	44.8	45.1	36.5	36.0	37.4
Influenza and pneumonia	79.3	74.0	64.9	72.1	73.0	71.3	64.3	66.0	67.3	69.6	43.7	48.6	45.4	38.0	47.7	36.1	40.3	35.8
Chronic liver disease and cirrhosis	85.6	72.4	56.1	57.5	52.9	57.4	48.4	43.9	43.9	42.8	44.1	44.8	44.5	40.0	35.8	38.3	43.6	44.3
Diabetes mellitus	83.1	74.0	63.5	65.9	63.1	69.6	83.5	90.8	84.4	82.7	80.3	77.0	83.8	76.4	79.9	78.3	78.1	80.8
Human immunodeficiency virus (HIV) disease	—	77.0	77.4	86.5	104.8	125.5	110.4	77.6	30.3	26.7	25.5	19.9	21.6	24.8	22.3	21.9	16.6	15.4
Unintentional injuries	742.7	636.6	510.8	535.1	516.5	516.1	525.7	497.7	507.5	439.5	420.5	425.7	431.4	431.1	429.6	415.0	413.7	411.0
Motor vehicle-related injuries	472.6	445.5	354.8	345.0	321.4	335.1	351.9	318.3	311.2	284.6	257.8	263.4	275.9	269.7	269.6	254.4	242.1	243.9
Suicide[f]	217.1	200.6	194.6	205.5	209.4	218.0	211.1	195.2	191.9	187.9	189.0	168.6	166.4	162.7	172.1	175.5	164.6	185.1
Homicide[f]	201.1	205.8	241.8	222.9	251.4	211.2	202.3	177.8	163.2	135.5	126.7	113.1	165.1	127.5	120.6	98.8	130.8	121.7
Hispanic or Latino[g, h]																		
All causes	—	7,963.3	7,759.2	7,597.6	7,592.3	7,555.7	7,426.7	6,884.1	6,362.6	6,135.8	6,067.1	6,037.6	5,982.2	5,865.9	5,910.0	5,654.0	5,757.9	5,601.9
Diseases of heart	—	1,082.0	1,022.7	1,025.0	988.2	970.2	962.0	936.8	914.1	897.3	871.7	821.3	791.6	796.9	767.7	733.1	727.0	686.8
Ischemic heart disease	—	756.6	724.8	713.1	690.2	677.8	665.8	650.6	621.2	607.0	604.7	564.6	539.1	540.1	501.3	483.3	483.2	445.2
Cerebrovascular diseases	—	238.0	240.5	222.1	235.7	228.8	232.0	228.5	225.0	228.0	206.3	207.8	201.4	193.4	187.3	187.9	184.9	184.5
Malignant neoplasms	—	1,232.2	1,219.6	1,198.0	1,165.6	1,191.9	1,172.0	1,146.7	1,138.6	1,127.6	1,108.4	1,098.2	1,099.1	1,052.9	1,056.5	1,013.7	1,017.5	987.7
Trachea, bronchus, and lung	—	193.7	193.7	174.7	174.3	177.5	173.9	172.0	168.7	163.2	159.7	152.1	154.9	150.5	144.9	136.3	138.1	125.0
Colorectal	—	100.2	101.5	99.4	100.7	102.6	97.9	93.7	96.5	97.4	97.0	101.4	95.8	96.7	100.1	91.2	86.4	91.5
Prostate[d]	—	47.7	55.6	58.6	58.9	63.9	60.8	59.1	47.6	56.1	48.7	42.9	49.4	44.1	43.4	38.8	41.7	43.8
Breast[e]	—	299.3	287.7	271.2	256.9	267.9	257.7	259.9	258.4	248.5	220.9	230.7	233.6	205.1	218.4	203.4	197.3	203.2
Chronic lower respiratory diseases	—	78.8	84.1	76.7	82.4	80.4	82.1	76.3	76.4	75.7	79.3	68.5	67.6	69.0	67.1	64.1	62.2	56.9
Influenza and pneumonia	—	130.1	122.7	113.1	129.9	116.4	108.5	106.5	107.2	100.7	67.1	76.0	66.1	65.5	76.4	67.8	69.5	65.1
Chronic liver disease and cirrhosis	—	329.1	321.2	303.2	302.2	305.2	281.4	279.2	262.2	250.8	248.9	252.1	247.7	237.9	221.8	212.5	210.3	201.4

TABLE 1.10

Years of potential life lost before age 75 for selected causes of death, by sex and race, selected years 1980–2006 [CONTINUED]

[Data are based on death certificates]

Sex, race, Hispanic origin, and cause of death[b]	1980	Age-adjusted[a] 1990	1991	1992	1993	1994	1995	1996	1997	1998	1999[c]	2000[c]	2001[c]	2002[c]	2003[c]	2004[c]	2005[c]	2006[c]
Diabetes mellitus	—	177.8	184.5	194.3	198.4	217.0	228.8	224.9	224.8	213.8	216.8	215.6	212.1	207.1	214.0	192.3	202.2	181.1
Human immunodeficiency virus (HIV) disease	—	800.1	665.5	730.7	750.5	864.6	865.0	587.6	293.4	211.7	225.8	209.4	190.3	179.1	175.4	154.9	139.3	129.0
Unintentional injuries	—	1,190.6	1,116.1	1,054.2	1,096.9	1,025.7	1,017.9	991.6	934.2	919.9	938.1	920.1	845.8	958.1	961.5	917.6	980.1	993.0
Motor vehicle-related injuries	—	740.8	674.7	614.8	625.5	606.5	593.0	576.0	540.3	516.1	515.0	540.2	554.0	569.6	563.6	547.7	569.2	564.7
Suicide[f]	—	256.2	259.6	249.0	255.8	252.2	245.1	232.7	207.0	192.9	183.8	188.5	185.1	185.6	188.3	200.3	193.2	185.1
Homicide[f]	—	720.8	729.3	700.2	667.1	625.7	575.4	481.0	417.9	366.8	343.2	335.1	365.2	330.2	345.0	328.8	343.0	335.3
White, not Hispanic or Latino[h]																		
All causes	—	8,022.5	7,823.6	7,615.5	7,690.7	7,686.6	7,607.5	7,317.5	7,104.1	6,977.4	6,943.3	6,960.5	6,970.9	6,997.9	6,961.6	6,832.9	6,853.3	6,813.8
Diseases of heart	—	1,504.0	1,460.0	1,417.2	1,416.0	1,393.1	1,368.2	1,330.3	1,300.7	1,255.1	1,209.3	1,175.1	1,144.4	1,143.8	1,114.7	1,064.8	1,046.4	1,024.0
Ischemic heart disease	—	1,127.2	1,083.3	1,047.0	1,034.2	1,013.1	988.7	960.8	917.8	876.5	854.2	824.7	794.7	781.3	755.8	713.8	694.4	673.5
Cerebrovascular diseases	—	210.1	200.7	197.3	197.7	198.5	199.6	198.6	194.7	187.7	178.9	183.0	170.6	169.4	162.8	161.1	155.5	152.5
Malignant neoplasms	—	1,974.1	1,930.7	1,886.0	1,866.9	1,852.7	1,814.2	1,782.0	1,741.2	1,703.0	1,685.3	1,668.4	1,652.3	1,629.7	1,590.6	1,549.7	1,534.3	1,505.9
Trachea, bronchus, and lung	—	566.8	546.8	536.8	530.4	518.0	507.0	498.4	483.6	474.8	456.5	460.3	451.9	443.7	433.5	425.1	416.3	402.4
Colorectal	—	162.1	157.9	152.5	150.8	150.6	147.8	141.6	140.8	138.7	138.6	136.2	138.5	137.6	127.7	123.4	120.8	121.8
Prostate[d]	—	89.2	84.4	81.9	78.2	77.0	73.6	71.5	65.6	61.9	58.3	54.9	53.2	51.7	51.0	49.2	47.3	47.6
Breast[e]	—	451.5	432.6	411.4	398.3	394.9	389.3	368.1	355.8	340.9	316.6	322.3	315.9	305.9	301.8	290.0	283.6	275.5
Chronic lower respiratory diseases	—	188.1	188.7	183.7	195.3	194.3	190.6	189.9	191.3	188.7	201.5	193.8	194.3	193.3	194.2	184.1	194.0	183.4
Influenza and pneumonia	—	112.3	111.5	102.4	109.0	106.8	105.8	104.6	105.4	104.0	73.8	76.4	72.9	75.8	82.1	71.3	76.8	70.4
Chronic liver disease and cirrhosis	—	162.4	155.6	153.1	152.1	152.8	151.4	149.8	148.1	145.1	148.0	150.0	153.0	152.1	153.2	148.3	147.8	147.4
Diabetes mellitus	—	131.2	130.8	130.9	135.1	141.0	142.8	146.8	141.1	143.3	148.0	150.2	151.0	155.8	154.9	152.0	151.5	150.1
Human immunodeficiency virus (HIV) disease	—	271.2	300.4	324.7	345.1	373.1	362.1	229.1	100.7	76.0	81.2	76.0	71.0	67.8	65.4	59.7	58.6	51.5
Unintentional injuries	—	1,114.7	1,050.9	984.1	1,004.8	1,017.4	1,026.1	1,012.5	1,009.6	1,006.4	1,023.6	1,041.4	1,057.2	1,117.4	1,135.3	1,170.6	1,199.6	1,246.4
Motor vehicle-related injuries	—	715.7	656.2	597.2	602.6	610.8	618.0	614.3	602.6	593.9	575.7	588.8	584.1	603.3	585.3	588.8	579.9	575.4
Suicide[f]	—	433.0	425.7	417.5	421.5	427.7	427.7	415.6	411.2	409.9	386.8	389.2	405.3	413.9	408.1	419.8	416.6	422.7
Homicide[f]	—	162.0	171.0	164.3	162.3	159.1	148.6	137.5	135.3	127.6	120.5	113.2	160.1	114.8	109.6	110.3	109.1	109.9

—Data not available.

[a]Age-adjusted rates are calculated using the year 2000 standard population. Prior to 2003, age-adjusted rates were calculated using standard million proportions based on rounded population numbers. Starting with 2003 data, unrounded population numbers are used to calculate age-adjusted rates.

[b]Underlying cause of death code numbers are based on the applicable revision of the International Classification of Diseases (ICD) for data years shown. For the period 1980–1998, causes were coded using ICD-9 codes that are most nearly comparable with the 113 cause list for ICD-10.

[c]Starting with 1999 data, cause of death is coded according to ICD-10.

[d]Rate for male population only.

[e]Rate for female population only.

[f]Figures for 2001 (in excel spreadsheet on the web) include September 11-related deaths for which death certificates were filed as of October 24, 2002.

[g]The race groups, white, black, Asian or Pacific Islander, and American Indian or Alaska Native, include persons of Hispanic and non-Hispanic origin. Persons of Hispanic origin may be of any race. Death rates for the American Indian or Alaska Native and Asian or Pacific Islander populations are known to be underestimated. Race, for a discussion of sources of bias in death rates by race and Hispanic origin.

[h]Prior to 1997, excludes data from states lacking an Hispanic-origin item on the death certificate.

Notes: Starting with Health, United States, 2003, rates for 1991–1999 were revised using intercensal population estimates based on the 2000 census. Rates for 2000 were revised based on 2000 census counts. Rates for 2001 and later years were computed using 2000-based postcensal estimates.

In 2003, seven states reported multiple-race data.

In 2004, 15 states reported multiple-race data.

In 2005, 21 states and the District of Columbia (D.C.) reported multiple-race data.

In 2006, 25 states and D.C. reported multiple-race data.

The multiple-race data for these states were bridged to the single-race categories of the 1977 Office of Management and Budget Standards for comparability with other states.

SOURCE: Adapted from "Table 29. Years of Potential Life Lost before Age 75 for Selected Causes of Death, by Sex, Race, and Hispanic Origin: United States, Selected Years 1980–2006," in *Health, United States, 2008. With Chartbook,* Centers for Disease Control and Prevention, National Center for Health Statistics, 2009, http://www.cdc.gov/nchs/data/hus/hus08.pdf (accessed December 12, 2009)

TABLE 1.11

Leading causes of death and numbers of deaths by age, 1980 and 2006

[Data are based on death certificates]

Age and rank order	1980 Cause of death	Deaths	2006 Cause of death	Deaths
Under 1 year				
—	All causes	45,526	All causes	28,527
1	Congenital anomalies	9,220	Congenital malformations, deformations and chromosomal abnormalities	5,819
2	Sudden infant death syndrome	5,510	Disorders related to short gestation and low birth weight, not elsewhere classified	4,841
3	Respiratory distress syndrome	4,989	Sudden infant death syndrome	2,323
4	Disorders relating to short gestation and unspecified low birthweight	3,648	Newborn affected by maternal complications of pregnancy	1,683
5	Newborn affected by maternal complications of pregnancy	1,572	Unintentional injuries	1,147
6	Intrauterine hypoxia and birth asphyxia	1,497	Newborn affected by complications of placenta, cord and membranes	1,140
7	Unintentional injuries	1,166	Respiratory distress of newborn	825
8	Birth trauma	1,058	Bacterial sepsis of newborn	807
9	Pneumonia and influenza	1,012	Neonatal hemorrhage	618
10	Newborn affected by complications of placenta, cord, and membranes	985	Diseases of circulatory system	543
1–4 years				
—	All causes	8,187	All causes	4,631
1	Unintentional injuries	3,313	Unintentional injuries	1,610
2	Congenital anomalies	1,026	Congenital malformations, deformations and chromosomal abnormalities	515
3	Malignant neoplasms	573	Malignant neoplasms	377
4	Diseases of heart	338	Homicide	366
5	Homicide	319	Diseases of heart	161
6	Pneumonia and influenza	267	Influenza and pneumonia	125
7	Meningitis	223	Septicemia	88
8	Meningococcal infection	110	Certain conditions originating in the perinatal period	65
9	Certain conditions originating in the perinatal period	84	In situ neoplasms, benign neoplasms and neoplasms of uncertain or unknown behavior	60
10	Septicemia	71	Cerebrovascular diseases	54
5–14 years				
—	All causes	10,689	All causes	6,149
1	Unintentional injuries	5,224	Unintentional injuries	2,258
2	Malignant neoplasms	1,497	Malignant neoplasms	907
3	Congenital anomalies	561	Homicide	390
4	Homicide	415	Congenital malformations, deformations and chromosomal abnormalities	344
5	Diseases of heart	330	Diseases of heart	253
6	Pneumonia and influenza	194	Suicide	219
7	Suicide	142	Chronic lower respiratory diseases	115
8	Benign neoplasms	104	Cerebrovascular diseases	95
9	Cerebrovascular diseases	95	Septicemia	84
10	Chronic obstructive pulmonary diseases	85	In situ neoplasms, benign neoplasms and neoplasms of uncertain or unknown behavior	76
15–24 years				
—	All causes	49,027	All causes	34,887
1	Unintentional injuries	26,206	Unintentional injuries	16,229
2	Homicide	6,537	Homicide	5,717
3	Suicide	5,239	Suicide	4,189
4	Malignant neoplasms	2,683	Malignant neoplasms	1,644
5	Diseases of heart	1,223	Diseases of heart	1,076
6	Congenital anomalies	600	Congenital malformations, deformations and chromosomal abnormalities	460
7	Cerebrovascular diseases	418	Cerebrovascular diseases	210
8	Pneumonia and influenza	348	Human immunodeficiency virus (HIV) disease	206
9	Chronic obstructive pulmonary diseases	141	Influenza and pneumonia	184
10	Anemias	133	Pregnancy, childbirth and puerperium	179

were a leading cause of death, followed by cancer and homicide.

Accidents were the leading cause of death in 2006 for young people aged 15 to 24. (See Table 1.11.) Homicide was the second-leading cause of death, followed by suicide.

Cancer was the fourth-leading cause of death among this age group.

Among adults aged 25 to 44 in 2006, accidents were the most frequent cause of death, and cancer was second. (See Table 1.11.) Heart disease and suicide were the third- and

TABLE 1.11

Leading causes of death and numbers of deaths by age, 1980 and 2006 [CONTINUED]

[Data are based on death certificates]

Age and rank order	1980		2006	
	Cause of death	Deaths	Cause of death	Deaths
25–44 years				
—	All causes	108,658	All causes	125,995
1	Unintentional injuries	26,722	Unintentional injuries	32,488
2	Malignant neoplasms	17,551	Malignant neoplasms	17,573
3	Diseases of heart	14,513	Diseases of heart	15,646
4	Homicide	10,983	Suicide	11,576
5	Suicide	9,855	Homicide	7,745
6	Chronic liver disease and cirrhosis	4,782	Human immunodeficiency virus (HIV) disease	5,192
7	Cerebrovascular diseases	3,154	Chronic liver disease and cirrhosis	2,867
8	Diabetes mellitus	1,472	Diabetes mellitus	2,767
9	Pneumonia and influenza	1,467	Cerebrovascular diseases	2,748
10	Congenital anomalies	817	Influenza and pneumonia	1,176
45–64 years				
—	All causes	425,338	All causes	466,432
1	Diseases of heart	148,322	Malignant neoplasms	151,788
2	Malignant neoplasms	135,675	Diseases of heart	103,572
3	Cerebrovascular diseases	19,909	Unintentional injuries	31,121
4	Unintentional injuries	18,140	Diabetes mellitus	17,124
5	Chronic liver disease and cirrhosis	16,089	Cerebrovascular diseases	16,859
6	Chronic obstructive pulmonary diseases	11,514	Chronic lower respiratory diseases	16,299
7	Diabetes mellitus	7,977	Chronic liver disease and cirrhosis	14,929
8	Suicide	7,079	Suicide	12,009
9	Pneumonia and influenza	5,804	Nephritis, nephrotic syndrome and nephrosis	6,613
10	Homicide	4,019	Septicemia	6,292
65 years and over				
—	All causes	1,341,848	All causes	1,759,423
1	Diseases of heart	595,406	Diseases of heart	510,542
2	Malignant neoplasms	258,389	Malignant neoplasms	387,515
3	Cerebrovascular diseases	146,417	Cerebrovascular diseases	117,010
4	Pneumonia and influenza	45,512	Chronic lower respiratory diseases	106,845
5	Chronic obstructive pulmonary diseases	43,587	Alzheimer's disease	71,660
6	Atherosclerosis	28,081	Diabetes mellitus	52,351
7	Diabetes mellitus	25,216	Influenza and pneumonia	49,346
8	Unintentional injuries	24,844	Nephritis, nephrotic syndrome and nephrosis	37,377
9	Nephritis, nephrotic syndrome, and nephrosis	12,968	Unintentional injuries	36,689
10	Chronic liver disease and cirrhosis	9,519	Septicemia	26,201

—Category not applicable.
Notes: For cause of death codes based on the International Classification of Diseases, 9th Revision (ICD-9) in 1980 and ICD-10 in 2006.

SOURCE: "Table 29. Leading Causes of Death and Numbers of Deaths, by Age: United States, 1980 and 2006," in *Health, United States, 2009. With Special Feature on Medical Technology*, Centers for Disease Control and Prevention, National Center for Health Statistics, 2010, http://www.cdc.gov/nchs/data/hus/hus09.pdf (accessed March 12, 2010)

fourth-leading causes, respectively, followed by homicide and HIV disease.

Among adults 45 to 64 years old, cancer and heart disease were ranked the first- and second-leading causes of death, respectively. (See Table 1.11.) Among those aged 65 and older, these two categories were reversed.

HEALTH CARE REFORM

The availability of insurance coverage may change for many Americans due to health care reform passed by Congress and signed into law by President Barack Obama (1961–) in March 2010. This legislation could have positive effects on infant mortality, life expectancy, and mortality rates because it provides insurance and preventive care to groups who were previously at higher risk due to lack of access of health care. The Patient Protection and Affordable Care Act (PPACA) and an amendment, titled the Health Care and Education Reconciliation Act of 2010, aim to implement changes over an eight-year period that would offer insurance to an estimated 32 million Americans who were uninsured when the legislation passed, as well as provide better access to health care, including preventative care. Among other reforms, the legislation would expand Medicaid; provide insurance premium subsidies for individuals and incentives to companies to offer employees health care; keep dependent children on their parents' insurance until age 26; prohibit insurance companies from dropping people when they get sick; and end the practice of denying people coverage due to pre-existing conditions. The Obama administration and Congress proposed to offset the costs for the reforms with methods that include taxes on upper income recipients of Medicare, businesses like tanning salons, and "Cadillac" (high-cost) health care plans; fees on some medical and pharmaceutical companies; and other cost-saving measures.

Yet the act was controversial and was fiercely opposed by Republicans in Congress. Democratic legislators who worked to pass the bill, as well as a few Republicans who opposed it, reported receiving death threats from angry constituents. The controversy and anger stemmed from several factors. Some critics were concerned about the cost to the country as it faced a steadily increasing federal deficit following the recession that began in December 2007. Despite a Congressional Budget Office report that estimated a $143-billion net reduction in the deficit in the decade following passage of the legislation, some critics asserted that the measures put in place by Congress would not be able to cover the costs of the reform, much less decrease the deficit. Another objection was that the PPACA requires people to obtain health insurance or pay a tax penalty. Some critics are also concerned that the plan could lead to health care rationing due to increased costs and that the country will not have enough health care professionals. There was also concern that the act undermines the sovereignty of the individual states. As of April 29, 2010, at least 19 states had considered or were planning to sue the federal government over the implementation of the legislation in its entirety or of parts with which they had particular concerns. A spokesperson for the Justice Department stated that the bill was constitutional.

SELF-ASSESSED HEALTH STATUS

The NCHS regularly asks respondents to the National Health Interview Survey to evaluate their health status. Figure 1.5 shows that from 1997 to June 2009 the percentage of people who considered their health to be excellent or very good was relatively unchanged, ranging from a high of 69.1% in 1998 but hovering around 66% for most years. From January to June 2009, 66.6% of respondents assessed their health as excellent or very good.

Overall, men were slightly more likely to rate their health as excellent. (See Figure 1.6.) However, for both men and women the percentage who considered their health as excellent or very good decreased with advancing age—83.9% for those younger than age 18, 64.8% for those aged 18 to 64, and 41.7% for those aged 65 and older. (See Figure 1.7.) Compared with the 70.6% of non-Hispanic white survey respondents who assessed their health as excellent or very good, fewer non-Hispanic African-American (57.3%) and Hispanic (57.9%) survey respondents rated their health status as excellent or very good. (See Figure 1.8.)

FIGURE 1.5

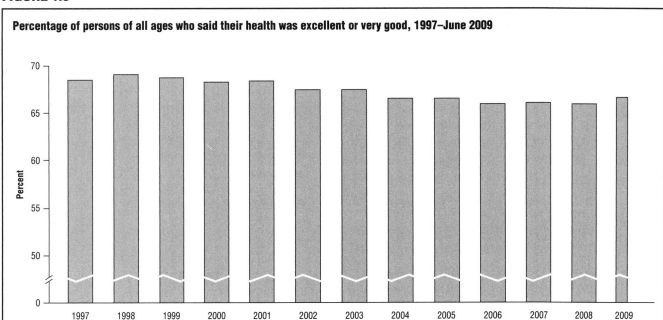

Percentage of persons of all ages who said their health was excellent or very good, 1997–June 2009

Notes: Health status data were obtained by asking respondents to assess their own health and that of family members living in the same household as excellent, very good, good, fair, or poor. The analyses excluded persons with unknown health status (about 0.2% of respondents each year). Beginning with the 2003 data, the National Health Interview Survey transitioned to weights derived from the 2000 census. In this Early Release, estimates for 2000–2002 were recalculated using weights derived from the 2000 census.

SOURCE: "Figure 11.1. Percentage of Persons of All Ages Who Had Excellent or Very Good Health: United States, 1997–June 2009," in *Early Release of Selected Estimates Based on Data from the January–June 2009 National Health Interview Survey*, Centers for Disease Control and Prevention, National Center for Health Statistics, December 2009, http://www.cdc.gov/nchs/data/nhis/earlyrelease/earlyrelease200912.pdf (accessed December 17, 2009)

FIGURE 1.6

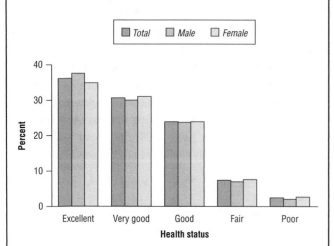

Percent distribution of respondent-assessed health status, by sex, for all ages, January–June 2009

Notes: Health status data were obtained by asking respondents to assess their own health and that of family members living in the same house hold as excellent, very good, good, fair, or poor. The analyses excluded 41 persons (0.1%) with unknown health status.

SOURCE: "Figure 11.2. Percent Distribution of Respondent-Assessed Health Status, by Sex, for All Ages: United States, January–June 2009," in *Early Release of Selected Estimates Based on Data from the January–June 2009 National Health Interview Survey*, Centers for Disease Control and Prevention, National Center for Health Statistics, December 2009, http://www.cdc.gov/nchs/data/nhis/earlyrelease/earlyrelease200912.pdf (accessed December 17, 2009)

FIGURE 1.7

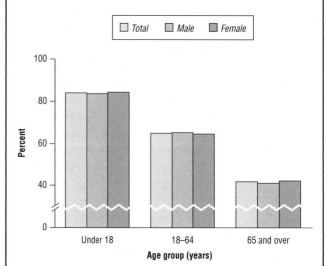

Percentage of persons of all ages who said their health was excellent or very good, by age group and sex, January–June 2009

Notes: Health status data were obtained by asking respondents to assess their own health and that of family members living in the same household as excellent, very good, good, fair, or poor. The analyses excluded 41 persons (0.1%) with unknown health status.

SOURCE: "Figure 11.3. Percentage of Persons of All Ages Who Had Excellent or Very Good Health, by Age Group and Sex: United States, January–June 2009," in *Early Release of Selected Estimates Based on Data from the January–June 2009 National Health Interview Survey*, Centers for Disease Control and Prevention, National Center for Health Statistics, December 2009, http://www.cdc.gov/nchs/data/nhis/earlyrelease/earlyrelease200912.pdf (accessed December 17, 2009)

FIGURE 1.8

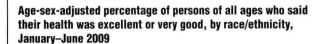

Age-sex-adjusted percentage of persons of all ages who said their health was excellent or very good, by race/ethnicity, January–June 2009

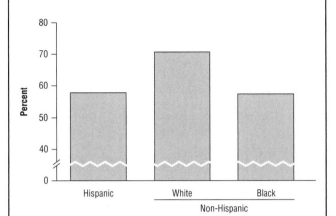

Notes: Health status data were obtained by asking respondents to assess their own health and that of family members living in the same household as excellent, very good, good, fair, or poor. The analyses excluded 41 persons (0.1%) with unknown health status. Estimates are age-sex adjusted using the projected 2000 U.S. population as the standard population and using three age groups: under 18 years, 18–64 years, and 65 years and over.

SOURCE: "Figure 11.4. Age-Sex-Adjusted Percentage of Persons of All Ages Who Had Excellent or Very Good Health, by Race/Ethnicity: United States, January–June 2009," in *Early Release of Selected Estimates Based on Data from the January–June 2009 National Health Interview Survey*, Centers for Disease Control and Prevention, National Center for Health Statistics, December 2009, http://www.cdc.gov/nchs/data/nhis/earlyrelease/earlyrelease200912.pdf (accessed December 17, 2009)

CHAPTER 2
PREVENTION OF DISEASE

Prevention is better than cure.

—Desiderius Erasmus

Preventing disease involves a wide range of interrelated programs, actions, and activities. Some prevention measures are sweeping global policy initiatives, such as national and state government actions to reduce health risks by limiting air pollution and other toxic exposures or to increase standards to ensure the safety of food and water supplies. Others are focused efforts of public health professionals and agencies, such as the National Institutes of Health's (NIH) Office of Disease Prevention, the Centers for Disease Control and Prevention (CDC), and the American Cancer Society (ACS), to reduce the incidence (occurrence of new cases) of specific diseases such as heart disease, diabetes, and lung cancer.

The effectiveness of local and global disease prevention programs largely depends on the extent to which individuals take personal responsibility for their own health by avoiding health risks such as tobacco use, substance abuse (misuse of alcohol and drugs), and unsafe sex. People who have a healthy diet; get adequate exercise and rest; wear seatbelts in automobiles and helmets on bicycles, motorcycles, and scooters; successfully manage stress; and maintain a positive outlook on life are on the front line of disease prevention. Similarly, individuals who effectively use health care resources by obtaining recommended immunizations, physical examinations, and health screenings are actively working to prevent disease and disability.

Prevention involves governments, professional organizations, public health professionals, health care practitioners (physicians, nurses, and allied health professionals), and individuals working at three levels to maintain and improve the health of communities. The first level, primary prevention, focuses on inhibiting the development of disease before it occurs. Secondary prevention, also called screening, refers to measures that detect disease before it is symptomatic. Tertiary prevention efforts focus on people already affected by disease and attempt to reduce resultant disability and restore functionality.

PRIMARY PREVENTION

Primary prevention measures fall into two categories. The first category includes actions to protect against disease and disability, such as getting immunizations, ensuring the supply of safe drinking water, applying dental sealants to prevent tooth decay, and guarding against accidents. Examples of primary prevention of accidents include government and state requirements for workplace safety to prevent industrial injuries and equipping automobiles with air bags and antilock brakes. Examples of primary prevention of mental health problems include measures to strengthen family and community support systems as well as to teach children communication and interpersonal skills, conflict management, and other relationship and life skills that foster emotional resiliency.

General action to promote health is the other category of primary prevention measures. Health promotion includes the basic activities of a healthy lifestyle: good nutrition and hygiene, adequate exercise and rest, and avoidance of environmental and health risks. Limiting exposure to sunlight, using sunscreen, and wearing protective clothing are examples of primary prevention measures to reduce the risk of developing skin cancer.

Health promotion also includes education about the other interdependent dimensions of health known as wellness. Examples of health education programs aimed at wellness include stress management, parenting classes, preparation for retirement from the workforce, and cooking classes.

Historically, public health programs in developed countries have emphasized the primary prevention of infectious diseases (illnesses caused by microorganisms) by making environmental changes, such as improving the safety and purity of food and water supplies, and providing immunizations. Figure 2.1 shows the 2009 recommended schedule of

FIGURE 2.1

Recommended childhood and adolescent immunization schedule, by vaccine and age, 2009

| | Range of recommended ages | Catch-up immunization | Certain high-risk groups |

Vaccine ▼ / Age ►	Birth	1 month	2 months	4 months	6 months	12 months	15 months	18 months	19–23 months	2–3 years	4–6 years
Hepatitis B	HepB	HepB	HepB		HepB	HepB	HepB	HepB			
Rotavirus			RV	RV	RV						
Diphtheria, tetanus, pertussis			DTaP	DTaP	DTaP		DTaP	DTaP			DTaP
Haemophilus influenzae type b			Hib	Hib	Hib	Hib	Hib				
Pneumococcal			PCV	PCV	PCV	PCV	PCV			PPSV	PPSV
Inactivated poliovirus			IPV	IPV	IPV	IPV	IPV	IPV			IPV
Influenza					Influenza (yearly)	Influenza (yearly)	Influenza (yearly)	Influenza (yearly)	Influenza (yearly)	Influenza (yearly)	Influenza (yearly)
Measles, mumps, rubella						MMR	MMR				MMR
Varicella						Varicella	Varicella				Varicella
Hepatitis A						HepA (2 doses)	HepA (2 doses)	HepA (2 doses)		HepA Series	HepA Series
Meningococcal										MCV	MCV

Vaccine ▼ / Age ►	7–10 years	11–12 years	13–18 years
Tetanus, diphtheria, pertussis		Tdap	Tdap
Human papillomavirus		HPV (3 doses)	HPV Series
Meningococcal	MCV	MCV	MCV
Influenza	Influenza (yearly)	Influenza (yearly)	Influenza (yearly)
Pneumococcal	PPSV	PPSV	PPSV
Hepatitis A	HepA Series	HepA Series	HepA Series
Hepatitis B	HepB Series	HepB Series	HepB Series
Inactivated poliovirus	IPV Series	IPV Series	IPV Series
Measles, mumps, rubella	MMR Series	MMR Series	MMR Series
Varicella	Varicella Series	Varicella Series	Varicella Series

Notes: PPV is pneumococcal polysaccharide vaccine and PCV is pneumococcal conjugate vaccine. MPSV4 is meningococcal polysaccharide vaccine and MCV4 is meningococcal conjugate vaccine. This schedule indicates the recommended ages for routine administration of currently licensed childhood vaccines, as of December 1, 2006 for children aged 0–18 years old. Any dose not administered at the recommended age should be administered at any subsequent visit, when indicated and feasible. Additional vaccines may be licensed and recommended during the year. Licensed combination vaccines may be used whenever any components of the combination are indicated and other components of the vaccine are not contraindicated and if approved by the Food and Drug Administration for that dose of the series. Providers should consult the Advisory Committee on Immunization Practices statement for detailed recommendations. Clinically significant adverse events that follow immunization should be reported to the Vaccine Adverse Event Reporting System (VAERS).

SOURCE: Adapted from "Figure 1. Recommended Immunization Schedule for Persons Aged 0 through 6 Years—United States, 2009," and "Figure 2. Recommended Immunization Schedule for Persons Aged 7 through 18 Years—United States, 2009," in *Morbidity and Mortality Weekly Report*, vol. 57, nos. 51 and 52, January 2, 2009, http://www.cdc.gov/mmwr/PDF/wk/mm5751.pdf (accessed December 18, 2009)

childhood and adolescent immunizations—a key primary prevention measure in the United States and other developed countries.

The most pressing health problems in developed countries in the 21st century are chronic diseases, such as heart disease, cancer, diabetes, and obesity. Primary prevention of chronic diseases is more challenging than primary prevention of infectious diseases because it requires changing health behaviors. Efforts to change deeply rooted and often culturally influenced patterns of behaviors—such as diet, alcohol and tobacco use, and physical inactivity—generally have been less successful than environmental health and immunization programs.

Primary prevention programs are developed in response to actual and potential threats to community public health. Recent primary prevention programs have examined ways to prevent youth violence, smoking, and acts of bioterrorism (the use of biological or chemical weapons). In 2009 and 2010 primary prevention programs to reduce the spread and incidence of influenza included intensified efforts to encourage H1N1 influenza and seasonal flu immunizations.

Primary Prevention of Youth Violence

Violence on U.S. high school campuses has focused media attention on the problem of violence during childhood, adolescence, and young adulthood. In "Youth Risk Behavior Surveillance—United States, 2007" (*Morbidity and Mortality Weekly Report*, vol. 57, no. SS-4, June 6, 2008), the CDC indicates that 5.2% of students interviewed said they had carried a firearm at least once during the past month, and 18% had carried a weapon such as a gun, knife, or club.

To develop programs that prevent violence and violent deaths among children and teens, the CDC follows a systematic public health approach that identifies and describes the problem, designs and evaluates measures to prevent the problem, and puts these measures in place in the community. The approach that public health professionals use to develop all prevention programs consists of the following steps, some of which may be conducted simultaneously:

- Surveillance—the first step is to collect and analyze data to determine the size and scope of the problem. To understand youth violence, researchers look at how many people were injured or killed as a result of youth violence. They look at the ages, attitudes, school performance, family histories, and other characteristics of the children and teens who committed violent acts. They also note when (day, night, weekends, summer, winter, spring, or fall) and where (school, home, or public parks) violence occurred.

- Determining the cause—by analyzing the data collected in the surveillance process, researchers can identify the underlying causes of the problem. Once public health professionals know who is at risk for a particular problem and why a certain group is at risk, they are better able to design actions to prevent it. Table 2.1, a list of potential participants for anti-youth violence interventions, notes risk factors and high-risk behaviors likely to lead to violence among children and adolescents.

- Develop and test preventive measures—using the results of the data analysis, public health professionals develop

TABLE 2.1

Potential participant groups for interventions to prevent youth violence

All children and adolescents in a community
All children in a specific age group, school, grade
Children and adolescents with risk factors such as—
    use of alcohol or other drugs
    history of early aggression
    social or learning problems
    exposure to violence at home, in their neighborhood, or in the media
    parental drug or alcohol use
    friends who engage in problem behavior
    academic failure or poor commitment to school
    poverty
    recent divorce, relocation, or other family disruption
    access to firearms
Children and adolescents with high-risk behaviors such as—
    criminal activity
    fighting or victimization
    drug or alcohol abuse
    selling drugs
    carrying a weapon
    membership in a gang
    dropping out of school
    unemployment
    homelessness
    recent immigration
Parents and other family members
Influential adults such as—
    teachers
    coaches
    child care providers
General population of a community

SOURCE: Timothy N. Thornton et al., eds., "Table 2. Potential Participant Groups for Interventions to Prevent Youth Violence," in *Best Practices of Youth Violence Prevention: A Sourcebook for Community Action*, rev. ed., Centers for Disease Control and Prevention, National Center for Injury Prevention and Control, June 2002, http://www.cdc.gov/ncipc/dvp/bestpractices/chapter1.pdf (accessed December 17, 2009)

prevention programs called interventions. These interventions target specific populations and may be conducted at specific locations. (See Table 2.2.) Before recommending widespread use of interventions, health professionals test the programs to find out if they work as effectively as hoped. Every intervention is evaluated to determine if it achieves its objectives. Table 2.3 is an example of a goal (reducing expulsions resulting from fights in middle schools) of an intervention and its measurable objectives.

- Implementation—during this phase the preventive measures found to be effective are communicated so they may be put into action. To communicate methods that prevent violence among children and teens, the CDC conducts training programs, publishes articles in journals for public health workers and health care practitioners, and produced *Best Practices of Youth Violence Prevention: A Sourcebook for Community Action* (June 2002, http://www.cdc.gov/ncipc/dvp/bestpractices.htm#Download), a book of recommended programs that was edited by Timothy N. Thornton et al. The book remains a seminal source and was still widely used in 2010.

TABLE 2.2

Possible settings for interventions to prevent youth violence

General population of young people	Young children
Schools	Child care centers
Churches	Homes
Playgrounds	Schools
Youth activity centers	**Parents**
Homes	
Shopping centers and malls	Homes
Movie theaters	Workplaces
High-risk youth	Churches
	Community centers
Alternative schools	
Juvenile justice facilities	
Social service facilities	
Mental health and medical care facilities	
Hospital emergency departments	
Recreation centers	

SOURCE: Timothy N. Thornton et al., eds., "Table 3. Possible Settings for Interventions to Prevent Youth Violence," in *Best Practices of Youth Violence Prevention: A Sourcebook for Community Action*, rev. ed., Centers for Disease Control and Prevention, National Center for Injury Prevention and Control, June 2002, http://www.cdc.gov/ncipc/dvp/bestpractices/chapter1.pdf (accessed December 17, 2009)

TABLE 2.3

Example of a goal and its objectives to prevent youth violence

Goal: Reduce expulsions resulting from fights in middle schools.

Objectives:

1. By 2000, offer a 25-lesson program in 6th-grade classes to help students develop social skills and learn nonaggressive responses appropriate for dealing with conflict.

   Who: Prevention specialists
   What: 1-hour sessions offered twice a week for one school year on topics such as self-understanding, conflict resolution, anger control, and prosocial actions
   How much: All 6th-grade classes
   When: By 2000
   Where: Columbia County schools

2. By 2001, implement a school-wide program to mediate behavior problems and disputes between adolescents.

   Who: Teachers and peer mediators
   What: Weekly mediation clinics
   How much: All 6th-, 7th-, and 8th-grade students
   When: By 2001
   Where: Columbia County schools

3. By 2002, reduce the number of fights among 8th-grade students from five per month to two per month.

   Who: Middle school students
   What: Incidents of physical aggression
   How much: Reduce by 60 percent
   When: By 2002
   Where: Columbia County schools

4. By 2004, reduce by half the number of middle school students (grades 6 through 8) expelled because of fights or other disruptive incidents in the schools.

   Who: Middle school students
   What: Expulsions related to fights in schools
   How much: Reduce from an average of two per month to one per month
   When: By 2004
   Where: Columbia County schools

SOURCE: Timothy N. Thornton et al., eds., "Table 4. Example of a Goal and Its Objectives," in *Best Practices of Youth Violence Prevention: A Sourcebook for Community Action*, rev. ed., Centers for Disease Control and Prevention, National Center for Injury Prevention and Control, June 2002, http://www.cdc.gov/ncipc/dvp/bestpractices/chapter1.pdf (accessed December 17, 2009)

TABLE 2.4

Mentoring activities

Social	Event-related (field trips)
Talking about life experiences	Camping or hiking
Having lunch together	Attending a concert or an art exhibit
Visiting the mentor's home	Attending a sporting event
Recreational	**Life skills-related**
Playing games or sports	Developing a fitness or nutrition plan
Doing arts and crafts	Attending a cooking class
Walking in the park	Discussing proper etiquette
Going to the mall	Participating in a public-speaking class
Academic	**Job- or career-related**
Working on homework	Visiting the mentor's workplace
Visiting the library	Developing a resume
Reading together	Talking about career options
Working on the computer	Practicing interview skills
Civic	
Helping in a community clean-up effort	
Working at a soup kitchen	

SOURCE: Timothy N. Thornton et al., eds., "Table 7. Mentoring Activities," in *Best Practices of Youth Violence Prevention: A Sourcebook for Community Action*, rev. ed., Centers for Disease Control and Prevention, National Center for Injury Prevention and Control, June 2002, http://www.cdc.gov/ncipc/dvp/bestpractices/chapter2b.pdf (accessed December 17, 2009)

- Evaluation—after preventive measures or interventions have been implemented, they are evaluated to see if they have effectively prevented the problem.

In *Best Practices of Youth Violence Prevention*, Thornton et al. include programs aimed at families, parents with infants and small children, and youth considered to be at risk. They recommend providing social services to strengthen families, improving communication skills, and mentoring. Mentoring pairs young people with adult role models who, by example, teach and support social skills. Table 2.4 shows some mentoring activities that Thornton et al. recommend.

Another example of effective primary prevention of youth violence is described by David A. Wolfe et al. in "A School-Based Program to Prevent Adolescent Dating Violence: A Cluster Randomized Trial" (*Archives of Pediatric and Adolescent Medicine*, vol. 163, no. 8, August 2009). The program consisted of interactive lessons about healthy relationships, sexual health, and substance use that included information about preventing dating violence. The program was delivered to 1,722 students aged 14 to 15 years old and intended to help students make decisions that favored safety in terms of their dating and other peer relationships. Over the course of two and a half years, students who participated in this primary prevention program reported fewer instances of physical dating violence, compared with a control group of students who did not receive this training.

SECONDARY PREVENTION

The goal of secondary prevention is to identify and detect disease in its earliest stages, before noticeable symptoms develop, when it is most likely to be treated successfully. With early detection and diagnosis, it may be possible to cure a disease, slow its progression, prevent or minimize complications, and limit disability.

Another goal of secondary prevention is to prevent the spread of communicable diseases (illnesses that can be transmitted from one person to another). In the community, early identification and treatment of people with communicable diseases, such as sexually transmitted diseases, provides not only secondary prevention for those who are infected but also primary prevention for people who come in contact with infected individuals.

Like primary prevention, individual health care practitioners and public health agencies and organizations perform secondary prevention. An example of secondary prevention that is conducted by many different professionals (physicians, nurses, and allied health professionals) in a variety of settings (medical offices, clinics, and health fairs) is blood pressure screening to identify people with hyper-

tension (high blood pressure). An example of mental health secondary prevention is the effort to identify young children with behavior problems to intervene early and prevent development of, or progression to, more serious mental disorders.

The U.S. Preventive Services Task Force (USPSTF; 2010, http://www.ahrq.gov/clinic/USpstfix.htm), an independent panel of experts "that systematically reviews the evidence of effectiveness and develops recommendations for clinical preventive services," stipulates the preventive measures that should be taken by healthy adult men, women, pregnant women, and children. (See Table 2.5.) The recommended preventive services include screening to detect and identify a wide range of conditions including high blood pressure, depression, obesity, and sexually transmitted diseases such as chlamydia and syphilis infection.

Secondary prevention plays an important role in diseases such as diabetes (a condition in which the body does not properly metabolize sugar), glaucoma (a disorder caused

TABLE 2.5

Recommended preventive services, 2009

The U.S. Preventive Services Task Force (USPSTF) recommends that clinicians discuss these preventive services with eligible patients and offer them as a priority. All these services have received an "A" or a "B" (recommended) grade from the Task Force.

Recommendation	Adults		Special populations	
	Men	Women	Pregnant women	Children
Abdominal aortic aneurysm, screening	✔			
Alcohol misuse screening and behavioral counseling interventions	✔	✔	✔	
Aspirin for the prevention of cardiovascular disease	✔	✔		
Asymptomatic bacteriuria in adults, screening			✔	
Breast cancer, screening		✔		
Breast and ovarian cancer susceptibility, genetic risk assessment and breast cancer (BRCA) mutation testing		✔		
Breastfeeding, primary care interventions to promote		✔	✔	
Cervical cancer, screening		✔		
Chlamydial infection, screening		✔	✔	
Colorectal cancer, screening	✔	✔		
Congenital hypothyroidism, screening				✔
Dental caries in preschool children, prevention				✔
Depression (adults), screening	✔	✔		
Diet, behavioral counseling in primary care to promote a healthy	✔	✔		
Gonorrhea, screening		✔	✔	
Gonorrhea, prophylactic medication				✔
Hearing loss in newborns, screening				✔
Hepatitis B virus infection, screening			✔	
High blood pressure, screening	✔	✔		
HIV, screening	✔	✔	✔	✔
Iron deficiency anemia, prevention			✔	✔
Iron deficiency anemia, screening			✔	
Lipid disorders in adults, screening	✔	✔		
Major depressive disorder in children and adolescents, screening				✔
Obesity in adults, screening	✔	✔		
Osteoporosis in postmenopausal women, screening		✔		
Phenylketonuria, screening				✔
Rh (D) incompatibility, screening			✔	
Sexually transmitted infections, counseling	✔	✔		✔
Sickle cell disease, screening				✔
Syphilis infection, screening	✔	✔	✔	
Tobacco use and tobacco-caused disease, counseling	✔	✔	✔	
Type 2 diabetes mellitus in adults, screening	✔	✔		
Visual impairment in children younger				

SOURCE: U.S. Preventive Services Task Force. *The Guide to Clinical Preventive Services 2009*, AHRQ Publication No. 09-IP006, March 2009. Agency for Healthcare Research and Quality, Rockville, MD. http://www.ahrq.gov/clinic/pocketgd09/pocketgd09.pdf (accessed December 19, 2009)

by too much fluid pressure inside the eyeball), breast cancer, and cancer of the cervix (the opening of the uterus). State and local health departments, voluntary health agencies, hospitals, medical clinics, schools, and physicians often conduct screenings for these conditions during which people with no signs or symptoms are tested to uncover these diseases in their earliest stages.

New USPSTF Screening Guidelines for Heart Disease, Depression, and Breast Cancer

In 2009 the USPSTF presented new screening guidelines for heart disease, depression, and breast cancer. The recommendations for heart disease screening advise against using biomarkers, such as measuring high-sensitivity C-reactive protein (hs-CRP) or homocysteine levels in healthy adults, as a way to screen for heart disease. In "Using Nontraditional Risk Factors in Coronary Heart Disease Risk Assessment" (October 2009, http://www.ahrq.gov/clinic/uspstf/uspscoronaryhd.htm), the USPSTF evaluates the relevant research and medical evidence and concludes "that the evidence is insufficient to assess the balance of benefits and harms of using the nontraditional risk factors discussed in this statement to screen asymptomatic men and women with no history of [coronary heart disease] CHD to prevent CHD events."

In "Screening for Depression in Adults" (December 2009, http://www.ahrq.gov/clinic/uspstf/uspsaddepr.htm), the USPSTF updates the 2002 depression screening guidelines by recommending "screening adults for depression when staff-assisted depression care supports are in place to assure accurate diagnosis, effective treatment, and follow-up" and by advising against routine screening for depression when such supports are not available. Concerning major depressive disorder in adolescents aged 12 to 18, the USPSTF puts forth in "Major Depressive Disorder in Children and Adolescents " (March 2009, http://www.ahrq.gov/clinic/uspstf/uspschdepr.htm) a similar recommendation by advising screening "when systems are in place to ensure accurate diagnosis, psychotherapy (cognitive-behavioral or interpersonal), and follow-up."

In November 2009 the USPSTF updated its breast cancer screening recommendations from doing annual mammography starting at the age of 40 to doing biennial (every two years) mammography starting at the age of 50. The new guidelines also advise against teaching breast self-examination. The USPSTF determined that the risks of this practice—in terms of unnecessary diagnostic tests and procedures such as fine-needle aspiration and biopsies (invasive procedures that remove some breast tissue cells for examination)—outweigh the benefits. Table 2.6 summarizes the USPSTF guidelines for the use of mammography and other screening tests in breast cancer screening by the age of the woman to be screened and describes the potential benefits, harms, and costs associated with screening.

NEW BREAST CANCER SCREENING RECOMMENDATIONS GENERATE DEBATE. Many health practitioners, professional associations, and breast cancer survivors assert that women's health will be harmed by adherence to the new recommendations. Others question whether the new guidelines justify rationing preventive services. Still others flatly reject the new guidelines. For example, as of March 2010, the ACS continued to advise annual screening using mammography and clinical breast examination for all women beginning at the age of 40. In the press release "American Cancer Society Responds to Changes to USPSTF Mammography Guidelines" (November 16, 2009, http://www.cancer.org/), the ACS states, "Our experts make this recommendation having reviewed virtually all the same data reviewed by the USPSTF, but also additional data that the USPSTF did not consider. When recommendations are based on judgments about the balance of risks and benefits, reasonable experts can look at the same data and reach different conclusions."

According to the American College of Radiology/American Roentgen Ray Society, in the press release "USPSTF Mammography Recommendations Will Result in Countless Unnecessary Breast Cancer Deaths Each Year" (November 16, 2009, http://www.eurekalert.org/pub_releases/2009-11/acor-umr111609.php), Carol H. Lee, the chair of the American College of Radiology Breast Imaging Commission, assails the new guidelines by averring that they "ignore the valid scientific data and place a great many women at risk of dying unnecessarily from a disease that we have made significant headway against over the past 20 years. Mammography is not a perfect test, but it has unquestionably been shown to save lives.... These new recommendations seem to reflect a conscious decision to ration care [and] could have deadly effects for American women."

In "Mammogram Math" (*New York Times*, December 13, 2009), John Allen Paulos observes that many people believe that because earlier and more frequent screening increases the odds of detecting cancer, it is always a good idea. However, he notes that the USPSTF guidelines are based on scientific evidence that the risks associated with more frequent mammography, including increased exposure to radiation, unnecessary biopsies, and aggressive treatment of slow-growing cancers unlikely to prove fatal, outweigh the benefits of more frequent screening.

Screening and Early Detection of Breast and Cervical Cancers

So, what does this mean if you are a woman in your 40s? You should talk to your doctor and make an informed decision about whether mammography is right for you based on your family history, general health, and personal values.

—Diana Petitti, vice chair of the U.S. Preventive Services Task Force, November 19, 2009

The ACS estimates in *Breast Cancer Facts and Figures 2009–2010* (September 2009, http://www.cancer.org/downloads/STT/F861009_final%209-08-09.pdf) that in 2009,

TABLE 2.6

Recommended screening for breast cancer, 2009

Population	Women aged 40–49 years	Women aged 50–74 years	Women aged ≥75 years
Recommendation	Do not screen routinely. Individualize decision to begin biennial screening according to the patient's context and values. Grade: C	Screen every 2 years. Grade: B	No recommendation. Grade: I (insufficient evidence)
Risk assessment	This recommendation applies to women aged ≥40 years who are not at increased risk by virtue of a known genetic mutation or history of chest radiation. Increasing age is the most important risk factor for most women.		
Screening tests	Standardization of film mammography has led to improved quality. Refer patients to facilities certified under the Mammography Quality Standards Act (MQSA), listed at www.fda.gov/cdrh/mammmograph/certified.html.		
Timing of screening	Evidence indicates that biennial screening is optimal. A biennial schedule preserves most of the benefit of annual screening and cuts the harms nearly in half. A longer interval may reduce the benefit.		
Balance of harms and benefits	There is convincing evidence that screening with film mammography reduces breast cancer mortality, with a greater absolute reduction for women aged 50 to 74 years than for younger women. Harms of screening include psychological harms, additional medical visits, imaging, and biopsies in women without cancer, inconvenience due to false-positive screening results, harms of unnecessary treatment, and radiation exposure. Harms seem moderate for each age group. False-positive results are a greater concern for younger women; treatment of cancer that would not become clinically apparent during a woman's life (overdiagnosis) is an increasing problem as women age.		
Rationale for no recommendation (I statement)			Among women 75 years or older, evidence of benefit is lacking.
Relevant USPSTF recommendations	USPSTF recommendations on screening for genetic susceptibility for breast cancer and chemoprevention of breast cancer are available at www.preventiveservices.ahrq.gov.		

Population	Women aged ≥40 years			
Screening method	Digital mammography	Magnetic Resonance Imaging (MRI)	Clinical Breast Examination (CBE)	Breast Self-Examination (BSE)
Recommendation		Grade: I (insufficient evidence)		Grade: D
Rationale for no recommendation or negative recommendation	Evidence is lacking for benefits of digital mammography and MRI of the breast as substitutes for film mammography.		Evidence of CBE's additional benefit, beyond mammography, is inadequate.	Adequate evidence suggests that BSE does not reduce breast cancer mortality.
Considerations for practice				
Potential preventable burden	For younger women and women with dense breast tissue, overall detection is somewhat better with digital mammography.	Contrast-enhanced MRI has been shown to detect more cases of cancer in very high-risk populations than does mammography.	Indirect evidence suggests that when CBE is the only test available, it may detect a significant proportion of cancer cases.	
Potential harms	It is not certain whether overdiagnosis occurs more often with digital than with film mammography.	Contrast-enhanced MRI requires injection of contrast material. MRI yields many more false-positive results and potentially more overdiagnosis than mammography.	Harms of CBE include false-positive results, which lead to anxiety, unnecessary visits, imaging, and biopsies.	Harms of BSE include the same potential harms as for CBE and may be larger in magnitude.
Costs	Digital mammography is more expensive than film.	MRI is much more expensive than mammography.	Costs of CBE are primarily opportunity costs to clinicians.	Costs of BSE are primarily opportunity costs to clinicians.
Current practice	Some clinical practices are now switching to digital equipment.	MRI is not currently used to screen women of average risk.	No standard approach or reporting standards are in place.	The number of clinicians who teach BSE to patients is unknown; it is likely that few clinicians teach BSE to all women.

USPSTF = U.S. Preventive Services Task Forces

SOURCE: U.S. Preventive Services Task Force. *Screening for Breast Cancer: Clinical Summary of U.S. Preventive Services Task Force Recommendation.* AHRQ Publication No.10-05142-EF-3, November 2009. Agency for Healthcare Research and Quality, Rockville, MD. http://www.ahrq.gov/clinic/uspstf09/breastcancer/brcansum.htm (accessed December 19, 2009)

254,650 women were diagnosed with breast cancer and 40,170 died of the disease. In *Cancer Facts and Figures 2009* (May 2009, http://www.cancer.org/downloads/STT/500809web.pdf), the ACS estimates that 11,270 new cases of cervical cancer were diagnosed in 2009 and that 4,070 women died of the disease. As with many other cancers, treatment for these types of cancer is most likely to be successful when the disease begins, before the cancer has metastasized (spread from its original site to other parts of the body).

In November 2009 the American College of Obstetrics and Gynecologists released new cervical cancer screening guidelines for the Papanicolaou test (also called Pap smear or Pap test). The Pap test is a screening examination for cancer of the cervix that can prevent practically all deaths from cervical cancer by detecting cervical cancer at an early stage, when it is most curable, or even preventing the disease if precancerous lesions found during the test are treated. The incidence of cervical cancer has decreased dramatically over the past 40 years largely due to screening and early treatment. The new guidelines indicate that women should have their first Pap test at age 21 and then should be screened every two years until the age of 30 as opposed to annually. Women aged 30 and older should be screened every three years.

According to Saundra Young, in "New Cervical Cancer Screening Guidelines Released" (CNN.com, November 20, 2009), this change in cervical cancer screening frequency did not generate the kind of controversy that surrounded the new mammography screening guidelines because Pap tests detect precancers that can take from 10 to 20 years to develop into cancers. Furthermore, this change was welcomed by professional associations such as the ACS, which "supports the guidelines and said it is reviewing new data and updating its own recommendations."

Even though a vaccine to immunize women against contracting the strain of human papillomavirus (HPV) that causes cervical cancer has been available since 2006, it is only effective for females who have not yet become sexually active and contracted the virus. For this reason, cervical cancer screening will continue to be important for several generations after widespread immunization has occurred.

In 1990 Congress passed the Breast and Cervical Cancer Mortality Prevention Act, establishing the CDC's National Breast and Cervical Cancer Early Detection Program (NBCCEDP). The NBCCEDP provides breast and pelvic examinations, screening mammography, and Pap tests to women at greater risk of death from breast or cervical cancer—racial and ethnic minorities, those who live below the poverty level, older women, and women with less than a high school education.

By June 2007 the NBCCEDP had screened over 3.2 million women, provided more than 7.8 million screening examinations, and diagnosed 35,090 breast cancers, 114,390 precancerous cervical lesions, and 2,161 cervical cancers. Figure 2.2 shows the number of women served by the NBCCEDP between July 2003 and June 2007. A significant component of the NBCCEDP effort is community education and outreach. Health educators must not only communicate the life-saving benefits of screening and early identification of disease but also

FIGURE 2.2

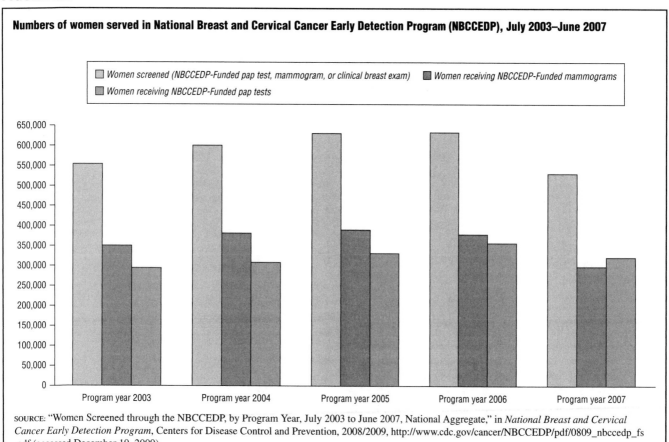

Numbers of women served in National Breast and Cervical Cancer Early Detection Program (NBCCEDP), July 2003–June 2007

SOURCE: "Women Screened through the NBCCEDP, by Program Year, July 2003 to June 2007, National Aggregate," in *National Breast and Cervical Cancer Early Detection Program*, Centers for Disease Control and Prevention, 2008/2009, http://www.cdc.gov/cancer/NBCCEDP/pdf/0809_nbccedp_fs .pdf (accessed December 19, 2009)

overcome barriers to access to care, such as the lack of transportation or child care.

The NBCCEDP also funds follow-up care for women who have abnormal screening results to enable them to receive needed services. These may include biopsy (surgical removal of a sample of cells for microscopic examination) to confirm the diagnosis and visits with surgeons and other medical specialists to receive timely treatment. The provision of follow-up care and treatment is a fundamental principle underlying screening programs.

Screening programs that do not provide facilities for diagnosis and treatment are unlikely to be effective, especially when they are serving populations unable to pay for medical care. Furthermore, many public health professionals believe it is unethical to offer screening without plans and provisions to care for disease identified through the screening process.

TERTIARY PREVENTION

Tertiary prevention programs aim to improve the quality of life for people with various diseases by limiting complications and disabilities, reducing the severity and progression of disease, and providing rehabilitation (therapy to restore functionality and self-sufficiency). Unlike primary and secondary prevention, tertiary prevention involves actual treatment for the disease and is conducted primarily by health care practitioners, rather than by public health agencies.

Tertiary prevention efforts demonstrate that it is possible to slow the natural course of some progressive diseases and prevent or delay many of the complications associated with chronic diseases such as arthritis (inflammation of the joints that causes pain, swelling, and stiffness), asthma (inflammation and obstruction of the airways that makes breathing difficult), heart disease, and diabetes.

Tertiary Prevention of Diabetes

Insulin is a hormone produced by the pancreas to control the amount of glucose (sugar) in the blood. Diabetes mellitus is a disease in which high blood glucose levels result from insufficient insulin production or action. When there is not enough insulin produced, the body is unable to metabolize (use, regulate, and store) glucose, and it remains in the blood.

Type 1 diabetes mellitus (also called insulin-dependent diabetes or juvenile-onset diabetes) occurs when pancreatic beta cells, the cells that make insulin, are destroyed by the body's own immune system. It usually develops in children and young adults. Because people with diabetes do not have enough insulin, they must be injected or inject themselves with insulin several times a day or receive insulin via a pump. In "National Diabetes Statistics, 2007" (June 2008, http://diabetes.niddk.nih.gov/dm/pubs/statistics/), the

National Institute of Diabetes and Digestive and Kidney Diseases (NIDDK) states that about 5% to 10% of all diagnosed cases of diabetes are Type 1.

Type 2 diabetes mellitus (also called noninsulin-dependent diabetes or adult-onset diabetes) occurs when the body becomes resistant to insulin. As a result of the cells being unable to use insulin effectively, the amount of glucose they can take up is sharply reduced and high levels of glucose accumulate in the blood. The NIDDK notes that approximately 90% to 95% of all diagnosed cases of diabetes are Type 2 diabetes.

Many people with Type 2 diabetes are able to control their blood sugar by losing excess weight, maintaining proper nutrition, and exercising regularly. Others require insulin injections or orally administered (taken by mouth) drugs to lower their blood sugar.

Other types of diabetes can occur as a result of pregnancy (gestational diabetes) or physiologic stress such as surgery, trauma, malnutrition, infections, and other illnesses. According to the NIDDK, these types of diabetes account for between 1% and 5% of all diagnosed cases of the disease.

The NIH reports in "New Survey Results Show Huge Burden of Diabetes" (January 26, 2009, http://www.nih.gov/news/health/jan2009/niddk-26.htm) that of the 13% of adults aged 20 and older who have diabetes, 40% are not aware that they have it. Another 30% of adults have prediabetes, a condition in which blood sugar is high but not yet in the diabetic range. Even though diabetes occurs infrequently in adolescents aged 12 to 19, the NIH finds that 16% have prediabetes.

COMPLICATIONS OF DIABETES. According to the NIDDK, in "National Diabetes Statistics, 2007," adults with diabetes suffer from heart disease at much higher rates—in fact, heart disease is the number-one cause of death among people with diabetes. Similarly, adults with diabetes have an increased risk for stroke (damage to the brain that occurs when its blood supply is cut off, frequently because of blockage in an artery that supplies the brain) and hypertension (75% of adults with diabetes have high blood pressure). Heart disease accounts for 68% of deaths in people with diabetes, and stroke accounts for 16% of deaths. Other serious complications of this disease include:

- Diabetic retinopathy—this is a condition that can cause blindness.

- Diabetic neuropathy—this condition causes damage to the nervous system that may produce pain or loss of sensation in the hands or feet and other nerve problems.

- Kidney disease—diabetes accounts for almost half of all new end-stage renal disease cases that require dialysis (mechanical cleansing of the blood of impurities) or kidney transplant.

- Amputation—diabetes is responsible for 60% of all lower-limb amputations (surgical removal of toes, feet, and the leg below the knee) performed in the United States.

- Dental disease—gum diseases are common among people with diabetes, and nearly one-third of all people with diabetes have severe periodontal (tooth and gum) diseases.

- Problems with pregnancy—diabetes may cause birth defects, miscarriage (spontaneous abortion), and excessively large babies that may create additional health risks for expectant mothers.

- Increased risk of infection—people with diabetes are more susceptible to infection and do not recover as quickly as people without diabetes.

Furthermore, poorly controlled or uncontrolled diabetes may produce life-threatening medical emergencies, such as diabetic ketoacidosis (excessive ketones—chemicals in the blood resulting from insufficient insulin and an excessive amount of counterregulatory hormones such as glucagon) or hyperosmolar coma (extremely high blood glucose, leading to dehydration).

Achieving optimal control of blood glucose levels can prevent many of the complications of diabetes and decrease the risk of death associated with the disease. Optimal control involves aggressive treatment of diabetes with close attention to the roles of diet, exercise, weight management, and pharmacology (proper use of insulin and other medication) in the self-management of the disease.

PREVENTING COMPLICATIONS OF DIABETES. In "National Diabetes Statistics, 2007," the NIDDK explains that even modest improvement in controlling blood glucose acts to help prevent diabetic retinopathy, neuropathy, and kidney disease. Reducing blood pressure can decrease cardiovascular complications (heart disease and stroke) by as much as 50% and can reduce the risk of retinopathy, neuropathy, and kidney disease by 33%. Lowering blood cholesterol (a waxy substance produced by the body and found in animal products), low-density lipoproteins (LDL), and triglycerides also reduces, by as much as 50%, the cardiovascular complications of diabetes. (Cholesterol, LDL, and triglycerides are lipids that may be measured in the blood.)

The NIDDK reports that early detection and treatment of diabetic eye disease can reduce by 50% to 60% the possibility of blindness or serious loss of vision. Similarly, early detection and treatment of kidney disease sharply reduces the risk of developing kidney failure, and careful attention to foot care reduces the risk of amputation by as much as 85%.

To help increase early detection of diabetes (secondary prevention) and reduce the morbidity (illnesses) and mortality (deaths) associated with it (tertiary prevention), the CDC and the NIDDK launched the National Diabetes Education Program (NDEP) in 1997. The NDEP's objectives are to increase public awareness of diabetes, improve self-management of people with diabetes, enhance health care providers' knowledge and treatment of diabetes, and promote health policies that improve access, availability, and quality of diabetes care. To meet these educational objectives, the NDEP, in working with a variety of other health organizations, develops and distributes teaching tools and resources.

In *The National Diabetes Education Program: Ten Years of Progress 1997–2007* (August 2007, http://ndep.nih .gov/media/NDEP_ProgressRpt07.pdf), the NDEP reports that between 1997 and 2007 it created news stories that were read by over 1 billion people. During this 10-year period, the NDEP produced television and radio public service announcements valued at more than $30 million, and its print advertising reached more than 53 million readers. Every month, the NDEP Information Clearinghouse responds to about 1,000 requests and disseminates 20,000 materials. Furthermore, it has distributed over 3.1 million publications. NDEP materials are available in 16 languages and its resources are also available online (http://www.ndep.nih.gov/, http://www.betterdiabetescare .nih.gov/, and http://www.diabetesatwork.org/).

The NDEP enumerates in the fact sheet "Changing the Way Diabetes Is Treated" (July 2009, http://ndep.nih .gov/media/NDEP_FactSheet.pdf) the strategies it employs to achieve the NDEP goal of reducing illness and death caused by diabetes and its complications. These strategies are intended to:

- Create program partnerships with organizations concerned about diabetes and the health status of their members.

- Develop and implement ongoing diabetes awareness and education campaigns for health care professionals and people with or at risk for diabetes.

- Identify, develop, promote, and disseminate educational tools and resources for people with diabetes and those at risk, including materials that address the needs of special populations.

- Disseminate guiding principles that promote quality diabetes care to health care professionals, payers, purchasers, and policymakers.

- Promote policies and activities to improve the quality of and access to care for people with and at risk for diabetes.

- Address the economic case for quality diabetes care to inform health care payers, purchasers, and policymakers.

EXEMPLARY MENTAL HEALTH PREVENTION PROGRAMS

This section presents a national mental health and suicide risk screening program for youth described in *Achieving the Promise: Transforming Mental Health Care in America* (July 2003, http://www.mentalhealthcommission.gov/reports/FinalReport/downloads/FinalReport.pdf) by the President's New Freedom Commission on Mental Health. It also offers recommendations and descriptions of interventions considered effective at preventing suicide from *Reducing Suicide: A National Imperative* (2002, http://www.nap.edu/books/0309083214/html/), which was edited by Sara K. Goldsmith et al.

Goldsmith et al. characterize current mental health prevention programs as rooted in the "universal, selective, and indicated prevention model." This model considers three defined populations: the entire population is included in universal programs, specific high-risk groups are targeted by selective programs, and indicated programs address specific high-risk individuals. Universal programming assumes a basically healthy population and generally aims at protection against developing a disorder by offering, for example, enhanced coping skills and resiliency training. Examples of universal programs are educational programs to heighten awareness of a problem and mass-media campaigns intended to increase understanding of and attitudes about a particular issue.

Population-based programs often produce greater gains than programs targeting individuals because there are higher rates of program participation. For example, all the students in a given grade will be exposed to school-based drug prevention programs. Selective programs target subsets of populations that have been identified as at risk but are not yet diagnosed with a specific problem or disorder—people who have a greater-than-average likelihood of developing mental disorders, such as adolescents with truancy or suspected substance abuse problems. Indicated programs are aimed at specific high-risk individuals who have presented early signs or symptoms of mental disorders, such as children diagnosed with attention deficit hyperactivity disorder, who may be at a greater risk of developing conduct disorders, or students who have engaged in disruptive or other disturbed behavior at school.

By recounting the histories, benefits, and scientific evaluation of mental health prevention programs, *Achieving the Promise* and *Reducing Suicide* offer a framework for developing and implementing mental health prevention programs and policies in a wide range of settings, including primary medical care practices and clinics, maternal and infant health and mental health programs, child care centers, school-based health centers, vocational training programs, social service agencies, parent education programs, and the media. Furthermore, these reports disseminate the methods and results of effective programs that have demonstrated efficacy, enabling mental health service providers and other stakeholders throughout the country to replicate these results in their local communities.

Adolescent Intervention Programs

One recommendation from *Achieving the Promise* is to "improve and expand school mental health programs." The commission cites research demonstrating that about 42% of students with serious emotional disturbances graduate from high school, compared with 57% of students with other disabilities. The commission believes this could be changed, because it finds ample evidence that school mental health programs improved academic achievement—with improved test scores, fewer absences, and less discipline problems—by detecting mental health problems early and providing timely referral to appropriate treatment.

The commission observes that the concerted effort needed to deliver quality mental health services in schools entails collaboration with parents and local providers of mental health care to support screening, assessment, and early intervention. It also asserts that mental health services must be integral parts of school health centers and that federal funds must be available to support the programs.

The commission lauds the Columbia University TeenScreen program as a model program of screening and early intervention. The program ensures mental health screening of all students before they leave high school and early identification of students at risk for suicide or those with symptoms of depression or other mental illness. Evaluation of the program found it to be remarkably effective—identifying more than 60% of students later found to have recurrent mental health problems or mental disorders. Table 2.7 summarizes the goals, features, outcomes, and principal challenges faced during implementation of the TeenScreen program.

Participants complete a 10-minute paper-and-pencil or computerized questionnaire. The questionnaire covers anxiety, depression, substance and alcohol abuse, and suicidal thoughts and behavior. The TeenScreen program does not recommend any particular type of treatment for the teens who are identified by the mental health screening. Parents of students identified as at possible risk are notified and offered information and referral to local mental health services where they can obtain further evaluation. No student is screened without parental consent, and the results of the screen are confidential. Screening occurs in a range of venues, including schools, clinics, physicians' offices, and juvenile justice facilities.

Screening increases the likelihood that students at risk for suicidal behavior will get into treatment. Madelyn S. Gould et al. indicate in "Service Use by At-Risk Youths after School-Based Suicide Screening" (*Journal of the American Academy of Child and Adolescent Psychiatry,*

TABLE 2.7

Columbia University teen mental health screening program

Program	Columbia University TeenScreen® Program
Goal	To ensure that all youth are offered a mental health check-up before graduating from high school. Teen-Screen® identifies and refers for treatment those who are at risk for suicide or suffer from an untreated mental illness.
Features	All youngsters in a school, with parental consent, are given a computer-based questionnaire that screens them for mental illnesses and suicide risk. At no charge, the Columbia University TeenScreen® Program provides consultation, screening materials, software, training, and technical assistance to qualifying schools and communities. In return, TeenScreen® partners are expected to screen at least 200 youth per year and ensure that a licensed mental health professional is on-site to give immediate counseling and referral services for youth at greatest risk. The Columbia TeenScreen® Program is a not-for-profit organization funded solely by foundations. When the program identifies youth needing treatment, their care is paid for depending on the family's health coverage.
Outcomes	The computer-based questionnaire used by TeenScreen® is a valid and reliable screening instruments.[a] The vast majority of youth identified through the program as having already made a suicide attempt, or at risk for depression or suicidal thinking, are not in treatments.[b] A follow-up study found that screening in high school identified more than 60% of students who, four to six years later, continued to have long-term, recurrent problems with depression and suicidal attempts.[c]
Biggest challenge	To bridge the gap between schools and local providers of mental health services. Another challenge is to ensure, in times of fiscal austerity, that schools devote a health professional to screening and referral.
How other organazitions can adopt	The Columbia University TeenScreen® program is pilot-testing a shorter questionnaire, which will be less costly and time-consuming for the school to administer. It is also trying to adapt the program to primary care settings.
Website	www.teenscreen.org
Sites where implemented	69 sites (mostly middle schools and high schools) in 27 states

[a]Shaffer, D., Fisher, P., Lucas, C. P., Dulcan, M. K., & Schwab-Stone, M. E. (2000). NIMH Diagnostic Interview Schedule for Children Version IV (NIMH DISC-IV): Description, differences from previous versions, and reliability of some common diagnoses. Journal of the American Academy of Child and Adolescent Psychiatry, 39, 28–38.
[b]Shaffer, D. & Craft, L. (1999). Methods of adolescent suicide prevention. Journal of Clinical Psychiatry, 60, Supplement 2, 70–74.
[c]Leslie McGuire, personal communication, June 24, 2003.

SOURCE: "Figure 4.2. Model Program: Screening Program for Youth," in *Achieving the Promise: Transforming Mental Health Care in America*, President's New Freedom Commission on Mental Health, 2003, http://www.mentalhealthcommission.gov/reports/FinalReport/FullReport-05.htm (accessed December 18, 2009)

vol. 48, no. 12, December 2009) that school-based mental health assessments effectively identify adolescents at risk for suicidal behavior and help ensure high rates of follow-up treatment. The researchers indicate that nearly 70% of adolescents identified by a school-based suicide screening effort followed through on referrals to treatment within one year. According to the TeenScreen National Center for Mental Health Checkups at Columbia University, in the press release "School-Based Mental Health Checkups Lead to High Rates of Follow-up Care for Teens" (November 20, 2009, http://www.teenscreen.org/school-based-mental-health-checkups), Laurie Flynn, the executive director of the TeenScreen National Center for Mental Health Checkups, said, "This study tells us adults, as parents and educators, that we are key players in improving our young peoples' access to care for mental illness. Dr. Gould's study affirms that mental health checkups are effective and that at-risk teens identified through school-based screenings are able to get help. As with any medical condition, the earlier you can identify illness and begin treatment, the better the outcome."

PREVENTING SUICIDE

In the landmark report *Mental Health: A Report of the Surgeon General* (1999, http://www.surgeongeneral.gov/library/mentalhealth/home.html), the Office of the Surgeon General states that suicide is a serious public health problem and recommends a three-pronged national strategy to prevent suicide, which includes programs to educate, heighten understanding, intervene, and advance the science of suicide prevention. Table 2.8 shows the components of AIM (awareness, intervention, and methodology)—the national strategy for suicide prevention—as well as the risk factors and protective factors for suicide.

According to the NIH, in "Suicide Facts at a Glance" (Summer 2009, http://www.cdc.gov/violenceprevention/pdf/Suicide-DataSheet-a.pdf), in 2006 more than 33,000 suicides occurred. There was one suicide for every 25 attempted suicides. In 2007, 14.5% of high school students (grades nine to 12) said they had seriously considered suicide in the previous 12 months, 6.9% of students reported trying to commit suicide at least once in the previous 12 months, and 2% of students had tried to commit suicide

TABLE 2.8

Suicide risk factors, protective factors, and national prevention strategy

- National Strategy for Suicide Prevention: AIM
  - Awareness: promote public awareness of suicide as a public health problem
  - Intervention: enhance services and programs
  - Methodology: advance the science of suicide prevention
- Risk factors
  - Male gender
  - Mental disorders, particularly depression and substance abuse
  - Prior suicide attempts
  - Unwillingness to seek help because of stigma
  - Barriers to accessing mental health treatment
  - Stressful life event/loss
  - Easy access to lethal methods such as guns
- Protective factors
  - Effective and appropriate clinical care for underlying disorders
  - Easy access to care
  - Support from family, community, and health and mental health care staff

SOURCE: Adapted from "Figure 4-1. Surgeon General's Call to Action to Prevent Suicide—1999," in *Mental Health: A Report of the Surgeon General*, U.S. Department of Health and Human Services, Substance Abuse and Mental Health Services Administration, Center for Mental Health Services, with the National Institute of Mental Health, 1999, http://www.mentalhealth.samhsa.gov/features/surgeongeneralreport/toc.asp (accessed December 21, 2009)

that resulted in an injury, poisoning, or overdose that required medical attention.

The CDC describes in "Preventing Suicide: Program Activities Guide" (January 2009, http://www.cdc.gov/violenceprevention/pdf/PreventingSuicide-a.pdf) activities in key prevention areas, including surveillance, research, capacity building, communication, partnership, and leadership. The CDC's violence prevention activities emphasize primary prevention, advancing the science of prevention, translating scientific advances into practical applications, and building on existing efforts to address community needs or gaps in preventive services. Ongoing activities include:

- Monitoring, tracking, and researching the problem. State and local agencies work together to gather data that enable policy and community leaders to make informed decisions about violence prevention programs and strategies. Other CDC research focuses on the relationship between different forms of violent behavior and suicide among adolescent and school-associated violent deaths.

- Supporting and enhancing prevention programs that are university- and school-based as well as multistate and national prevention and education initiatives that promote awareness of suicide as a preventable public health problem.

- Providing prevention resources, such as a toll-free hotline, a Web site, or a fax-on-demand service that supplies prevention information and print publications.

- Encouraging research and development on violence, injury, and suicide prevention in specific populations such as adolescents making the transition to early adulthood, urban youth, and youth identified as at risk for suicidal behavior by screening programs.

ACTIVE MILITARY AND VETERANS ARE AT RISK FOR SUICIDE

According to Robin B. McFee, in "Gulf War Servicemen and Servicewomen: The Long Road Home and the Role of Health Care Professionals to Enhance the Troops' Health and Healing" (*Disease-a-Month*, vol. 54, no. 5, May 2008), returning from war presents a wide range of physical and psychological risks, injuries, and therapeutic challenges. Troops must reenter society after experiencing the horrors of war, the loss of friends, injuries, and deprivation not encountered in the United States. Unlike earlier wars, such as World War II (1939–1945) or the Korean War (1950–1953), most U.S. citizens are not involved with the wars in Iraq and Afghanistan on a daily basis, and as a result many communities lack support for returning veterans.

In "Rising Military Suicides" (November 25, 2009, http://www.congress.org/news/2009/11/25/rising_military_suicides), John Donnelly observes that "more U.S. military personnel have taken their own lives so far in 2009 than have been killed in either the Afghanistan or Iraq wars." Between January and November 2009, 334 members of the U.S. military had committed suicide, compared with 297 killed in Afghanistan and 144 killed in Iraq. Of the 334 military personnel who committed suicide, 211 were in the U.S. Army, 47 were in the U.S. Navy, 34 were in the U.S. Air Force, and 42 were in the U.S. Marine Corps (active duty only). These numbers are alarming because members of the U.S. military have generally had much lower rates of suicide than the U.S. population, which according to the CDC is about 20 per 100,000 among men aged 20 to 29. For example, the army reported just 9 suicides per 100,000 active duty troops in 2001, and the Marine Corps reported 12.5 per 100,000 in 2002. By 2008 the army rate had risen to 20.2 per 100,000 and the Marine Corps rate was 19.5 per 100,000. Even though it may not be the sole contributing factor to the rising number, Donnelly observes that "the rising number of suicides has coincided with U.S. military forces redeploying frequently to Iraq and Afghanistan."

Identifying Troops and Veterans at Risk for Suicide

The U.S. Department of Veterans Affairs (VA) identifies in "How to Recognize When to Ask for Help" (March 5, 2010, http://www.mentalhealth.va.gov/suicide_prevention/index.asp) veteran-specific risks for suicide, including:

- Frequent deployments

- Deployments to hostile environments

- Exposure to extreme stress

- Physical/sexual assault while in the service (not limited to women)

- Length of deployments

- Service-related injury

The VA also instructs health professionals about how to identify and respond to risk for suicide. Table 2.9 enumerates the warning signs for suicide risk.

In "The Need for Outreach in Preventing Suicide among Young Veterans" (*PLoS Medicine*, vol. 6, no. 3, March 3, 2009), Jitender Sareen and Shay-Lee Belik note that suicide is the second-most common cause of death in the U.S. military and that most service members with mental health problems do not seek or receive treatment. One study finds that just one out of five veterans who committed suicide had any contact with a mental health professional. Sareen and Belik describe five major areas of suicide prevention:

TABLE 2.9

Warning signs for suicide risk

Look for the warning signs
- Threatening to hurt or kill self
- Looking for ways to kill self
- Seeking access to pills, weapons or other means
- Talking or writing about death, dying or suicide

Presence of any of the above warning signs requires immediate attention and referral. Consider hospitalization for safety until complete assessment may be made.

Additional warning signs
- Hopelessness
- Rage, anger, seeking revenge
- Acting reckless or engaging in risky activities, seemingly without thinking
- Feeling trapped—like there is no way out
- Increasing alcohol or drug abuse
- Withdrawing from friends, family and society
- Anxiety, agitation, unable to sleep or sleeping all the time
- Dramatic changes in mood
- No reason for living, no sense of purpose in life

For any of the above refer for mental health treatment or assure that follow-up appointment is made.

SOURCE: "Look for the Warning Signs," in *Suicide Risk Assessment Guide*, U.S. Department of Veterans Affairs, December 11, 2009, http://www.mentalhealth.va.gov/College/docs/Suicide_PocketCard_Magnet.pdf (accessed December 21, 2009)

1. Education and awareness programs for the general public and professionals

2. Screening methods for high-risk people

3. Treatment of psychiatric disorders

4. Restricting access to lethal means

5. Safe media reporting of suicide to minimize the risk of so-called copycat suicides, especially in youth

The VA Suicide Prevention Program Expands

The VA states in "How to Recognize When to Ask for Help" that its National Suicide Prevention Lifeline "has directly saved more than 5,000 lives from suicide and provided counseling for more than 185,000 veterans and their loved ones at home and overseas." The lifeline, which is available 24 hours per day, seven days per week, is staffed by trained mental health counselors.

In July 2009 the VA launched an online chat service that provides a forum where veterans, their families, and friends can chat anonymously with a trained VA counselor. Should the counselor identify the veteran's problem as a crisis or emergency, he or she can provide immediate assistance by connecting the person online to the VA Suicide Prevention Hotline for counseling and crisis intervention services. The online service is an outreach program intended to communicate with and inform all veterans—not only those enrolled in the VA health care system—and offer them immediate online access to peer support and trained counselors who can provide anonymous suicide prevention services.

The U.S. Air Force Suicide Prevention Program

The suicide prevention program initiated by the U.S. Air Force is comprehensive and acts to increase knowledge and change attitudes within a community, dispel barriers to treatment, and improve access to support and intervention. According to General Carrol H. Chandler, in "Suicide Prevention: A Leadership Challenge for All" (June 26, 2009, http://www.af.mil/news/story.asp?id=123150937), the program resulted in a 28% decline in suicide rates between 2000 and 2009.

The Air Force Suicide Prevention Program is a population-based, community approach to suicide risk prevention and behavioral health promotion. It integrates human, medical, and mental health services by uniting a coalition of community agencies from within and outside the health care delivery system to significantly reduce suicide among air force personnel, which had risen to an all-time high during the mid-1990s.

The program attempts to reduce risk factors, such as problems with the law, finances, intimate relationships, mental health, job performance, substance abuse, social isolation, and poor coping skills. It simultaneously seeks to strengthen protective factors such as effective coping skills, a sense of social connectedness, support, and policies and norms that encourage effective help-seeking behaviors. To stimulate help-seeking behaviors, the program stresses the urgent need for air force leaders, supervisors, and frontline workers to support one another during times of heightened life stress. It exhorts members of the air force to seek help from mental health clinics and observes that seeking help early is likely to enhance careers rather than hinder them. The program instructs commanders and supervisors to support and protect those who seek mental health care and eliminates policies that previously served as barriers to seeking and obtaining mental health care.

To improve surveillance, a Web-based database is used to capture demographic, risk factor, and protective factor information about individuals who attempted or completed suicide. This extremely secure tool protects privacy and permits timely detection of changes in patterns in suicidal behavior that can be used to strengthen policies and enhance practices throughout the air force community. To improve crisis management, critical incident stress management teams are assembled and poised for deployment to installations hit hard by potentially traumatizing events such as combat deployments, serious aircraft accidents, natural disasters, and suicides within the units.

The air force experience is not necessarily applicable to the general population, because the air force is a tightly controlled and relatively homogenous community with identifiable leaders readily able to influence community norms and priorities. Regardless, it can still serve as a model for comparable hierarchical organizations and offer insight into prevention program planning. The program's overarching principles, such as engaging community leaders to change cultural norms, improving coordination of diverse human and health services, and providing educational programs to community members, can inform national efforts and may be replicable in other populations.

PREVENTION RESEARCH AND GOALS

In 1986 Congress funded the first Prevention Research Centers. In "Prevention Research Centers—Building the Scientific Research Base with Community Partners: At a Glance 2010" (December 17, 2009, http://www.cdc.gov/ chronicdisease/resources/publications/AAG/ prc.htm), the CDC indicates that as of 2009, 35 such centers were affiliated with medical schools or schools of public health. The centers explore and research a wide range of public health problems and test strategies to address these problems. In 2009 hundreds of funded projects were examining programs addressing myriad prevention efforts such as childhood obesity, reducing smoking, promoting healthy aging, and workplace safety.

Primary prevention research and programming in the past aimed to prevent illness by more effectively encouraging people to avoid behaviors (such as smoking, abusing drugs, engaging in unsafe sexual practices, or overeating) linked to health risk. By March 2010, prevention research and education also emphasized avoiding or reducing environmental exposures (such as sun, water pollution, radon, ozone, pesticides, and hazardous chemicals) that increase health risk.

SATISFYING WORK, SOCIAL ACTIVITIES, AND PERSONAL RELATIONSHIPS ARE KEY TO HEALTH AND WELLNESS

Family, friends, active interests, and community involvement may do more than simply help people enjoy their life. Social activities and relationships may actually enable people to live longer by preventing or delaying the development of many diseases, including dementia. During the past two decades research has demonstrated that social experiences, activities, relationships, and work stress are related to health, well-being, and longevity. The kind of work stress that causes the greatest harm to physical and mental health is effort-reward imbalance— when great effort is made and the effort is neither recognized nor rewarded. Even though women appear more vulnerable to work stress, men's health seems more dependent on the availability of social relationships and emotional support.

Several studies, such as the landmark RAND Corporation's "Health, Marriage, and Longer Life for Men" (1998, http://www.rand.org/pubs/research_briefs/RB5018/ index1.html), show that marriage or living with a partner has greater health benefits for men than for women, because traditionally women are caregivers. More recent findings, such as a comparison of blood pressure and mental health among people who are happily married, unhappily married, and single, question whether the nurturing qualities of women are solely responsible for married men's improved health. Julianne Holt-Lunstad, Wendy Birmingham, and Brandon Q. Jones find in "Is There Something Unique about Marriage? The Relative Impact of Marital Status, Relationship Quality, and Network Social Support on Ambulatory Blood Pressure and Mental Health" (*Annals of Behavioral Medicine*, vol. 35, no. 2, April 2008) that both marital status and marital quality influence health status. Married people reported greater satisfaction with life and blood pressure dipping than single individuals. Among married people, those who deemed their marital quality "higher" had lower blood pressure, lower stress, less depression, and reported higher levels of overall satisfaction with life. Holt-Lunstad, Birmingham, and Jones also observe that men and women living alone had better health than those with unsatisfactory relationships with their partner.

Cheryl A. Frye of the University at Albany, State University of New York, finds in "Neurosteroids' Effects and Mechanisms for Social, Cognitive, Emotional, and Physical Functions" (*Psychoneuroendocrinology*, vol. 34, supp. 1, December 2009) that social supports—their presence or absence—may influence the course of age-related changes in physical, mental, and emotional health and well-being. The loss of close relationships, especially among older adults, is one of the greatest risk factors for mental and physical decline. Emerging research suggests that these changes may be hormonally mediated, and Frye indicates that "further understanding of these neurobiological and/or behavioral factors may lead to findings that ultimately can promote health and prevent disease."

Along with personal relationships, social activities also seem to protect against disease and increase longevity, even when the activities do not involve physical exercise. In "The Quality of Dyadic Relationships, Leisure Activities, and Health among Older Women" (*Health Care for Women International*, vol. 30, no. 12, December 2009), Tanya R. Fitzpatrick of McGill University examines the influence of social relationships and leisure activities on the health of older women and finds that the quality of interpersonal relationships "has a strong influence on mental health measured by spirit, happiness, and an interesting life." Fitzpatrick also observes that leisure activities not only predict but also improve physical health as measured by self-report and the number of chronic health conditions. There is also evidence that close relationships can substitute for other close relationships. This is a key concern because the death of a spouse or a close friend may increase the survivor's risk for social isolation. The observation that strong connections with children, relatives, and friends can substitute for relationships with spouses or partners is especially significant for widowed, divorced, or never-married older adults.

There is mounting evidence of the health benefits of socialization. The National Social Life, Health, and Aging Project (NSHAP) considers indicators of social connectedness, social participation, social support, and loneliness among older adults. In "Measuring Social Isolation among Older Adults Using Multiple Indicators from the NSHAP Study" (*Journals of Gerontology Series B: Psychological Sciences and Social Sciences*, vol. 64, supp. 1, November 2009), Erin York Cornwell and Linda J. Waite analyze two aspects of social isolation: social disconnectedness (defined as physical separation from others) and perceived isolation. The researchers find that, in general, social disconnectedness does not vary across age groups, but that the oldest older adults (aged 75 and older) do feel more isolated than younger older adults (aged 65 to 75). Furthermore, Cornwell and Waite reconfirm the association between social supports and health outcomes reported in earlier studies, in that social disconnectedness and perceived isolation are greater among those who have worse health.

Pets Are More Than Best Friends; They Can Help Keep People Healthy

Research conducted during the late 1990s found that pet ownership was associated with better health. At first it was believed that the effects were simply increased well-being—the obvious delight of hospital and nursing home patients petting puppies, watching kittens play, or viewing fish in an aquarium clearly demonstrated pets' abilities to enhance mood and stimulate social interactions.

However, in March 1999 Parminder Raina et al. reported in "Influence of Companion Animals on the Physical and Psychological Health of Older People: An Analysis of a One-Year Longitudinal Study" (*Journal of the American Geriatrics Society*, vol. 47, no. 3) that attachment to a companion animal was linked to maintaining or slightly improving the physical and psychological well-being of older adults. The researchers followed 1,054 older adults for one year and found that pet owners were better able to perform the activities of daily living and were more satisfied with their physical health, mental health, family relationships, living arrangements, finances, and friends. These findings were confirmed by Karen Allen, Jim Blascovich, and Wendy B. Mendes in "Cardiovascular Reactivity and the Presence of Pets, Friends, and Spouses: The Truth about Cats and Dogs" (*Psychosomatic Medicine*, vol. 64, no. 5, September–October 2002).

Other research reveals the specific health benefits of human interaction with animals. Erika Friedmann et al.

examine in "Relation between Pet Ownership and Heart Rate Variability in Patients with Healed Myocardial Infarcts" (*American Journal of Cardiology*, vol. 91, no. 6, March 2003) the differences in survival between pet owners and nonowners who suffered heart attacks over a two-year period. The researchers find that subjects without pets had reduced heart rate variability, which was associated with an increased risk of cardiac disease and mortality. Several researchers observe that petting dogs and cats actually lowers blood pressure. The physiologic mechanisms responsible for these health benefits are as yet unidentified; however, some researchers think that pets connect people to the natural world, enabling them to focus on others, rather than simply on themselves. Other researchers observe that dog owners walk more than people without dogs and credit pet owners' improved health to exercise. Nearly all agree that the nonjudgmental affection pets offer boosts health and wellness.

Erika Friedmann and Heesook Son assert in "The Human-Companion Animal Bond: How Humans Benefit" (*Veterinary Clinics of North America Small Animal Practice*, vol. 39, no. 2, March 2009) that pet ownership, or just the presence of a companion animal, is associated with health benefits, including improvements in mental, social, and physiologic health status. In "The Benefits of Human-Companion Animal Interaction: A Review" (*Journal of Veterinary Medical Education*, vol. 35, no. 4, winter 2008), a review of research published since 1980 about the benefits of human-companion animal bonds, Sandra B. Barker and Aaron R. Wolen conclude that many studies support the health benefits of interacting with companion animals. The researchers call for more rigorous research to increase the understanding of the dynamics of these interactions and how they exert benefits on human health.

Healthy People 2020

Since 1979 the U.S. Department of Health and Human Services has been compiling scientific insights and advances in medicine from each decade to develop 10-year national objectives for promoting health and preventing disease. *Healthy People 2020* (November 3, 2009, http://www.healthypeople.gov/hp2020/default.asp), like the previous public health objectives, "will reflect assessments of major risks to health and wellness, changing public health priorities, and emerging issues related to our nation's health preparedness and prevention." Its overarching goals are to:

- Eliminate preventable disease, disability, injury, and premature death.

- Achieve health equity, eliminate disparities, and improve the health of all groups.

- Create social and physical environments that promote good health for all.

- Promote healthy development and healthy behaviors across every stage of life.

Nearly all the *Healthy People 2020* goals and objectives will involve one or more of the three levels of prevention discussed in this chapter. Figure 2.3 displays the model action plan that *Healthy People 2020* will use to improve the nation's health.

FIGURE 2.3

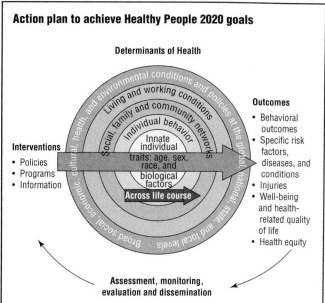

Action plan to achieve Healthy People 2020 goals

SOURCE: "Exhibit A. Action Model to Achieve Healthy People 2020 Overarching Goals," in *The Secretary's Advisory Committee on National Health Promotion and Disease Prevention Objectives for 2020 Phase I Report: Recommendations for the Framework and Format of Healthy People 2020*, U.S. Department of Health and Human Services, October 28, 2008, http://www.healthypeople.gov/HP2020/advisory/phasel/phasel.pdf (accessed December 22, 2009)

CHAPTER 3
DIAGNOSING DISEASE: THE PROCESS OF DETECTING AND IDENTIFYING ILLNESS

"Diagnosis" means finding the cause of a disorder, not just giving it a name.

—Sydney Walker III, *A Dose of Sanity: Mind, Medicine, and Misdiagnosis* (1996)

The practice of medicine is often considered to be both science and art because identifying the underlying causes of disease and establishing a diagnosis require that health care practitioners (physicians, nurses, and allied health professionals) use a combination of scientific method, intuition, and interpersonal (communication and human relations) skills. Diagnosis relies on the powers of observation; listening and communication skills; analytical ability; knowledge of human anatomy (structure and parts of the human body) and physiology (the functions and life processes of body systems); and an understanding of the natural course of illness.

The editors of the 17th edition of *Harrison's Principles of Internal Medicine* (2008) explain that diagnosis requires a logical approach to problem solving involving analysis and synthesis. In other words, health care practitioners must systematically break down the information they obtain from a patient's medical history, physical examination, and laboratory test results and then reassemble it into a pattern that fits a well-defined syndrome (a group of symptoms that collectively describe a disease).

MEDICAL HISTORIES

Obtaining a complete and accurate medical history is the first step in the diagnostic process. In fact, many health care practitioners believe that the patient's medical history is the key to diagnosis and that the physical examination and results of any diagnostic testing (laboratory analyses of blood or urine, x-rays, or other imaging studies) simply serve to confirm the diagnosis made on the basis of the medical history.

A medical history is developed using data collected during the health care practitioner's interview with the patient. The medical history may also include data from a health history form or health questionnaire completed by the patient before the visit with the practitioner. The objectives of taking a medical history are to:

- Obtain, develop, and document (in writing) a clear, accurate, and chronological account of the individual's medical history (including a family history, employment history, social history, and other relevant information) and current medical problems.

- List, describe, and assign priority to each symptom, complaint, and problem presented.

- Observe the patient's emotional state as reflected in voice, posture, and demeanor.

- Establish and enhance communication, trust, understanding, and comfort in the physician-patient (or nurse-patient) relationship.

Besides eliciting a history of all the patient's previous medical problems and illnesses, the health care practitioner asks questions to learn about the history of the present illness or complaint—how and when it began, the nature of symptoms, aggravating and relieving factors, its effect on function, and any self-care measures the patient has taken.

The medical history also includes a review of physiological systems—such as the cardiovascular (related to heart and circulation), gastrointestinal (GI; digestive disorders), psychiatric (mental and emotional health), and neurologic (brain and nerve disorders) systems—through which the patient may experience symptoms of disease. The review of physiological systems frequently helps the practitioner obtain information to help assess the severity of the present problem and confirm the diagnosis.

Because it relies on the patient's assessment of the severity, duration, and other characteristics of symptoms, as well as the patient's memories and interpretation of past illnesses, the medical history provides the practitioner with subjective information. With the objective findings of the physical examination and other diagnostic tests, it helps the practitioner to identify disease correctly.

PHYSICAL EXAMINATION

The National Institutes of Health's U.S. National Library of Medicine (February 23, 2009, http://www.nlm.nih.gov/medlineplus/ency/article/002274.htm) notes that during a physical examination, "a health care provider studies a patient's body to determine the presence or absence of physical problems." It includes inspection (looking), palpation (feeling), auscultation (listening), and percussion (tapping to produce sounds).

Vital Signs

In a clinic or office-based medical practice, the physical examination may begin with a nurse or medical assistant measuring the patient's vital signs: temperature, respiration, pulse, and blood pressure. Temperature is measured using a thermometer. Normal oral temperature (measured by mouth) is 98.6 degrees Fahrenheit (37 degrees Celsius). Temperature may also be measured rectally, under the arm (axillary), or aurally with an electronic thermometer placed in the ear.

Respiration is measured by observing the patient's rate of breathing. Besides determining the rate of respiration (the average adult takes 12 to 20 breaths per minute), the practitioner also notes any difficulties in breathing.

Pulse rate and rhythm are assessed by compressing the resting patient's radial artery at the wrist. The normal resting pulse rate is between 60 and 100 beats per minute, and the rhythm should be regular, with even spaces between beats. Pulse rates higher than 100 beats per minute are called tachycardia, and rates lower than 60 beats per minute are called bradycardia. Some variations in pulse rates are considered normal and do not signify disease. Athletes who engage in high levels of physical conditioning often have pulse rates of less than 60 beats per minute at rest. Similarly, pulse rates increase naturally in response to exercise or emotional stress.

Blood pressure is measured using an inflatable blood pressure cuff, also known as a sphygmomanometer. Blood pressure is measured in millimeters of mercury (mm Hg). Two readings are recorded: systolic pressure and diastolic pressure. Systolic pressure is the top number of a blood pressure reading and represents the pressure at which beats are first heard in the artery; diastolic pressure is the bottom number and is the pressure at which the beat can no longer be heard. As with pulse rates, blood pressure varies in response to exercise and emotional stress. Normally, the systolic blood pressure of an adult is less than 140 mm Hg and diastolic blood pressure is less than 90 mm Hg. Repeated blood pressure readings higher than 140/90 mm Hg lead to a diagnosis of hypertension (high blood pressure).

Head and Neck

Physical examination of the head and neck involves inspection of the head (including the skin and hair), ears, nose, throat, and neck. An instrument called an otoscope is used to examine the ear canal and tympanic membrane for swelling, redness, lesions, drainage, discharge, or deformity. When examining the throat, the practitioner looks for abnormalities and, by depressing the tongue, can inspect the mouth, oropharynx, and tonsils.

The practitioner notes any scars, asymmetry, or masses (lumps or thickenings) in the neck and systematically palpates (presses) to examine the chains of lymph nodes (also called lymph glands, which are clusters of cells that filter fluid known as lymph) that run in front and behind the ear, near the jaw, and at the base of the neck. The practitioner also inspects and palpates the thyroid gland (the largest gland in the endocrine system, located where the larynx and trachea meet).

Eye Examination

An eye examination consists of a vision test and visual inspection of the eye and surrounding areas for abnormalities, deformities, and signs of infection. Two numbers describe visual acuity (vision). The first number is the distance (in feet) that the patient is standing from the test chart, and the second number is the distance that the eye can read a line of letters from the test chart. Because 20/20 is considered normal vision, a person with 20/60 vision can read a line of letters from 20 feet (6.1 m) away that a person with normal vision can read from a distance of 60 feet (18.3 m) away from the test chart. Using an ophthalmoscope, the practitioner examines the inner structures of the eye by looking through the pupil.

Chest and Lungs

The examination of the chest and lungs focuses on identifying disorders of breathing, which consists of inspiration and expiration (inhaling and exhaling). Changes in the length of either action could be a sign of disease. For example, prolonged expiration may be the result of an obstruction in the airway due to asthma.

Percussion is a tapping technique used to produce sounds on the chest wall that may be distinguished as normal, dull, or hyperresonant. Dull sounds may indicate the presence of pneumonia (infection of the lungs), whereas hyperresonant sounds may be signs of pneumothorax (collapsed lung) or emphysema (a disease in which the alveoli—microscopic air sacs—of the lung are destroyed).

The practitioner listens to breath sounds with a stethoscope. Listening with the stethoscope is called auscultation. Decreased breath sounds may be signs of emphysema or pneumothorax, whereas high-pitched wheezes are associated with asthma. Another device used to monitor the breathing of patients with asthma is a peak flow meter. After taking a deep breath, the patient exhales into the peak flow meter, which measures the velocity of exhaled breath.

Back and Extremities

The examination of the back and extremities (arms and legs) focuses on the anatomy of the musculoskeletal system. Major muscle groups and all joints are examined, and pulses on the arms, legs, and feet (radial, posterior tibial, and dorsalis pedis, respectively) are checked to be certain that blood flow to the extremities is adequate. Monitoring capillary refill time is another way to assess the adequacy of blood flow. To do this, the practitioner presses the patient's fingernail or toenail until it pales and then observes how long it takes to regain color once the pressure is released. Longer capillary refill time may be a sign of peripheral vascular disease or blocked arteries.

Cardiovascular System

The examination of the cardiovascular system focuses on the rate and rhythm of radial and carotid artery pulses (located at the wrist and neck), blood pressure, and the sounds associated with blood flow through the carotid arteries and the heart. After measuring and recording the rate and rhythm of radial and carotid pulses, the practitioner may listen with a stethoscope for abnormal sounds in the carotid arteries. Rushing sounds, called bruits, may indicate a narrowing of the arteries and an increased risk for stroke.

Examination also entails assessment of jugular vein pressure and listening with a stethoscope to heart sounds. Heart murmurs, clicks, and extra sounds are abnormal heart sounds associated with the functioning of heart valves. Some murmurs are considered innocent (normal variations), whereas others are indicators of serious malfunctioning of heart valves.

Abdominal Examination

Inspection of the abdomen focuses on the shape of the abdomen and the presence of scars, lesions, rashes, and hernias (protrusion of an organ through a wall that usually encloses it). Using a stethoscope, the practitioner listens to the arteries that supply blood to the kidneys, listens to the aorta (the main artery that supplies blood to all the organs except the lungs), and listens for bowel sounds.

Percussion of the abdomen that produces a dull sound may indicate an abnormality, such as an abdominal mass. Percussion is also used to determine the size of the liver (the largest gland in the body, which produces bile to aid in the digestion of fats) that measures 2.5 to 5 inches (6 to 12 cm) in a healthy adult. An expanse of dullness around the liver or spleen (an organ on the left side of the body, below the diaphragm, that filters and stores blood) may indicate that these organs are enlarged.

Breast and Pelvic Examination

Visual inspection of the breast focuses on symmetry, dimpling, swelling, or discoloration of the skin and position of the nipple. Manual breast examination is performed by slowly and methodically palpating breast tissue in overlapping vertical strips using small circular movements from the midline to the axilla (armpit). The practitioner presses the nipple to observe whether there is any discharge (fluid) and palpates the axilla for the presence of lymph nodes.

A pelvic examination is often performed after the breast examination, during a woman's physical examination. At this time, a sample of tissue is usually obtained for a Papanicolaou (Pap) test, which is examined microscopically by the cytology laboratory for cervical cancer cells.

Neurologic and Mental Status Examinations

Neurologic examination considers mental status, cranial nerves (the 12 cranial nerves are olfactory, optic, oculomotor, trochlear, trigeminal, abducens, facial, acoustic, glossopharyngeal, vagus, accessory, and hypoglossal), muscle strength, coordination and gait, reflexes, and the senses. Figure 3.1 shows the nervous system and describes each of the four

FIGURE 3.1

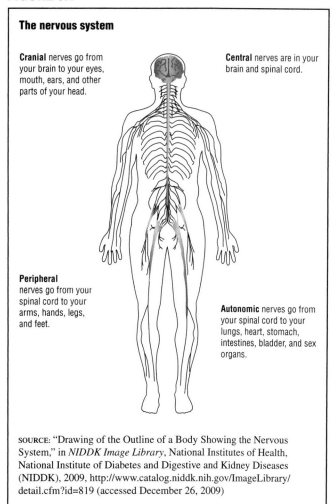

The nervous system

Cranial nerves go from your brain to your eyes, mouth, ears, and other parts of your head.

Central nerves are in your brain and spinal cord.

Peripheral nerves go from your spinal cord to your arms, hands, legs, and feet.

Autonomic nerves go from your spinal cord to your lungs, heart, stomach, intestines, bladder, and sex organs.

SOURCE: "Drawing of the Outline of a Body Showing the Nervous System," in *NIDDK Image Library*, National Institutes of Health, National Institute of Diabetes and Digestive and Kidney Diseases (NIDDK), 2009, http://www.catalog.niddk.nih.gov/ImageLibrary/detail.cfm?id=819 (accessed December 26, 2009)

types of nerves. The cranial nerves connect the brain to the eyes, mouth, ears, and other parts of the head. The central nerves are in the brain and spinal cord. The peripheral nerves go from the spinal cord to the arms, hands, legs, and feet. The autonomic nerves go from the spinal cord to internal organs—lungs, heart, stomach, intestines, bladder, and sex organs.

Generally, the cranial nerves are assessed by observation as the health care practitioner asks the patient to demonstrate their use. For example, the facial nerve may be tested by watching patients open their mouth and clench their teeth. The practitioner also tests sensation to the parts of the face supplied by branches of the trigeminal nerve by applying sharp and dull objects to these areas and asking the patient to distinguish between them. Finally, the practitioner touches the patient's cornea lightly to observe whether the corneal reflex is functioning properly; if it is, the patient will blink.

Evaluating the motor system involves the assessment of muscle symmetry, tone, strength, gait, and coordination. Patients are observed performing different skills and walking. Reflexes are tested and graded as normal, hypoactive, or hyperactive. An example of reflex testing is when the practitioner strikes the patellar tendon just below the kneecap to observe contraction of the quadriceps muscle in the thigh and extension of the knee.

The sensory system test determines whether there is a loss of sensation in any body part. The practitioner may use the vibrations from a tuning fork or hot, cold, or sharp objects to evaluate patients' abilities to perceive sensation accurately. The practitioner may also test discrimination (the ability to accurately interpret touch and position) by tracing a number on the patient's palm and asking the patient to name the number.

A preliminary evaluation of mental status aims to determine the patient's orientation, immediate and short-term memory, and ability to follow simple verbal and written commands. Patients are considered "oriented" if they can identify time, place, and person accurately. Immediate and short-term memories are tested when the practitioner poses simple questions for the patient to answer, and the ability to follow commands is assessed by observing the patient perform tasks in response to verbal or written instructions.

Weighing the Value of Annual Physicals

In recent years the American Medical Association and other medical professional societies have played down the importance of traditional "head-to-toe" annual physical examinations. Instead, they favor a periodic health examination—an individualized screening and examination based on the patient's age, health status, lifestyle, and risk factors.

In "Preventive Health Examinations and Preventive Gynecological Examinations in the United States" (*Archives of Internal Medicine*, vol. 167, no. 17, September 24, 2007), Ateev Mehrotra, Alan M. Zaslavsky, and John Z. Ayanian report the results of their research, which analyzed 8,413 physician visits for preventive medical examinations conducted between 2002 and 2004. They find that about 21% of Americans had preventive physical exams each year and about 18% of adult women obtained an annual preventive gynecological examination. The number of adults varied geographically—people living in the Northeast had a 60% greater chance of having a physical exam than those living on the West Coast.

Mehrotra, Zaslavsky, and Ayanian also find that Americans received most of their preventive medical care when they visited physicians for reasons other than an annual physical examination, so the relatively low percentage of annual physical examinations did not mean that preventive care was not obtained. The researchers opine that the value of annual physical examinations has not been confirmed by research and observe that critical preventive care is often received during other visits.

DIAGNOSTIC TESTING

Once the history and physical examination have been completed, the health care practitioner is often relatively certain about the cause of illness and the diagnosis. However, occasions occur when the history and physical examination point to more than one possible diagnosis. In such instances, the practitioner develops a differential diagnosis (a list of several likely diagnoses). The practitioner may then order specific diagnostic tests to narrow the list of possibilities. The results of these tests are evaluated in the context of the patient's history and physical examination.

There are scores of diagnostic tests—including blood tests, x-rays, computed tomography (CT) scans, ultrasounds, and magnetic resonance imaging (MRI) scans—to help the health care practitioner identify the cause of disease. It is important for practitioners to choose tests that not only improve their understanding of the disease but also affect treatment decisions. The decision to order a specific diagnostic test takes into account the test's reliability, validity, sensitivity, and specificity besides its risks to the patient and costs in terms of time and dollars.

The Reliability and Validity of Diagnostic Tests

The reliability of diagnostic testing refers to the test's ability to be repeated and to produce equivalent results in comparable circumstances. A reliable test is consistent and measures the same way each time it is used with the same patients in the same circumstances. For example, a well-calibrated balance scale is a reliable instrument for measuring body weight.

Validity is the accuracy of the diagnostic test. It is the degree to which the diagnostic test measures the disease, blood level, or other quality or characteristic it is intended to detect. A valid diagnostic test is one that can distinguish between those who have the disease from those who do not. There are two components of validity: sensitivity and specificity.

THE SENSITIVITY AND SPECIFICITY OF DIAGNOSTIC TESTS. Sensitivity refers to a test's ability to identify people who have the disease. By contrast, specificity refers to a test's ability to identify people who do not have the disease. Ideally, diagnostic tests would be highly sensitive and highly specific, thereby accurately classifying all people tested as either positive or negative. In practice, however, sensitivity and specificity are frequently inversely related—most tests with high levels of sensitivity have low specificity, and the reverse is also true.

The likelihood that a test result will be incorrect can be gauged based on the sensitivity and specificity of the test. For example, if a test's sensitivity is 95%, then when 100 patients with the disease are tested, 95 will test positive and five will test "false negative"—they have the disease but the test has failed to detect it.

However, if a test is 90% specific, when 100 healthy, disease-free people are tested, 90 will receive negative test results and 10 will be given "false-positive" results—they do not have the disease but the test has inaccurately classified them as positive.

The advantages of highly sensitive tests are that they produce few false-negative results, and people who test negative are almost certain to be truly negative. Highly sensitive tests may be useful as preliminary screening measures for diseases where early detection is vitally important, such as the enzyme-linked immunosorbent assay (ELISA) screening test for the human immunodeficiency virus (HIV), the virus that produces the acquired immunodeficiency syndrome (AIDS).

In contrast, highly specific tests produce few false-positive results and those who test positive are nearly certain to be positive. Highly specific tests are useful when confirming a diagnosis and in cases where the risks of treatment are high, such as the Western blot test to confirm the presence of HIV after it has been detected by the highly sensitive, but less specific, ELISA test.

Laboratory Tests

The editors of *Harrison's Principles of Internal Medicine* observe that the growing number and availability of laboratory tests has encouraged physicians and other health care practitioners to become increasingly reliant on them as diagnostic tools. Laboratory tests are easy, convenient screening measures because multiple tests may be performed on a single sample of blood and abnormal test results can provide valuable clues for diagnosis.

For screening purposes (to detect disease at its earliest stage, before it produces symptoms), the health care practitioner may order a complete blood count (a measurement of the size, number, and maturity of the different blood cells in a specific volume of blood), as well as a variety of other blood tests, including:

- Fasting blood glucose—this is a screening and diagnostic test for diabetes; values consistently greater than 126 milligrams per deciliter (mg/dl) indicate diabetes. Fasting blood glucose levels between 100 mg/dl and 125 mg/dl are considered impaired and are called prediabetes.

- Calcium—blood levels of calcium can be elevated as a result of hyperactive parathyroid glands.

- Lipids—elevated cholesterol, triglycerides, and low-density lipoproteins are associated with an increased risk of heart disease.

- Thyroid stimulating hormone (TSH)—high levels of TSH indicate hypothyroidism (underactivity of the thyroid gland), and abnormally low levels indicate hyperthyroidism (overly active thyroid gland).

- Venereal Disease Research Laboratory or rapid plasma reagin—these tests screen for syphilis, a sexually transmitted disease.

- HIV—it is important to screen for the presence of this virus.

- Prostate specific antigen—this blood test is used to screen for prostate cancer and to monitor treatment of the disease.

- Stool occult blood (also called fecal occult blood test)—this tests for the presence of blood in the stool, which could be an indicator of colon cancer.

Diagnostic Imaging Techniques

Imaging studies are another form of diagnostic testing. In the past all diagnostic imaging studies were obtained using ionizing radiation (x-rays) and recorded on transparent film. Modern imaging studies such as ultrasound and MRI use nonionizing radiation and can be recorded digitally, viewed on computer monitors, sent via e-mail, and stored on compact discs, digital tape, or transparent film. Most imaging studies are painless and pose little risk to patients apart from minimal exposure to radiation.

X-RAYS AND ULTRASOUND. The images produced by x-rays are the result of varying radiation absorption rates of different body tissues—the calcium in bone has the highest x-ray absorption, soft tissue such as fat absorbs less, and air absorbs the least. Chest x-rays, which offer images of the lungs, ribs, heart, and diaphragm, are among the most frequently ordered imaging studies.

To view tissues normally invisible on x-ray, contrast agents, such as barium and iodine, may be introduced into the body. For example, contrast agents are often used for imaging studies of the GI tract to diagnose digestive disorders.

Another common use of diagnostic x-rays is the measurement of bone density. Bone mass measurement (also called bone mineral density) is performed to evaluate the risk of bone fractures. Bone density is usually measured in the spine, hip, and/or wrist because these are the most common sites of fractures resulting from osteoporosis, a disease in which bones become weak, thin, fragile, and more likely to break.

Mammography also relies on x-ray technology to detect and pinpoint changes or abnormalities in the breast tissue that are too small to be felt by hand. Another imaging technique for breast examination is ultrasound, which can accurately distinguish solid tumors (lumps or masses) from fluid-filled cysts.

Ultrasound images are produced using the heat reflected from body tissues in response to high-frequency sound waves. Whereas x-ray is ideal for examining bone, ultrasound is used to examine soft tissue, such as the ovaries, uterus, breast, and prostate. It is not suitable for looking at bones, because calcium-containing tissues such as bone absorb, rather than reflect, sound waves.

COMPUTED TOMOGRAPHY, MAGNETIC RESONANCE IMAGING, AND POSITRON EMISSION TOMOGRAPHY. For conventional flat x-rays, the patient, x-ray source, and camera remain fixed and immobile. CT scans use a mobile x-ray source and generate a series of cross-section pictures, or slices, that are assembled by computer into images. Because CT distinguishes differences in soft tissue more effectively and with higher resolution than conventional x-rays, it is often used to examine internal organs in the abdomen, such as the liver, pancreas, spleen, kidneys, and adrenal gland, and the aorta and vena cava (large blood vessels that pass through the abdomen).

MRI scans generate images based on interaction between a large magnet, radio waves, and hydrogen atoms in the body. Stimulated by ordinary radio waves within the powerful magnetic field, these atoms give off weak signals that a computer builds into images. MRI is frequently used to create images of the brain, spinal cord, heart, abdomen, bone marrow, and knee.

CT and MRI scans generate images of the body's structure (anatomy), whereas positron emission tomography (PET) scans offer insight into body function or processes (physiology). To create PET images, positron-emitting atoms are injected into the body, where they travel and strike other electrons, producing gamma rays. The gamma rays are then interpreted into images by a computer. Unlike CT and MRI scans, PET scans are rarely used for screening or diagnostic purposes. Instead, they are used to track the progress and treatment of patients with diagnosed diseases such as cancer.

Diagnostic Procedures

Other diagnostic tests commonly performed to screen for the presence of disease include:

- Throat culture—this test is used to determine whether streptococcus pyrogenes (commonly called strep) bacteria are the cause of a sore throat. To obtain a sample of the mucus in the throat, the health care practitioner swabs the back of the throat and places the swab in a tube. The swab is transferred into a culture in the laboratory, where it is examined for bacterial growth. The results of this test are available in two to three days. A rapid strep test that produces results in minutes is also available.

- Urinalysis and urine culture—chemical and microscopic examination of urine allow the identification of infection, diabetes, and the presence of blood in the urine.

- Colonoscopy—using a long tube fitted with a lens, the health care practitioner is able to look at the entire colon; identify and remove polyps; detect cancer; and diagnose other causes of blood in the stool, abdominal pain, and digestive disorders. To prepare for a colonoscopy, patients must empty their intestines completely before the examination.

- Flexible sigmoidoscopy—this test is similar to the colonoscopy, in that it uses a tube fitted with a camera to examine the colon. However, because the instrument is shorter than a colonoscope, it does not enable views of the entire colon. Through the flexible sigmoidoscope, the practitioner can examine only the sigmoid (lower portion) of the colon to detect polyps and cancers.

- Electrocardiogram—this test assesses the electrical function of the heart, detects abnormal heart rhythms, and aids in the diagnosis of myocardial infarction (heart attack) and other heart diseases.

Prenatal Diagnostic Testing

Ultrasound is routinely used to monitor the progress of pregnancy; evaluate the size, health, and position of the fetus; and detect some birth defects. Fetal ultrasound assists in the prediction of multiple births (more than one baby) and sometimes provides information about the gender of the unborn child.

Chorionic villus sampling (CVS) enables obstetricians and perinatologists (physicians specializing in the evaluation and care of high-risk expectant mothers and babies) to assess the progress of pregnancy during the first trimester (the first three months). A physician passes a small, flexible tube called a catheter through the cervix to extract chorionic villi tissue—cells that will become the placenta and are genetically identical to the baby's cells. The cells are examined in the laboratory for indications of genetic disorders such as cystic fibrosis (an inherited disease characterized by chronic respiratory and digestive problems), Down syndrome (a genetic condition caused by having an extra copy of chromosome 21), Tay-Sachs disease (a fatal disease that generally affects children of east European Jewish ancestry), and thalassemia (an inherited disorder of hemoglobin in red blood cells). The results of the testing are available within seven to 14 days. CVS provides the same diagnostic information as amniocentesis; however, the risks (miscarriage, infection, vaginal bleeding, and birth defects) associated with CVS are slightly higher.

Amniocentesis involves analyzing a sample of the amniotic fluid that surrounds the fetus in the uterus. The fluid is obtained when a physician inserts a hollow needle through the abdominal wall and the uterine wall. Like CVS, amniocentesis samples and analyzes cells derived from the baby to enable parents to learn of chromosomal abnormalities and the gender of the unborn child. Results are usually available about two weeks after the test is performed.

Blood tests are also available to help diagnose fetal abnormalities. The enhanced alpha-fetoprotein test (also called a triple screen) measures the levels of protein and hormones produced by the fetus and can identify some birth defects, such as Down syndrome and neural tube defects. Two of the most common neural tube defects are anencephaly (absence of the majority of the brain) and spina bifida (incomplete development of the back and spine). Test results are available within two to three days. Women with abnormal results are often advised to undergo additional diagnostic testing, such as CVS or amniocentesis.

DIAGNOSING MENTAL ILLNESS

Unlike physical health problems and medical conditions, there are no laboratory tests such as blood and urine analyses or x-rays to assist practitioners to definitively diagnose mental illnesses. Instead, practitioners generally rely on listening carefully to patients' complaints and observing their behavior to assess their moods, motivations, and thinking. Sometimes mental health disorders may accompany physical complaints or medical conditions. The presence of more than one disease or disorder is called comorbidity.

Even though there are varying opinions about the personality traits and characteristics that taken together constitute optimal mental health, historically it has been somewhat easier to define and identify mental illness—deviations from, or the absence of, mental health. Within the broad diagnosis of mental illness, there is more consensus about the origins, nature, and symptoms of mental disorders—serious and often long-term conditions in which changes in cognition (thought processes), behavior, or mood impair functioning—than exists about mental health

problems—shorter term, less intense conditions that often resolve spontaneously and without treatment.

Because many mental health disorders are identified by primary-care physicians (general practitioners, family practitioners, internists, and pediatricians), the World Health Organization (WHO) developed educational materials and guidelines to assist practitioners in general medical settings—as opposed to psychiatric or other mental health settings—to assess and treat the mental health problems and disorders of patients in their care. The guidelines call for an assessment interview, during which a series of screening questions are asked. If a patient provides predominantly positive answers, the patient has an "identified mental disorder." If a patient responds positively to many questions but not enough to fulfill the diagnostic criteria for a disorder, the patient has a "subthreshold disorder." These disorders are defined by the WHO's 10th revision of the *International Classification of Diseases: Classification of Mental and Behavioural Disorders* (*ICD-10*), the European guide for the diagnosis of mental disorders. In North America the fourth edition of the *Diagnostic and Statistical Manual of Mental Disorders* (*DSM-IV*) by the American Psychiatric Association (APA) is used for the same purpose as the *ICD-10*. Practitioners are encouraged to ask open-ended questions that enable patients to freely express their emotions, to ensure confidentiality, to acknowledge patients' responses, and to closely observe their body language and tone of voice.

Changing Criteria for Mental Illness

There are many controversies in mental health diagnosis, beginning with the definitions and classification of mental illnesses. Which criteria distinguish conditions as mental illness rather than as normal variations in thinking and behavior? Should conditions such as attention deficit hyperactivity disorder (ADHD) be classified as learning problems or mental disorders? Should practitioners distinguish between neurological conditions that cause brain dysfunction and cognitive impairment such as Alzheimer's disease (a type of dementia that causes confusion, memory failure, speech disturbances, and an inability to function) and mental illness involving brain dysfunction such as depression that may result from an imbalance of chemicals in the brain?

DSM-IV is the authoritative encyclopedia of diagnostic criteria for mental disorders. This definitive guide, which expands on the *ICD-10*, is the most widely used psychiatric reference in the world and catalogs more than 300 mental disorders.

An examination of past versions of the *DSM* reveals that the definitions of mental illnesses have changed dramatically from one edition to another. People diagnosed with a specific mental disorder based on diagnostic criteria in one edition might no longer be considered mentally ill according to the next edition. Critics of the *DSM*, which has expanded more than 10-fold since its inception in 1952, claim that diseases are added arbitrarily by the APA and that even though some entries represent changing ideas about mental health and illness, others are politically motivated. For example, homosexuality was once considered a mental illness, but in the 21st century, largely in response to changing societal attitudes, it is no longer considered an illness.

Skeptics also question the sharp increase in the number of diagnoses and the number of Americans receiving these diagnoses. Does the increasing number of diagnoses reflect rapid advances in mental health diagnostic techniques? Have mental health professionals (psychiatrists, psychologists, clinical social workers, marriage and family therapists, and other mental health practitioners) simply improved their diagnostic skills? Are the stresses of 21st-century life precipitating an epidemic of mental illness in the United States? Or are mental health professionals simply labeling more behaviors and aspects of everyday life as pathological (diseased)?

Furthermore, there is dissent even within the mental health field about diagnosis that is rooted in the ongoing debate about the origins of mental illness. After taking into account all the relevant medical research, the Office of the Surgeon General concludes in *Mental Health: A Report of the Surgeon General* (1999, http://www.surgeongeneral .gov/library/mentalhealth/home.html) that for most mental illnesses there is no demonstrable physiological cause. This means there is no laboratory test, imaging study (x-ray, MRI, or PET), or abnormality in brain tissue that has been definitively identified as causing mental illness. As of March 2010, there were no published studies refuting this contention. As such, the majority of people suffering from mental illness apparently have normal brains, and those with abnormal brain structure or function are diagnosed with neurological disorders rather than with mental illnesses.

Finally, there are those who view mental illness as a social condition rather than as one requiring medical diagnosis. They observe that even the surgeon general's report, which favors biological explanations of the origin, diagnosis, and treatment of mental illness, concedes that mental health is poorly understood and defined differently across cultures. If mental health and illness are rooted in cultural mores and values, then they are likely socioeconomic and political in origin. The proponents of societal causes of mental illness contend that if mental illness is in part defined as a functional impairment, and during the course of their life an estimated 26.2% of Americans will be impaired (according to the National Institute of Mental Health [NIMH], in "The Numbers Count: Mental Disorders in America" [August 10, 2009, http://www.nimh.nih.gov/publicat/numbers.cfm]), then perhaps it is not the individual who is ailing, but the society.

Despite the challenges of diagnosing mental illnesses, the NIMH notes in the press release "Mental Illness Exacts Heavy Toll, Beginning in Youth" (June 6, 2005, http://www.nimh .nih.gov/science-news/2005/mental-illness-exacts-heavy-toll-beginning-in-youth.shtml) that "while approximately 80 percent of all people in the U.S. with a mental disorder *eventually* seek treatment, there are public health implications from such long delays in treatment. Untreated psychiatric disorders can lead to more frequent and more severe episodes, and are more likely to become resistant to treatment. In addition, early-onset mental disorders that are left untreated are associated with school failure, teenage childbearing, unstable employment, early marriage, and marital instability and violence." In the press release "New Research to Help Youth with Mental Disorders Transition to Adulthood" (September 5, 2007, http://www.nimh.nih.gov/science-news/2007/new-research-to-help-youth-with-mental-disorders-transition-to-adulthood.shtml), the NIMH indicates that in September 2007 it launched research to help young people with mental disorders transition from adolescence to adulthood. The research is intended to help these young people manage their disorders, become independent, and avoid substance abuse, gambling, dangerous driving, unsafe sex, and interactions with the criminal justice system.

ONLY HALF OF CHILDREN AND TEENS WITH MENTAL HEALTH DISORDERS SEEK TREATMENT. Kathleen Ries Merikangas et al. find in "Prevalence and Treatment of Mental Disorders among US Children in the 2001–2004 NHANES" (*Pediatrics*, vol. 125, no. 1, January 2010) that an estimated 13% of American children and young teens have at least one mental health disorder and nearly 2% have more than one disorder, but just half have been seen by a mental health professional. The researchers report that based on a sample of 3,042 children aged eight to 15 years, 8.6% had ADHD, 3.7% suffered from depression, 2.1% had conduct disorder, 0.7% had an anxiety disorder (generalized anxiety or panic disorder), and 0.1% had an eating disorder.

Boys were more likely than girls to have ADHD and girls were more likely to suffer from depression. Children and teenagers of lower socioeconomic status were more likely to report any mental health disorder, particularly ADHD, whereas those of higher socioeconomic status were more likely to report having an anxiety disorder. Concerning race and ethnicity, Mexican-Americans had significantly higher rates of mood disorders than whites or African-Americans. Noting that African-Americans and Mexican-Americans were much less likely to seek treatment than whites, Merikangas et al. call for increased efforts to "identify and remove barriers to treatment for minority youth."

Technological Advances Offer New Diagnostic Tools

In "Integration of Diagnostic and Communication Technologies" (*Journal of Telemedicine and Telecare*, vol. 15, no. 7, 2009), Nafees N. Malik of the University of Cambridge describes key areas of diagnostics that have benefited from advances in communication and computer technologies, including point-of-care testing (analysis of clinical specimens such as blood at the site where care is delivered such as the patient's bedside), microelectromechanical systems (technology that combines computers with tiny mechanical devices such as sensors embedded in semiconductor chips), and the discovery of additional biomarkers (biological molecules found in blood or other body fluids that indicate or predict normal or abnormal processes or that detect a condition or disease). Malik observes that a growing number of people are able to send data (such as blood glucose readings, changes in body weight and diet, and medication logs) from their home to their physicians using their telephones and the Internet. The widespread availability of broadband enables patients to interact in real-time videoconferences with physicians and other health professionals and also allows physicians immediate access to specialists around the world.

Malik notes that many patients are already monitoring their heart rates and blood pressure at home and sending the results using communication technologies to their physicians, who can promptly review the information to diagnose problems. As diagnostic and communication technologies converge, it will be possible for patients to transmit increasingly complex health care data to their physicians, who will then be able to promptly identify problems and institute timely treatment to prevent complications of patients' medical conditions. These advances promise to improve patient care in a wide range of health care settings, from improving the proportion of the population that makes use of preventive measures such as screenings to management of acute medical conditions and chronic diseases.

CHAPTER 4
GENETICS AND HEALTH

Even at birth the whole individual is destined to die, and perhaps his organic disposition may already contain the indication of what he is to die from.

—Sigmund Freud, "The Dissolution of the Oedipus Complex" (1924)

Genetics, which is the branch of biology that studies heredity, concerns the biochemical instructions that convey information from generation to generation. To appreciate the role of genetics in health and illness, it is important to understand the interaction of genes, chromosomes, and genomes and to learn how deoxyribonucleic acid (DNA) functions as the information molecule of living organisms.

Genes are units of hereditary information that are made of DNA and located on chromosomes, which are separate strands of DNA wrapped in a double helix (two intertwined three-dimensional spirals) around a core of proteins contained in the nuclei of cells. Genes contain the instructions for the production of proteins, which make up the structure of cells and direct their activities. They exist in corresponding pairs, and a genome is a complete set of paired genes for an organism. The Human Genome Project explains in "The Science behind the Human Genome Project" (March 26, 2008, http://www.ornl.gov/sci/techresources/Human_Genome/project/info.shtml) that humans have 46 chromosomes arranged in 23 pairs and that the human genome contains between 20,000 and 25,000 genes and 600,000 pairs of DNA. Changes in the number, size, shape, or structure of chromosomes can result in a variety of physical and mental abnormalities and diseases.

GENETIC INHERITANCE

The inheritance of simple genetic traits involves two inherited copies of the gene that determines the phenotype (the observable characteristic) for that trait. When genes for a particular trait, such as eye color or hair color, exist in two or more different forms that may differ between individuals and populations, they are called alleles. For every gene, the offspring receives two alleles, one from each parent. The specific combination of inherited alleles is known as the genotype of the organism, and its expression, which can be observed, is its phenotype.

For many traits the phenotype results from an interaction between the genotype and environmental influences. For example, many readily apparent traits in humans, such as height, weight, and skin color, result from interactions between genetic and environmental factors. Height and weight are strongly influenced by nutrition as well as by genetic predisposition, and skin color may be influenced by exposure to ultraviolet radiation from sunlight. Along with these easily observed traits, there are other complex phenotypes that involve multiple gene-encoded proteins and the alleles of these particular genes that are influenced by a subtle and intricate interplay of genetic or environmental factors. So even though the presence of specific genes indicates a susceptibility or a likelihood to develop a certain trait, it does not guarantee expression of the trait.

For a specific trait, some alleles may be dominant whereas others are recessive. The phenotype of a dominant allele is always expressed, but the phenotype of a recessive allele is expressed only when both alleles are recessive. Recessive genes are passed from one generation to the next, and they can only be expressed in individuals who do not inherit a copy of the dominant gene for the specific trait.

In some instances, known as incomplete dominance, one allele does not completely dominate over the other, and the resulting phenotype is a blend of both traits. For example, skin color is a trait often governed by incomplete dominance, with offspring appearing to be a blend of the skin tones of each parent. Furthermore, some traits are multigenic or polygenic, which means that they are determined by a combination of several genes, and the resulting phenotype is determined by the final combination of alleles of all the genes that govern the particular trait.

Some multigenic traits are governed by many genes, and each contributes equally to the expression of the trait. In cases such as these, a defect in a single gene pair may have little impact on the expression of the trait. Other multigenic traits are predominantly directed by one major gene pair and only mildly influenced by the effects of other gene pairs. For these traits, the impact of a defective gene pair depends on whether it is the major pair governing expression of the trait or one of the minor pairs influencing its expression.

Genetic inheritance can be quite complex, and a broad array of other factors enters into whether a trait will appear and the extent to which it is expressed. For example, different individuals may express a trait with different levels of intensity or severity. When this occurs, it is known as variable expressivity.

The Influence of Heredity on Health

It has long been understood that heredity exerts a profound influence on health. Genetic inheritance explains how and why certain traits such as the propensity to obesity, eye color, and blood types run in families. Genomics (the study of more than single genes) considers the functions and interactions of all the genes in the genome. Genomics is a relatively recent discipline, because it has only been about two decades since the human genome was fully elaborated, but it already has important applications in advancing an understanding of health and disease.

Genomics relies on knowledge of and access to the entire genome and has already been applied to understanding the causes of many serious and increasingly prevalent diseases such as breast and colorectal cancer, Parkinson's disease (a disease affecting the part of the brain associated with movement), and Alzheimer's disease (a type of dementia that causes confusion, memory failure, speech disturbances, and an inability to function). Furthermore, genomics has also played a key role in understanding susceptibility to, and treatment of, infectious diseases, which were, until recently, thought to be caused exclusively by environmental factors. Examples of infectious diseases in which multiple genes and environmental exposures influence the risk of developing the disease include infection with the human immunodeficiency virus (HIV; the virus that produces the acquired immunodeficiency syndrome, or AIDS) and tuberculosis. Genetic variations may confer protection against disease or may have a causative role in the expression of disease.

Even though most conditions involve an interplay in which genetics and environmental factors make important, though not necessarily equal, contributions, it is nonetheless conventional to classify diseases as primarily genetic in origin or largely attributable to environmental causes.

As understanding of genomics advances and scientists identify genes involved in more diseases, the distinction between these two classes of disorders is blurring. This chapter considers genetic testing, some of the disorders believed to be predominantly genetic in origin, and some that are the result of genes acted on by environmental factors.

GENETIC DISORDERS

There are two types of genes: dominant and recessive. When a dominant gene is passed on to offspring, the feature or trait it determines will appear independent of the characteristics of the corresponding gene on the chromosome inherited from the other parent. If the gene is recessive, the feature it determines cannot appear in the offspring unless both of the parents' chromosomes contain the recessive gene for that characteristic. Similarly, among diseases and conditions primarily attributable to a single gene or multiple genes, there are autosomal (a non-sex-related chromosome) dominant disorders and autosomal recessive disorders. Figure 4.1 shows an example of how X-linked recessive inheritance of one such condition, Duchenne muscular dystrophy (DMD; this is the most common form of muscular dystrophy in children), occurs.

Another way to characterize genetic disorders is by their pattern of inheritance, as single gene, multifactorial, chromosomal, or mitochondrial. Single-gene disorders (also called Mendelian or monogenic) are caused by mutations in the DNA sequence of one gene. According to the U.S. National Library of Medicine, in "Genetics" (February 23, 2010, http://www.nlm.nih.gov/medlineplus/ency/article/002048.htm), there are about 18,000 known single-gene disorders. Examples are cystic fibrosis (an inherited disease characterized by chronic respiratory and digestive problems), sickle-cell anemia (an inherited disease producing abnormal hemoglobin in the blood), Huntington's disease, and hereditary hemochromatosis. Hemochromatosis is a disorder in which the body absorbs too much iron from food. Instead of excreting the excess iron, the body stores it throughout the body, and this buildup of iron eventually damages the pancreas, liver, skin, and other tissues. Single-gene disorders are the result of either autosomal dominant, autosomal recessive, or X-linked inheritance (involving a gene on the X chromosome passed down through the family).

Multifactorial disorders (also called polygenic disorders) involve a complex interaction of environmental factors and mutations in multiple genes. For example, different genes that influence breast cancer susceptibility have been found on different chromosomes, rendering it more difficult to analyze than single-gene or chromosomal disorders. Until 2009, it was thought that breast cancer risk was associated with genes on seven chromosomes. However, in May 2009 Shahana Ahmed et al. identified in "Newly Discovered

FIGURE 4.1

An example of X-linked recessive inheritance

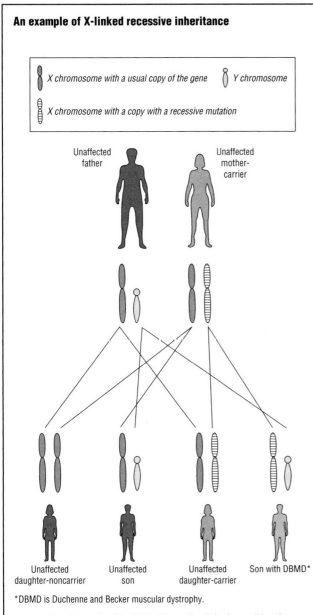

Unaffected
daughter-noncarrier

Unaffected
son

Unaffected
daughter-carrier

Son with DBMD*

*DBMD is Duchenne and Becker muscular dystrophy.

SOURCE: "An Example of X-Linked Recessive Inheritance," in *About X-Linked Conditions*, Centers for Disease Control and Prevention, National Center on Birth Defects and Developmental Disabilities, August 28, 2006, http://www.cdc.gov/ncbddd/single_gene/x-link.htm (accessed December 27, 2009)

Breast Cancer Susceptibility Loci on 3p24 and 17q23.2" (*Nature Genetics*, vol. 41, no. 5) new genetic variations in two regions of DNA—on chromosomes 1 and 14—that may be associated with the risk of developing breast cancer. Many common chronic diseases such as heart disease, Alzheimer's disease, arthritis, diabetes, and cancer are multifactorial in origin.

Chromosomal disorders result from abnormalities in chromosome structure, missing or extra copies of chromosomes, or errors such as the movement of a chromosome section from one chromosome to another, which is called translocation. Down syndrome is a chromosomal disorder that results when an individual has an extra copy, or a total of three copies, of chromosome 21. Mitochondrial disorders, which occur infrequently compared with other inherited disorders, result from mutations in the nonchromosomal DNA of mitochondria, which are organelles involved in cellular respiration.

The possibility of preventing and changing genetic legacies appears within reach of modern medical science in the 21st century. Genomic medicine has the capacity to predict the risk of disease—from disorders that are highly probable as in the case of some of the well-established single-gene disorders to those in which increased susceptibility may be triggered by environmental factors. The promise of genomic medicine is to make preventive medicine more powerful and to individualize and customize treatment for each individual. Such treatment takes into account an individual's genetic susceptibilities and the characteristics of the specific disease or disorder.

GENETIC TESTING

A genetic test analyzes DNA, ribonucleic acid (RNA), chromosomes, and proteins to detect heritable diseases for the purposes of diagnosis, treatment, and other clinical decision making. A simple blood sample, which allows the extraction of the DNA from white blood cells, enables most genetic tests to be performed, but other body fluids and techniques may also be used for genetic testing. Genetic tests are used to screen for and diagnose genetic disease in newborns, children, and adults; to identify future health risks; to predict drug responses; and to assess the risk of disease in future generations.

Genetic tests performed to screen for disease are different from those used to establish a diagnosis. Diagnostic tests are intended to definitively determine whether a patient has a particular problem. Such tests are generally quite complex and often require sophisticated analysis and interpretation. Because they are complex, require highly trained personnel to interpret them, and may be expensive, they are usually performed only on people believed to be at risk, such as patients who already have symptoms of a specific disease.

By contrast, screening is performed on healthy people with no symptoms of disease and may often be applied to the entire population or people considered to be at risk of developing a specific disorder. By definition, a good screening test is relatively inexpensive, easy to use and interpret, and assists to identify which individuals in the population are at higher risk for a specific disease. Screening tests identify people who require further testing or people who should take special preventive measures or precautions. For example, people deemed especially susceptible to genetic conditions with specific environmental triggers, such as people with life-threatening allergic sensitivities, are advised to avoid specific environmental triggers.

Commonly used genetic tests include screening people of Ashkenazi Jewish heritage (the east European Jewish population primarily from Germany, Poland, and Russia, as opposed to the Sephardic Jewish population, which is primarily from Spain, parts of France, Italy, and North Africa) for Tay-Sachs disease; screening African-Americans for sickle-cell disease; and screening expectant mothers over the age of 35 whose fetuses are at an increased risk for Down syndrome. Table 4.1 lists some of the more than 1,000 DNA-based genetic tests that are currently available.

The most common form of genetic testing is the screening of newborn infants for genetic abnormalities. This screening is accomplished by testing blood obtained from a prick of the newborn's heel within the first few days of life. Newborn infants are screened for specific genetic disorders such as phenylketonuria, an inherited error of metabolism resulting from a deficiency of an enzyme called phenylalanine hydroxylase. If left undiagnosed and untreated, the deficiency of this enzyme can cause mental retardation, organ damage, and postural problems.

Genetic screening aims to identify disorders that require early detection and benefit from timely treatment to prevent serious illness, disability, or death. The determination of which disorders to include in screening programs is made by each state; as such, the tests conducted vary from state to state. To determine which disorders to screen for, states generally consider criteria such as how often the disorder occurs in the population, whether screening is effective, and whether the disease or disorder is treatable. Figure 4.2 shows a method developed by the Health Resources and Services Administration's (HRSA) Maternal and Child Health Bureau that may be used to score and evaluate conditions to determine whether they should be included in routine newborn screening. The American College of Medical Genetics (ACMG) explains in *Newborn Screening: Toward a Uniform Screening Panel and System* (March 2005, ftp://ftp.hrsa.gov/mchb/genetics/screeningdraftforcomment.pdf) that it used this method to conduct, at the behest of the HRSA, an analysis of the scientific literature on the effectiveness of newborn screening and consider expert opinion to develop recommendations about the conditions to include in newborn screening. The ACMG was also asked to develop a uniform condition panel to help standardize screening.

The March of Dimes notes in the press release "States Expand Newborn Screening for Life-Threatening Disorders" (February 18, 2009, http://www.marchofdimes.com/printableArticles/22684_51920.asp) that "all 50 states and the District of Columbia now require that every baby be screened for 21 or more of the 29 serious genetic or functional disorders on the uniform panel recommended by the American College of Medical Genetics (ACMG) and endorsed by the March of Dimes." By 2009, 24 states and the District of Columbia required screening for all

TABLE 4.1

Currently available DNA-based gene tests

Alpha-1-antitrypsin deficiency (AAT; emphysema and liver disease)

Amyotrophic lateral sclerosis (ALS; Lou Gehrig's Disease; progressive motor function loss leading to paralysis and death)

Alzheimer's disease* (APOE; late-onset variety of senile dementia)

Ataxia telangiectasia (AT; progressive brain disorder resulting in loss of muscle control and cancers)

Gaucher disease (GD; enlarged liver and spleen, bone degeneration)

Inherited breast and ovarian cancer* (BRCA 1 and 2; early-onset tumors of breasts and ovaries)

Hereditary nonpolyposis colon cancer* (CA; early-onset tumors of colon and sometimes other organs)

Central core disease (CCD; mild to severe muscle weakness)

Charcot-Marie-Tooth (CMT; loss of feeling in ends of limbs)

Congenital adrenal hyperplasia (CAH; hormone deficiency; ambiguous genitalia and male pseudohermaphroditism)

Cystic fibrosis (CF; disease of lung and pancreas resulting in thick mucous accumulations and chronic infections)

Duchenne muscular dystrophy/Becker muscular dystrophy (DMD; severe to mild muscle wasting, deterioration, weakness)

Dystonia (DYT; muscle rigidity, repetitive twisting movements)

Emanuel syndrome (severe mental retardation, abnormal development of the head, heart and kidney problems)

Fanconi anemia, group C (FA; anemia, leukemia, skeletal deformities)

Factor V-Leiden (FVL; blood-clotting disorder)

Fragile X syndrome (FRAX; leading cause of inherited mental retardation)

Galactosemia (GALT; metabolic disorder affects ability to metabolize galactose)

Hemophilia A and B (HEMA and HEMB; bleeding disorders)

Hereditary demochromatosis (HFE; excess iron storage disorder)

Huntington's disease (HD; usually midlife onset; progressive, lethal, degenerative neurological disease)

Marfan syndrome (FBN1; connective tissue disorder; tissues of ligaments, blood vessel walls, cartilage, heart valves and other structures abnormally weak)

Mucopolysaccharidosis (MPS; deficiency of enzymes needed to break down long chain sugars called glycosaminoglycans; corneal clouding, joint stiffness, heart disease, mental retardation)

Myotonic dystrophy (MD; progressive muscle weakness; most common form of adult muscular dystrophy)

Neurofibromatosis type 1 (NF1; multiple benign nervous system tumors that can be disfiguring; cancers)

Phenylketonuria (PKU; progressive mental retardation due to missing enzyme; correctable by diet)

Polycystic kidney disease (PKD1, PKD2; cysts in the kidneys and other organs)

Adult polycystic kidney disease (APKD; kidney failure and liver disease)

Prader Willi/Angelman syndromes (PW/A; decreased motor skills, cognitive impairment, early death)

Sickle cell disease (SS; blood cell disorder; chronic pain and infections)

Spinocerebellar ataxia, type 1 (SCA1; involuntary muscle movements, reflex disorders, explosive speech)

Spinal muscular atrophy (SMA; severe, usually lethal progressive muscle-wasting disorder in children)

Tay-Sachs Disease (TS; fatal neurological disease of early childhood; seizures, paralysis)

Thalassemias (THAL; anemias—reduced red blood cell levels)

Timothy syndrome (CACNA1C; characterized by severe cardiac arrhythmia, webbing of the fingers and toes called syndactyly, autism)

SOURCE: "Some Currently Available DNA-Based Gene Tests," in *Gene Testing*, U.S. Department of Energy Office of Science, Office of Biological and Environmental Research, Human Genome Program, September 19, 2008, http://www.ornl.gov/sci/techresources/Human_Genome/medicine/genetest.shtml (accessed December 27, 2009)

FIGURE 4.2

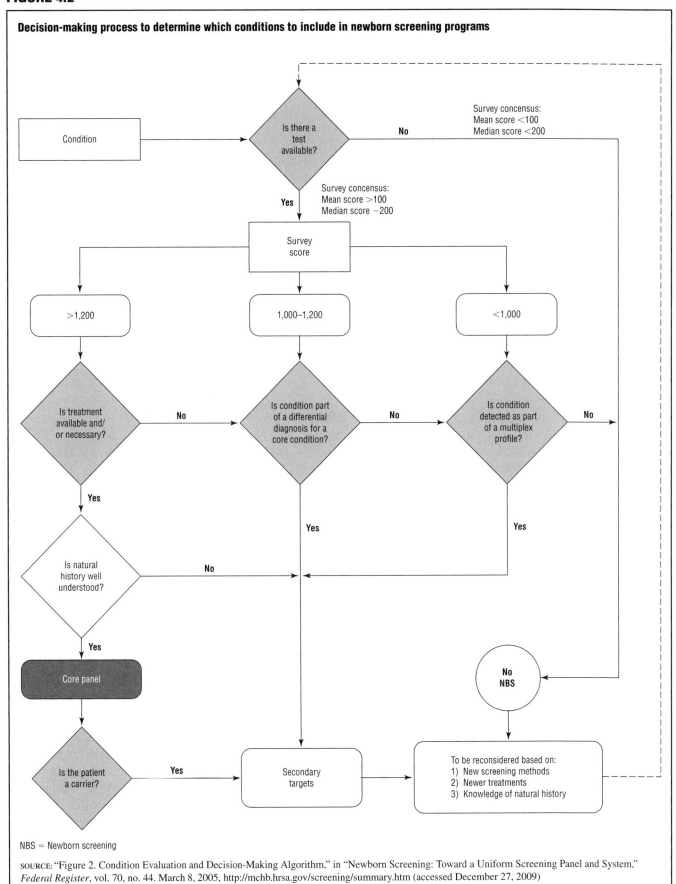

Decision-making process to determine which conditions to include in newborn screening programs

NBS = Newborn screening

SOURCE: "Figure 2. Condition Evaluation and Decision-Making Algorithm," in "Newborn Screening: Toward a Uniform Screening Panel and System," *Federal Register*, vol. 70, no. 44. March 8, 2005, http://mchb.hrsa.gov/screening/summary.htm (accessed December 27, 2009)

29 disorders, and 46 states and the District of Columbia screened for 26 or more of these conditions.

GENETIC TESTING AND HUMAN REPRODUCTION

By March 2010 thousands of genetic diseases, both frequently occurring disorders and extremely rare ones, had been identified that may be conveyed from one generation to the next. As genetic research advances, many more genetic diseases will be uncovered and additional tests will be developed to screen parents at risk of passing on genetic disease to their children and to identify embryos, fetuses, and newborns that suffer from genetic diseases.

Carrier Identification

Carrier identification is used to determine whether a healthy individual has a gene that may cause disease if passed on to his or her offspring. It is nearly always performed on populations deemed to be at a higher than average risk, such as those of Ashkenazi Jewish descent. Carrier testing is important because many people have just one copy of a gene for an autosomal recessive trait and because they are unaffected by the trait or disorder and are unaware that they may pass it on to their children. Only an individual with two copies of the gene will actually have the disorder. So even though it is generally assumed that everyone is an unaffected carrier of at least one autosomal recessive gene, it only becomes a problem in terms of genetic inheritance when both parents are carriers—meaning that mother and father both have the same recessive disorder gene. When both parents are carriers, the offspring each have a one in four chance of receiving a defective copy of the gene from each parent and developing the disorder. (See Figure 4.3.)

Another example of carrier identification is the test for a deletion in the dystrophin gene, which results in DMD. Carriers may avoid having an affected child by preventing pregnancy or by undergoing prenatal testing for DMD, with the option of ending the pregnancy if the fetus is found to be affected.

Using genetic testing to detect carriers poses some challenges. Typically, a carrier has inherited a mutant gene from one parent and a normal gene from another parent. If, however, the carrier harbors a mutation that is only found in germ cells (the sperm or eggs), and only in some of these germ cells, then conventional genetic testing, which is performed on white blood cells, will miss the mutation.

Preimplantation Genetic Diagnosis

Preimplantation genetic diagnosis (PGD) permits prospective parents using in vitro fertilization (fertilization that takes place outside the body) to screen an embryo for

FIGURE 4.3

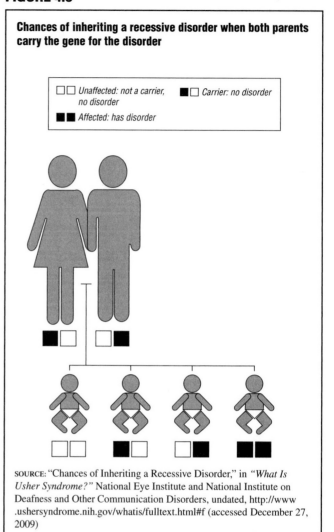

Chances of inheriting a recessive disorder when both parents carry the gene for the disorder

□□ Unaffected: not a carrier, no disorder   ■□ Carrier: no disorder

■■ Affected: has disorder

SOURCE: "Chances of Inheriting a Recessive Disorder," in *"What Is Usher Syndrome?"* National Eye Institute and National Institute on Deafness and Other Communication Disorders, undated, http://www.ushersyndrome.nih.gov/whatis/fulltext.html#f (accessed December 27, 2009)

specific genetic mutations before it is implanted in the uterus—when it is no larger than six or eight cells. One advantage of PGD is that it can screen any congenital disorder for which the causative gene is known and may be used by couples who wish to avoid traditional prenatal diagnosis and the possibility of termination of pregnancy.

Prenatal Genetic Testing

Most prenatal genetic tests examine blood or other tissue from the mother to detect abnormalities in the fetus. The most common prenatal genetic blood test is the triple-marker screen, which measures the levels of three substances in the blood—alpha fetoprotein, human chorionic gonadotropin, and unconjugated estriol—and can identify selected birth defects such as Down syndrome and neural tube defects. (Two common neural tube defects are anencephaly—absence of the majority of the brain—and spina bifida—incomplete development of the back and spine.) The results of triple-marker screens are available within several days, and women with abnormal results are often advised to undergo further diagnostic testing such as

TABLE 4.2

Prenatal tests

Amniocentesis	This test takes a small sample of the amniotic fluid surrounding the baby.	This test can be given after 14 weeks or during the third trimester. The former checks for genetic defects like Down Syndrome; the latter checks for abnormal lung development.
Chorionic Villus Sampling (CVS)	This test withdraws a small sample of tissue from just outside the amniotic sac in which the baby grows.	Taken between 10 and 12 weeks, this test checks for the possibility of such genetic diseases as Huntington's Disease and Duchenne muscular dystrophy.
Quad-screen test	This is a blood test taken from the mother that checks several different components.	This test is usually performed in the second trimester (15–20 weeks). The screening looks for several things, particularly the risk of Down Syndrome.
Rh incompatibility	This test determines whether the mother and baby have incompatible blood types.	This test can be done before pregnancy or at the first prenatal visit. If there is Rh incompatibility, treatments can help prevent later complications.
Ultrasound	This test uses high frequency sound waves to show internal organs and the growing baby within the womb.	Ultrasound can be used during the first, second, and third trimesters to show the gender, status, position, health, and growth of the baby.

SOURCE: "Understanding Prenatal Tests," in *Medline Plus*, vol. 3, no. 1, Winter 2008, http://www.nlm.nih.gov/medlineplus/magazine/issues/winter08/articles/winter08pg22.html (accessed December 27, 2009)

chorionic villus sampling (CVS), amniocentesis, or percutaneous umbilical blood sampling. Table 4.2 describes five prenatal diagnostic procedures and when they are performed in terms of the weeks or trimesters of pregnancy.

CVS permits physicians who specialize in evaluation and care of high-risk expectant mothers and infants to monitor the progress of pregnancy during the first trimester (the first three months). Laboratory examination of cells obtained via CVS can detect chromosomal abnormalities that produce genetic disorders such as Down syndrome, Tay-Sachs disease, cystic fibrosis, and thalassemia (an inherited disorder of the hemoglobin in red blood cells). Some test results are available within a few days and others take one to two weeks, depending on the complexity of the laboratory analysis. CVS provides comparable diagnostic information as amniocentesis; however, the risks (miscarriage, infection, vaginal bleeding, and birth defects) associated with CVS are slightly higher. CVS may also be performed earlier in pregnancy, at 10 to 12 weeks, than amniocentesis, which is generally performed at 15 to 20 weeks. Approximately one out of 100 pregnancies is miscarried as a result of CVS.

Amniocentesis involves taking a sample of the fluid that surrounds the fetus in the uterus for chromosome analysis. Like CVS, amniocentesis samples and analyzes cells derived from the baby to enable parents to learn of chromosomal abnormalities and the gender of the unborn child. The results are available in about two weeks after the test is performed. The risk of miscarriage (about one out of 200 pregnancies) resulting from amniocentesis is lower than the risk associated with CVS.

Down syndrome is the genetic disease most often identified by amniocentesis or CVS. Down syndrome is rarely inherited; most cases arise from an error in the formation of the egg or sperm, which results in the addition of an extra chromosome 21 at conception. Like most prenatal diagnoses for inherited genetic diseases, this use of genetic testing is intended to help prospective parents

TABLE 4.3

Prevalence of Down Syndrome, 1979–2003

Interval	Prevalence
1979–1983	9.5
1984–1988	10.3
1989–1993	10.8
1994–1998	11.0
1999–2003	11.8

SOURCE: "Down Syndrome at Birth per 10,000 Live Births, 1979–2003," in *Down Syndrome Cases at Birth Increased*, Centers for Disease Control and Prevention, National Center on Birth Defects and Developmental Disabilities, Division of Birth Defects, December 23, 2009, http://www.cdc.gov/Features/dsDownSyndrome/ (accessed December 27, 2009)

make informed decisions about the viability of a pregnancy. The CDC reports in "Down Syndrome Cases at Birth Increased" (December 23, 2009, http://www.cdc.gov/Features/dsDownSyndrome/) that the prevalence of Down syndrome has increased since 1979. Between the interval 1979–83 and the interval 1999–2003 the prevalence of Down syndrome increased by 24.2%, from 9.5 per 10,000 live births to 11.8 per 10,000 live births. (See Table 4.3.) The number of infants born with Down syndrome was nearly five times higher among older mothers (38.6 per 10,000 live births) than among births to younger mothers (7.8 per 10,000 live births).

Periumbilical blood sampling (PUBS) is the most invasive prenatal genetic test. Using a high-resolution ultrasound, a physician inserts a needle through the expectant mother's abdominal wall to extract a sample of fetal blood from the umbilical cord. PUBS may be performed from approximately 16 weeks' gestation to term. PUBS poses a high risk to the fetus—one out of 50 procedures results in miscarriage. Because it is an invasive, relatively high-risk procedure, it is primarily used when a diagnosis must be made quickly. For example, when an expectant mother is exposed to an infectious agent with the potential to produce birth defects, it may be used to detect infection in the blood of the fetus.

GENETIC TESTING IN CHILDREN AND ADULTS

Genetic testing may also be performed to find out which children and adults are at an increased risk of developing specific diseases. Predictive genetic testing can identify which individuals are at risk for many heritable diseases including cystic fibrosis, Tay-Sachs disease, Huntington's disease, and amyotrophic lateral sclerosis (a degenerative neurologic condition commonly known as Lou Gehrig's disease), as well as some cancers (including some cases of breast, colon, and ovarian cancer).

The presence of a defective or altered gene is considered a "positive" result from predictive genetic testing. However, a positive result does not guarantee that the person will develop the disease; it simply identifies the individual as genetically susceptible and at an increased risk for developing the disease. Also, like other types of diagnostic medical testing, genetic tests are not 100% predictive—the results rely on the quality of laboratory procedures and the accuracy of interpretations—and there is always the chance of obtaining false-positive and false-negative test results.

Health professionals and researchers are optimistic that positive test results will motivate people at higher-than-average risk of developing a disease to be particularly attentive to disease prevention activities and to seek regular and periodic screening to detect the disease early, when it is most successfully treated. There is an expectation that genetic information will increasingly be used in routine population screening to determine individual susceptibility to common disorders such as heart disease, diabetes, and cancer. This type of screening will identify groups at risk so that primary prevention efforts such as diet and exercise or secondary prevention efforts such as early detection can be directed to them.

Symptomatic Genetic Testing

Even though the majority of genetic testing is performed on people who are healthy and symptom-free to determine if they are carriers or to assess their risk of developing a specific disease or disorder, some testing is performed on people with symptoms of a disease to clarify or to establish the diagnosis and calculate the risk of developing the disease for other family members. This type of testing is known as symptomatic genetic testing (it is also called diagnostic genetic testing or predictive genetic testing).

Symptomatic genetic testing is used to predict the likelihood that a healthy person with a family history of a disorder will develop the disease. Testing positive for a specific genetic mutation indicates an increased susceptibility to the disorder but does not confirm the diagnosis. For example, a woman may opt to undergo testing to learn whether she has a genetic mutation (BRCA1 or BRCA2, respectively) that would indicate the likelihood of developing hereditary breast or ovarian cancer. If she tests positive for the genetic mutation, she may then choose to undergo some form of preventive treatment. Preventive measures may include increased surveillance such as more frequent mammography and breast ultrasound examinations, chemoprevention (prescription drug therapy intended to reduce risk), or surgical prophylaxis, such as mastectomy (surgical removal of one or both breasts) and/or oophorectomy (surgical removal of one or both ovaries).

Interestingly, researchers have discovered that these preventive measures are not as widely used as might be expected. For example, chemoprevention for breast cancer can cause serious side effects such as increased risk of developing endometrial cancer (cancer of the lining of the uterus) and increased risk of developing cataracts. In "Women's Decisions Regarding Tamoxifen for Breast Cancer Prevention: Responses to a Tailored Decision Aid" (*Breast Cancer Research and Treatment*, vol. 119, no. 3, February 2010), Angela Fagerlin et al. note that women considered to be at high risk for developing the disease were apprised of the risks and benefits of chemoprevention. Just 29% of the study subjects said they intended to seek more information or talk to their physician about chemoprevention, and only 6% thought they would use it. Many of the subjects said the benefits of chemoprevention did not outweigh the risks.

Symptomatic genetic testing may also assist in directing the treatment for symptomatic patients in whom a mutation in a single gene (or in a gene pair) accounts for a disorder. Cystic fibrosis and myotonic dystrophy (the most common adult form of muscular dystrophy) are examples of disorders that may be confirmed or ruled out by diagnostic genetic testing and other methods (the sweat test for cystic fibrosis or a neurologic evaluation for myotonic dystrophy).

One issue involved in symptomatic genetic testing is the appropriate frequency of testing in view of rapidly expanding genetic knowledge and identification of genes linked to disease. Physicians frequently see symptomatic patients for whom there is neither a definitive diagnosis nor a genetic test. The as yet unanswered question is: Should such people be recalled for genetic testing each time a new test becomes available? Even though clinics that perform genetic testing counsel patients to maintain regular contact so they may learn about the availability of new tests, there is no uniform guideline or recommendation about the frequency of testing.

Testing Children for Adult-Onset Disorders

In 2000 the American Academy of Pediatrics Committee on Genetics recommended genetic testing for people under the age of 18 only when testing offers immediate medical benefits or when there is a benefit to another family member and there is no anticipated harm to the person being tested. Rebekah Hamilton of the University of Illinois, Chicago, observes in "Genetics: Breast Cancer as an Exemplar" (*Nursing Clinics of North America*, vol. 44, no. 3, September 2009) that genetic counseling before and after testing for adult-onset diseases is an essential component of the process.

The American Academy of Pediatrics Committee on Bioethics and Newborn Screening Task Force recommends that genetic tests included in the newborn-screening battery should be based on scientific evidence. The committee also advocates informed consent for newborn screening. (As of March 2010, most states did not require informed consent.) The committee does not endorse carrier screening in people under the age of 18, except in the case of a pregnant teenager. It also recommends against predictive testing for adult-onset disorders in people under 18 years.

The American College of Medical Genetics, the American Society of Human Genetics, and the World Health Organization (WHO) have also weighed in about genetic testing of asymptomatic (exhibiting no symptoms of illness or disease) children, asserting that decision making should emphasize the children's well-being. One issue involves the value of testing asymptomatic children for genetic mutations associated with adult-onset conditions such as Huntington's disease. Because no treatment can be begun until the onset of the disease, and presently there is no treatment to alter the course of the disease, it may be ill advised to test for it. Another concern is testing for the carrier status of autosomal-recessive or X-linked conditions such as cystic fibrosis or DMD. Experts caution that children might confuse carrier status with actually having the condition, which in turn might provoke needless anxiety.

There are, however, circumstances in which genetic testing of children may be appropriate and useful. Examples are children with symptoms of suspected hereditary disorders or those at risk for cancers in which inheritance plays a primary role. In "Developmental Defects and Childhood Cancer" (*Current Opinions in Pediatrics*, vol. 21, no. 6, December 2009), Thomas P. Slavin and Georgia L. Wiesner observe that genetic testing is available for many disorders and that guidelines for screening are evolving rapidly. The researchers assert that genetic testing can help improve diagnostic accuracy and "allow for targeted surveillance in appropriate individuals; for example, presymptomatic genetic testing in a family with a known cancer-predisposing mutation." They caution, however, that in children with no known family mutation, gene testing may not be fully predictive because some children with certain cancer syndromes may not have identifiable genetic defects.

Regardless, Michael Parker of the University of Oxford notes in "Genetic Testing in Children and Young People" (*Familial Cancer*, vol. 9, no. 1, 2010) that nearly all recommendations for genetic testing of children concur "that where there are no 'urgent medical reasons,' presymptomatic and predictive testing for adult-onset disorders, and carrier testing should be postponed until a child is able to give his or her own consent." Parker explains that there are "situations in which this requirement can be in tension with genetics professionals' and others' judgement of what is in the child's best interests."

ETHICAL CONSIDERATIONS AND GENETIC TESTING

Rapid advances in genetic research since the 1990s have challenged scientists, health care professionals, ethicists, government regulators, legislators, and consumers to stay abreast of new developments. Understanding the scientific advances and their implications is critical for everyone involved in making informed decisions about the ways in which genetic research and information will affect the lives of current and future generations. As of March 2010, consideration of these ethical issues had not produced simple or universally applicable answers to the many questions posed by the increasing availability of genetic information. Ongoing public discussion and debate are intended to inform, educate, and assist people in every walk of life to make personal decisions about their health and participate in decisions that concern others.

In "Ethical and Policy Issues in Newborn Screening" (*NeoReviews*, vol. 10, no. 2, 2009), Lainie Friedman Ross of the University of Chicago reviews the controversies and as yet unresolved questions and ethical considerations of newborn screening. Some of the issues she addresses are obtaining informed consent from parents, whether to disclose incidental discoveries such as carrier status, whether an effective treatment must exist as a rationale for screening, and when to screen—determining whether specific tests should be universal or whether testing should target selected populations.

As researchers learn more about the genes responsible for a variety of illnesses, they can design more tests with ever-increasing accuracy and reliability to predict whether an individual is at risk of developing specific diseases. However, the ethical issues involved in genetic testing have turned out to be far more complicated than originally anticipated. Physicians and researchers initially believed that at-risk families would welcome a test to determine in advance who would develop or escape a disease. They would be able to plan more realistically about having children, choosing jobs, obtaining insurance, and living their life. Nevertheless, many people with family histories of a genetic disease have decided that not knowing is better than anticipating a grim future and an agonizing, slow death. They prefer to live with the hope that they will not develop the disease rather than having the certain knowledge that they will.

The discovery of genetic links and the development of tests to predict the likelihood or certainty of developing a disease raise ethical questions for people who carry a defective gene. Should women who are carriers of Huntington's disease or cystic fibrosis have children? Should a fetus with a defective gene be carried to term or aborted? There is already some evidence that prenatal screening has influenced parents' decisions about continuing pregnancies when as yet unborn children will be born with specific genetic diseases. For example, Marilynn Marchione reports in "Genetic Disease Testing Leads Some Adults Not to Have Kids" (Associated Press, February 17, 2010) that "Kaiser Permanente, a large health maintenance organization, offered prenatal screening. From 2006 through 2008, 87 couples with cystic fibrosis mutations agreed to have fetuses tested, and 23 were found to have the disease. Sixteen of the 17 fetuses projected to have the severest type of disease were aborted, as were four of the six fetuses projected to have less severe disease."

Concerns persist about privacy and the confidentiality of medical records, as well as the possibility that the results of genetic testing can lead to stigmatization despite legislation passed in 2008 that prevents such discrimination. Some people remain reluctant to be tested because they still fear they may lose their health, life, and disability insurance, or even their jobs, if they are found to have an increased risk of developing a chronic disease that is costly to treat or that may produce significant disability.

Historically, the fear of stigmatization and discrimination by insurance companies and employers when they learn the results of genetic testing was often justified. An insurance carrier might deny coverage or charge an individual a higher rate on the basis of test results, and an employer might choose not to hire or to deny an affected employee a promotion. Most medical professional associations agreed that people should not be forced to forgo taking a genetic test that could provide lifesaving information to retain their health insurance coverage or to save their job.

Until May 21, 2008, when the Genetic Information Nondiscrimination Act (GINA) became law, Americans' dissemination of genetic information was protected by an uneven array of federal and state regulations. Considered to be the first major civil rights bill of the 21st century, GINA prevents health insurers from denying coverage, adjusting premiums on the basis of genetic test results, or requesting that an individual undergo genetic testing. The law prohibits employers from using genetic information to make hiring, firing, or promotion decisions. It also sharply restricts an employer's right to request, require, or purchase workers' genetic information.

COMMON GENETICALLY INHERITED DISEASES

Even though many diseases, disorders, and conditions are called genetic, classifying a disease as genetic simply means that there is an identified genetic component to either its origin or expression. Many medical geneticists contend that most diseases cannot be classified as strictly genetic or environmental. Environmental factors can greatly influence the way disease-causing genes express themselves. They can even prevent the genes from being expressed at all. Similarly, environmental (infectious) diseases may not be expressed because of some genetic predisposition to immunity. Each disease, in each individual, exists along a continuum between a genetic disease and an environmental disease.

A multitude of diseases are believed to have strong genetic contributions, including:

- Heart disease—coronary atherosclerosis (a disease in which cholesterol and other deposits build up on the inner walls of the arteries, limiting the flow of blood), hypertension (high blood pressure), and hyperlipidemia (elevated blood levels of cholesterol and other lipids)

- Diabetes

- Cancer—retinoblastomas (cancer of the eye), colon, stomach, ovarian, uterine, lung, bladder, breast, skin (melanoma), pancreatic, and prostate

- Neurological disorders—Alzheimer's disease, amyotrophic lateral sclerosis, Gaucher's disease (a disease of fat processing linked to the lack of an enzyme), Huntington's disease, multiple sclerosis, narcolepsy (a neurological disorder marked by a sudden recurrent uncontrollable compulsion to sleep), neurofibromatosis (a hereditary disorder characterized by widespread abnormalities in the nervous system, skin, and bones), Parkinson's disease (disease affecting the part of the brain associated with movement), Tay-Sachs disease, and Tourette's syndrome (a neurological disorder characterized by repeated, involuntary movements and uncontrollable vocal sounds)

- Mental illnesses, mental retardation, and behavioral conditions—alcoholism, anxiety disorders, attention deficit hyperactivity disorder, eating disorders, Lesch-Nyhan's syndrome (a rare disorder that disrupts the ability to build and break down purines and can produce self-destructive behavior), manic depression, and schizophrenia

- Other disorders—cleft lip and cleft palate, clubfoot, cystic fibrosis, DMD, hemophilia (a genetic blood disorder in which blood does not clot properly), Hurler's syndrome (a rare disorder in which the enzyme that breaks down long chains of sugar molecules is absent), Marfan's syndrome (a disease characterized by elongated bones, especially in limbs and digits, and abnormalities of the eyes and circulatory system), phenylketonuria, sickle-cell disease, and thalassemia

- Medical and physical conditions with genetic links— alpha-1-antitrypsin deficiency (the lack of this liver protein may result in emphysema and liver and skin disease), arthritis, asthma, baldness, congenital adrenal hyperplasia (lack of an enzyme necessary to make the hormones cortisol and aldosterone), migraine headaches, obesity, periodontal disease, porphyria (a genetic abnormality of metabolism causing abdominal pains and mental confusion), and selected speech disorders

Cystic Fibrosis

Cystic fibrosis (CF) is the most common inherited fatal disease of children and young adults in the United States. The National Library of Medicine's Genetics Home Reference reports in "Genetic Conditions: Cystic Fibrosis" (March 7, 2010, http://ghr.nlm.nih.gov/condition=cysticfibrosis) that CF occurs in about 1 out of 2,500 to 3,500 whites, 1 out of 17,000 African-Americans, and 1 out of 31,000 Asian-Americans. In "Learning about Cystic Fibrosis" (December 21, 2009, http://www.genome.gov/10001213), the National Institutes of Health's National Human Genome Research Institute (NHGRI) observes that one out of 31 Americans—about 10 million people—are symptom-free carriers of the CF gene. Because it is a recessive genetic disorder, a child must receive the CF gene from both parents to inherit CF.

The CF gene was identified in 1989 and was cloned and sequenced in 1991. The gene was originally called cystic fibrosis transmembrane conductance regulator because it encodes a cell membrane protein that controls the movement of chloride ions across the plasma membrane of cells. Chloride transport is crucial because chloride is a component of salt involved in fluid absorption and volume regulation, and this seemingly minor defect can cause disease that affects organs and tissues throughout the body, provoking abnormal, thick secretions from glands and epithelial cells. Over time, a thick, viscous mucus fills the lungs and pancreas, which produces difficulty in breathing and interference with digestion. Eventually, affected children die of respiratory failure.

CF is usually diagnosed by the time an affected child is three years old. Often, the only signs are a persistent cough, a large appetite but poor weight gain, an extremely salty taste to the skin, and large, foul-smelling bowel movements. A simple sweat test is the standard diagnostic test for CF. The test measures the amount of salt in the sweat; abnormally high levels are the hallmark of CF.

The U.S. Food and Drug Administration (FDA) reports in *Aztreonam for Inhalation Solution (NDA 50-814) for Improvement of Respiratory Symptoms in Cystic Fibrosis Patients* (December 10, 2009, http://www.fda.gov/downloads/AdvisoryCommittees/CommitteesMeetingMaterials/Drugs/Anti-InfectiveDrugsAdvisoryCommittee/UCM193023.pdf)

that aztreonam, an inhaled drug used to treat life-threatening lung infections in CF patients in Europe and Canada, is safe and effective and recommends that it be approved for sale in the United States. The drug combats lung infections caused by pseudomonas aeruginosa bacteria, for which there are few inhaled antibiotics available.

Huntington's Disease

Huntington's disease (HD) is one of the more common hereditary diseases. It is an inherited, progressive brain disorder that causes the degeneration of cells in a pair of nerve clusters deep in the brain that affect both the body and the mind. HD is caused by a single dominant gene and affects men and women of all races and ethnic groups.

According to Genetics Home Reference, in "Genetic Conditions: Huntington Disease" (March 7, 2010, http://ghr.nlm.nih.gov/condition=huntingtondisease), HD affects 3 to 7 per 100,000 people of European ancestry. It seems to be less common in other populations, including people of Japanese, Chinese, and African descent. In "Learning about Huntington's Disease" (October 9, 2009, http://www.genome.gov/10001215), the NHGRI reports that 30,000 people in the United States have HD, an additional 35,000 display some symptoms, and 75,000 carry the gene mutation that will cause them to develop the disease.

The gene mutation responsible for HD was mapped to chromosome 4 in 1983 and was cloned in 1993. The mutation occurs in the DNA that codes for the protein called huntingtin. The number of repeated triplets of nucleotides—cytosine (C), adenine (A), and guanine (G), known as CAG (nucleotides are nitrogen-containing molecules that link together to form strands of DNA and RNA)—is inversely related to the age when the individual first experiences symptoms: the more repeated triplets, the younger the age at which the disease first appears.

HD generally begins during the third and fourth decades of life; however, there is a form of the disease that can affect children and adolescents. It is easy to overlook early symptoms, such as forgetfulness, a lack of muscle coordination, or a loss of balance, and as a result the diagnosis is often delayed. The disease progresses gradually, usually over a 10- to 25-year period.

As HD progresses, patients develop involuntary movement (chorea) of the body, limbs, and facial muscles; speech becomes slurred; and swallowing becomes increasingly difficult. HD patients' cognitive abilities decline and there are distinct personality changes—depression and withdrawal, sometimes countered with euphoria. By the late stages of the illness, nearly all patients must be institutionalized, and they usually die as a result of choking or infections.

PREDICTION TEST. In 1983 researchers identified a DNA marker that made it possible to offer a test to determine, before symptoms appear, whether an individual has inherited the HD gene. It is even possible to make a prenatal diagnosis by testing DNA from fetal cells removed via CVS or amniocentesis. However, some people prefer not to know whether or not they carry the defective gene.

PROMISING RESEARCH FINDINGS. According to the National Institute of Neurological Disorders and Stroke, in "NINDS Huntington's Disease Information Page" (March 11, 2010, http://www.ninds.nih.gov/disorders/huntington/huntington.htm), in August 2008 the FDA approved tetrabenazine to treat the involuntary writhing movements characteristic of HD; the drug is the first approved for use in the United States to treat the disease. In "Tetrabenazine as Anti-chorea Therapy in Huntington Disease: An Open-Label Continuation Study" (*BMC Neurology*, vol. 9, December 2009), Samuel Frank and the Huntington Study Group TETRA-HD Investigators report the results of research concerning the long-term safety and efficacy of the new drug. The study followed 45 patients for 80 weeks and concluded that the drug effectively suppressed HD-related involuntary movements and was generally well tolerated but did produce some undesirable side effects such as sleep disturbances, depression, and anxiety.

Muscular Dystrophy

Muscular dystrophy (MD) is a term that describes a group of hereditary muscle-destroying disorders. The CDC estimates in "Prevalence of Duchenne/Becker Muscular Dystrophy among Males Aged 5–24 Years—Four States, 2007" (*Morbidity and Mortality Weekly Report*, vol. 58, no. 40, October 16, 2009) that DMD is diagnosed in 1 out of 3,500 (2.9 per 10,000) male births and Becker MD (like DMD but with later onset and slower progression) is diagnosed in 1 out of 18,518 (0.5 per 10,000) male births. All forms of the disease are caused by defects in genes that play key roles in the growth and development of muscles. The gene is passed from the mother to her children. Females who inherit the defective gene generally do not display symptoms—instead they become carriers, and their children have a 50% chance of inheriting the disease.

Because the proteins produced by the defective genes are abnormal, the muscles begin to atrophy (waste away). As the muscle cells die, they are replaced by fat and connective tissue. The symptoms of MD often progress slowly, so they may not be noticed until as much as 50% of the muscle tissue has been affected.

Even though all the various forms of MD cause progressive weakening and wasting of muscle tissues, they vary in terms of the usual age when symptoms appear, the rate of progression, and the initial group of muscles affected. The most common childhood type, DMD, affects young boys, who exhibit symptoms in early childhood and generally die from respiratory weakness or damage to the heart before adulthood. Other forms of MD develop later in life and are usually not fatal.

In 1992 scientists discovered the defect in the gene that causes myotonic dystrophy, the most common adult form of MD. In people with this disorder, a segment of the gene is enlarged and unstable. This finding helps physicians to diagnose myotonic dystrophy. Researchers have since identified genes linked to other types of MD, including DMD, Becker MD, limb-girdle MD, and Emery-Dreifuss MD.

TREATMENT AND HOPE. Even though there is no cure for MD, treatment modalities such as physical therapy, exercise programs, and orthopedic devices (special shoes, braces, or powered wheelchairs) can help patients maintain mobility and independence as long as possible.

Many researchers believe that genetic research holds the key to development of effective treatments, and even cures, for these diseases. Because defective or absent proteins cause MD, researchers hope that experimental treatments to transplant normal muscle cells into wasting muscles will replace the diseased cells. Muscle cells, unlike other cells in the body, fuse together to become giant cells. It is hoped that by introducing cells with healthy genes the muscle cells will start to produce the deficient or entirely absent proteins.

The challenge is to get the body to accept the new muscle cells without mounting an immune attack on them. Researchers are experimenting with new delivery methods called vectors to help the healthy genes gain access to the body. One such vector implants a healthy gene into a virus that has been stripped of all its harmful properties. The modified virus containing the gene is then injected into a patient. Researchers hope this will sharply reduce the patient's immune system response, which will enable the healthy gene to restore the missing muscle protein.

In "The Contribution of Human Synovial Stem Cells to Skeletal Muscle Regeneration" (*Neuromuscular Disorders*, vol. 20, no. 1, January 2010), Jinhong Meng et al. assert that because human stem cells have some ability to regenerate muscle fibers, stem cell therapy, in which undifferentiated cells are used to repair and renew tissues, holds promise for treating muscle diseases such as MD. Stem cell therapy may also be able to repair damaged muscle cells and revive their ability to make the correct form of dystrophin, the protein that is defective in DMD.

Sickle-Cell Disease

Sickle-cell disease (SCD) is a group of inherited blood disorders (including sickle-cell anemia, sickle-hemoglobin C disease, sickle beta-plus thalassemia, and sickle beta-zero thalassemia) that affects red blood cells.

In SCD the red blood cells contain an abnormal type of hemoglobin, called hemoglobin S, which is responsible for hemolysis (the premature destruction of red blood cells). It also causes the red blood cells to stiffen and change shape; they become sickle, or crescent shaped, particularly in parts of the body where the amount of oxygen is relatively low. These abnormally shaped cells have shorter life spans than normal red blood cells and they have difficulty passing through the smaller blood vessels and capillaries. Unlike normal red blood cells, they tend to clog the vessels, which prevents blood and oxygen from reaching vital tissues. The lack of oxygen damages the tissue, which in turn causes more sickling and more damage. Figure 4.4 shows how a mutation in an amino acid produces the abnormal hemoglobin, which in turn can produce the sickled cells that cause illness.

SYMPTOMS OF SCD. SCD produces symptoms comparable to those of anemia, including fatigue, weakness, fainting, and palpitations or an increased awareness of the heartbeat. The palpitations result from the heart's

attempts to compensate for the anemia by pumping blood faster than normal.

Sickle-cell patients experience periodic sickle-cell crises—attacks of pain in the bones and stomach. Blood clots may also develop in the lungs, kidneys, brain, and other organs. A severe crisis or several acute crises can damage the organs of the body by impeding blood flow. The frequency of these crises varies from patient to patient. Sickle-cell crises are, however, more likely to occur during times of stress, such as when the body is combating an infection or after an accident or injury. Cumulative damage can lead to death from heart failure, kidney failure, or stroke.

WHO CONTRACTS SCD? SCD occurs most frequently in people of African, Native American, and Hispanic descent. However, it also occurs in Portuguese, Spanish, French-Corsicans, Sardinians, Sicilians, mainland Italians, Greeks, Turks, and Cypriots. There are also occurrences of SCD in the Middle East and Asia. According to the WHO, in "Genes and Human Disease: Monogenic Diseases" (2010, http://www.who.int/genomics/public/geneticdiseases/en/index2.html#SCA), SCD is the most common inherited blood disorder in the United States, affecting an estimated 72,000 Americans, most of whom have African ancestry. SCD occurs in approximately 1 out of 500 African-American births and in 1 out of 1,000 to 1,400 Hispanic-American births.

When one parent has the sickle-cell gene, the offspring will carry the trait, but only when both the mother and the father have the trait can they produce a child with SCD. Figure 4.5 shows the inheritance pattern for the sickle-cell trait. The sickle-cell trait is present in one out of 12 African-Americans, or about 2 million people.

Examining amniotic fluid or tissue taken from the placenta as early as the first trimester of pregnancy enables detection of the likelihood the unborn child will have the sickle-cell trait or SCD. A genetic counselor evaluates the results and can inform the expectant parents of the chances that their child will have the sickle-cell trait or SCD.

BENEFITS OF UNIVERSAL SCREENING. The National Heart Lung and Blood Institute notes in "What Is Sickle Cell Anemia?" (August 2008, http://www.nhlbi.nih.gov/health/dci/Diseases/Sca/SCA_WhatIs.html) that SCD screening of all newborns is important because early diagnosis and treatment significantly improves future health. Early diagnosis and timely treatments such as penicillin have reduced the number of deaths attributable to SCD and enabled most children born with SCD to live well into adulthood.

THE CURE FOR SCD. According to the CDC, in "Sickle Cell Disease: 10 Things You Need to Know" (June 9, 2009, http://www.cdc.gov/features/sicklecell/),

FIGURE 4.4

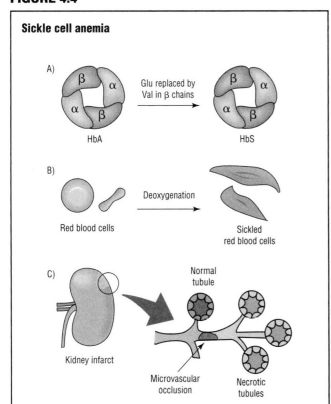

Sickle cell anemia

A) Hemoglobin is made up of 4 chains: 2 α and 2 β. In sickle cell anemia, a point mutation causes the amino acid glutamic acid (Glu) to be replaced by valine (Val) in the β chains of HbA, resulting in the abnormal HbS.
B) Under certain conditions, such as low oxygen levels, red blood cells with HbS distort into sickled shapes.
C) These sickled cells can block small vessels producing microvascular occlusions which may cause necrosis (death) of the tissue.

SOURCE: "Anemia, Sickle Cell," in *Genes and Disease*, National Institutes of Health, National Center for Biotechnology Information, 2007, http://www.ncbi.nlm.nih.gov/books/bv.fcgi?call=bv.View ..ShowSection&rid=gnd.section.98 (accessed December 28, 2009)

FIGURE 4.5

Inheritance of sickle cell trait

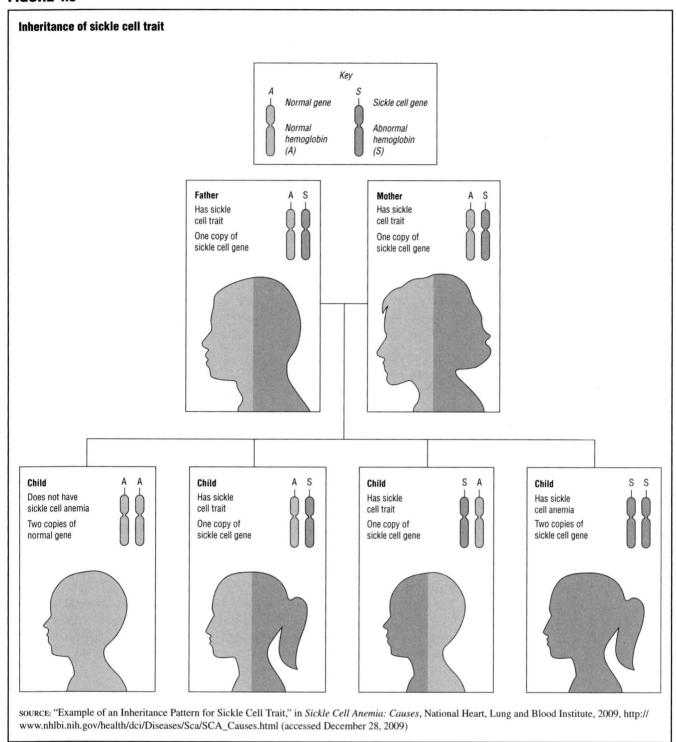

SOURCE: "Example of an Inheritance Pattern for Sickle Cell Trait," in *Sickle Cell Anemia: Causes*, National Heart, Lung and Blood Institute, 2009, http://www.nhlbi.nih.gov/health/dci/Diseases/Sca/SCA_Causes.html (accessed December 28, 2009)

bone marrow transplant and stem cell treatment can cure SCD. Bone marrow is the spongy tissue in the cavities of bones that creates and contains blood cells. A bone marrow/stem cell transplant procedure extracts blood stem cells (the cells that form blood) from a healthy donor and places them into a person whose bone marrow is not functioning properly. Bone marrow/stem cell transplants carry significant risks, which even include death of the recipient. To be optimally effective, the bone marrow must be a close match and the ideal donor is most often a sibling. Because of the associated risks, bone marrow/stem cell transplants are reserved for children with severe cases of SCD.

Tay-Sachs Disease

Tay-Sachs disease (TSD) is a fatal genetic disorder in children that causes the progressive destruction of the central nervous system. It is named for Warren Tay

(1843–1927), a British ophthalmologist, and Bernard Sachs (1858–1944), an American neurologist, the physicians who first identified and described the disease. It is caused by insufficient activity of, or the complete absence of, an important enzyme called hexosaminidase A (hex-A). Without hex-A, a fatty substance called ganglioside GM2 builds up abnormally in the cells, particularly the brain's nerve cells. Ultimately, this buildup causes these cells to degenerate and die. This destructive process begins well before birth, but the disease is usually not diagnosed until the baby is several months old.

SYMPTOMS OF TSD. A baby with TSD appears healthy at birth and usually develops normally during the first months of life, but then development slows. The child begins to regress and loses skills one by one—the ability to crawl, to sit, to reach out, and to turn over. The victim gradually becomes blind, deaf, and unable to swallow. Muscles atrophy, and paralysis sets in. Mental retardation occurs, and the child is unable to interact with the outside world. There is no cure for this disease. Even with optimal medical care and treatment, death from infection usually occurs by age four.

HOW IS TSD INHERITED? TSD is transmitted from parent to child the same way eye or hair color is inherited. It is an autosomal recessive genetic disorder caused by mutations in both alleles of the HEXA gene on chromosome 15. Both parents must be carriers of the TSD gene to give birth to a child with the disease.

People who carry the TSD gene have no signs of the disease and are generally unaware that they have the potential to pass this disease on to their offspring. When just one parent is a carrier, the offspring will not have TSD, but there is a 50% chance of having a child who is a carrier. When both parents carry the recessive TSD gene, there is a 25% chance of having a child with the disease and a 50% chance of bearing a child who is a carrier. Prenatal diagnosis early in pregnancy, using CVS or amniocentesis, can accurately predict if the fetus is affected by TSD.

WHO IS AT RISK? Like SCD, TSD occurs most frequently in specific populations. People of east European (Ashkenazi) Jewish descent have the highest risk of being carriers of TSD. According to the National Tay-Sachs and Allied Diseases Association (2007, http://www.tay-sachs .org/taysachs_disease.php), approximately one out of 27 Jews in the United States is a carrier of the TSD gene. French-Canadians and Cajuns also have the same carrier rate as Ashkenazi Jews, and one out of 50 Irish-Americans is a carrier. The Pennsylvania Dutch population as well as people of British Isle and Italian descent also have a higher carrier rate than that observed in the general population, where the carrier rate is 1 out of 250.

CHAPTER 5
CHRONIC DISEASES: CAUSES, TREATMENT, AND PREVENTION

The Centers for Disease Control and Prevention (CDC) defines chronic diseases as prolonged illnesses that do not resolve spontaneously and are rarely cured completely. According to the CDC, in "Chronic Diseases and Health Promotion" (December 17, 2009, http://www.cdc.gov/nccdphp/overview.htm), chronic illnesses such as cardiovascular disease, cancer, respiratory disease, cerebrovascular disease, and diabetes account for 70% of all deaths in the United States and are among the most common and potentially preventable of all health problems in the United States.

CARDIOVASCULAR DISEASES

Cardiovascular disease, which includes coronary heart diseases, arrhythmias, diseases of the arteries, congestive heart failure, rheumatic heart disease, cerebrovascular disease (stroke), and congenital heart defects, was the leading cause of death in the United States in 2006. (See Figure 5.1.) In *NHLBI Fact Book, Fiscal Year 2008* (April 7, 2009, http://www.nhlbi.nih.gov/about/factbook/FactBookFinal.pdf), the National Heart Lung and Blood Institute (NHLBI) reports that in 2005 cardiovascular disease accounted for 864,000 deaths—35% of all deaths—and cerebrovascular disease, the third-leading cause of death after cancer, accounted for 144,000 deaths. In terms of death rate and years of potential life lost, heart disease is second only to all cancers combined.

According to Donald Lloyd-Jones of Northwestern University et al. in "Heart Disease and Stroke Statistics—2010 Update" (*Circulation*, February 23, 2010), if all forms of major cardiovascular disease were eliminated, life expectancy in the United States would rise by almost seven years. If all forms of cancer were eliminated, the estimated gain would be three years.

Heart Attack and Angina Pectoris

A heart attack, or myocardial infarction (MI), occurs when the blood supply from a coronary artery to the heart muscle (the myocardium) is cut off abruptly. This happens when one of the coronary arteries that supply blood to the heart is obstructed (blocked). When the blood supply is eliminated, the heart's muscle cells are deprived of oxygen and die. Disability or death can result, depending on how much of the heart muscle has been damaged.

Angina pectoris is not a disease; it is a symptom and the name for chest pain or pressure that occurs when poor blood flow through a partially occluded (blocked) artery to the heart quickly and temporarily reduces its supply of oxygen. When the blood flow is restored, the pain subsides. A common condition, angina is often a warning of the risk of heart attack. Its dull, constricting pain typically occurs when an individual is physically active or excited but subsides when activity ceases. In men, angina usually occurs after the age of 50, whereas women tend to develop angina later in life. Lloyd-Jones et al. note that in 2005 an estimated 10.2 million people in the United States suffered from angina.

WARNING SIGNALS OF A HEART ATTACK. In "Heart Attack Symptoms and Warning Signs" (2009, http://www.americanheart.org/presenter.jhtml?identifier=4595), the American Heart Association (AHA) lists several warning signs of a heart attack:

- An uncomfortable pressure, squeezing, fullness, or pain in the center of the chest behind the breastbone

- Pain that spreads to the shoulders, neck, or arms

- Chest discomfort accompanied by sweating, nausea, shortness of breath, or a feeling of weakness

IMMEDIATE CARE IS CRUCIAL. Immediate medical care dramatically improves the odds of surviving a heart attack. Treatments are most effective if given within an hour of when the attack begins. According to the AHA, intensive emergency care in the first 12 hours after a heart attack improves the patient's chance of survival and recovery.

FIGURE 5.1

Ten leading causes of death and their death rates, 2006

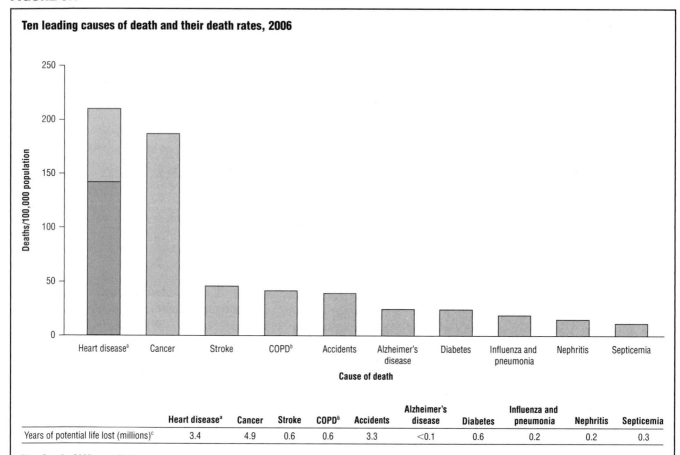

	Heart disease[a]	Cancer	Stroke	COPD[b]	Accidents	Alzheimer's disease	Diabetes	Influenza and pneumonia	Nephritis	Septicemia
Years of potential life lost (millions)[c]	3.4	4.9	0.6	0.6	3.3	<0.1	0.6	0.2	0.2	0.3

Note: Data for 2006 are preliminary.

[a]Includes 141.9 deaths per 100,000 population from coronary heart disease (CHD).

[b]Chronic obstructive pulmonary disease (COPD) and allied conditions (including asthma); the term in the Internal Classification of Diseases (ICD)/10 is "chronic lower respiratory diseases."

[c]Based on the average remaining years of life up to age 77 years.

SOURCE: "Ten Leading Causes of Death: Death Rates, U.S., 2006," in *NHLBI Factbook, Fiscal Year 2008*, National Institutes of Health, National Heart, Lung, and Blood Institute, April 2009, http://www.nhlbi.nih.gov/about/factbook/FactBookFinal.pdf (accessed December 29, 2009)

Researchers believe that patients who suffer heart attacks benefit from early intensive treatment—such as improved monitoring of their conditions and aggressive use of pharmacologic (drug) therapy, including appropriate reperfusion therapies and "clot-busting" medications—initiated with as little delay as possible. There are a variety of drugs that dissolve clots, but tissue plasminogen activator, which was approved by the U.S. Food and Drug Administration (FDA) in 1996, is currently used most often.

Treatments for Heart Disease

Once it is clear that a person is having a heart attack, immediate treatment usually includes administering drugs to help open the blocked artery, which restores blood flow to the heart and prevents clots from forming again. If the patient gets to an emergency room quickly, reperfusion might be done. Drugs may be administered to decrease workload of the heart, relieve chest pain, reduce blood pressure, and thin blood to prevent clot formation in the arteries and promote reperfusion. Patients with heart disease may also undergo other procedures, including:

- Balloon angioplasty or percutaneous transluminal coronary angioplasty to widen narrowed arteries with an inflated balloon

- Placement of wire mesh tubes, called stents, into arteries after angioplasty to prevent later collapse or restenosis (renarrowing)

- Coronary artery bypass graft (CABG) surgery to improve blood supply to parts of the heart muscle that have decreased blood flow

Once emergency care and immediate treatment is completed, most communities have cardiac rehabilitation programs to help people recover from a heart attack and reduce the chances of having another one.

Bypass Surgery

CABG, commonly known as bypass surgery, can improve blood flow to the heart, relieve chest pains, and help the heart pump more efficiently. Generally, a segment of a large healthy vein, usually taken from the patient's leg, is spliced between the aorta (the main vessel carrying blood from the left side of the heart to all the arteries of the body and limbs) and the blocked coronary arteries. The coronary bypass operation thus supplies blood to the area of the heart that had a deficient blood supply. During the operation the patient is placed on a heart-lung machine that takes over the function of the heart and lungs while the surgery is proceeding. Usually, patients recovering from CABG surgery spend two or three days in the intensive care unit and several days to one week in the hospital following the surgery. Lloyd-Jones et al. report that in 2007, coronary artery bypass surgeries were performed on 176,138 patients in the United States.

Lloyd-Jones and his colleagues also note that from 1996 to 2006 the total number of cardiovascular operations and procedures increased by 33% from 5.4 million to 7.2 million per year. During this period, CABG surgery volume declined, and the numbers of selected procedures such as cardiac catheterizations also decreased slightly. In contrast, the numbers of other kinds of catheter-based interventions increased as did the use of newer techniques such as minimally invasive direct coronary bypass surgery. In this procedure the surgeon makes one or more small incisions (about three inches long) in the chest wall and works directly on the clogged artery while the heart is beating. Some surgeons use fiber-optic techniques similar to those used in gallbladder and other procedures. Anesthesiologists slow the heartbeat with drugs such as calcium channel blockers and beta-blockers to allow surgeons more control. Another technique actually stops the heartbeat and uses a modified heart-lung machine connected to a large artery in the groin while the surgeon operates through small incisions using a video camera and long-handled instruments.

Research studies, such as "Eight-Year Experience with Minimally Invasive Cardiothoracic Surgery" by Alexander Iribarne et al. of Columbia University Medical Center (*World Journal of Surgery*, April 2010), find that minimally invasive procedures have delivered the anticipated benefits including shorter recovery times, less time spent in the hospital, and the possibility of combining the new procedure with angioplasty or other procedures. Iribarne and his collaborators followed more than 900 patients for an average of eight years, and concluded that "minimally invasive approaches were effective and reproducible with acceptable operating time duration and low morbidity and mortality rates."

Catheter-Based Interventions

A growing number of patients are candidates for much simpler procedures called catheter-based interventions because the procedures are performed via a thin tube inserted into an artery, rather than operating on the coronary artery by cutting through the chest wall. One

such catheter-based intervention, performed under a local anesthetic, is percutaneous coronary intervention (PCI; this procedure is also called percutaneous transluminal coronary angioplasty). A physician punctures an artery in the patient's groin and threads a balloon-tipped catheter into the artery. The tip of the catheter is slowly advanced up through the arterial system and positioned in the coronary artery at the point of the blockage or stenosis (narrowing). The small, sausage-shaped balloon on the end of the catheter is then inflated, flattening the fatty plaque and widening the artery. The balloon is sometimes inflated and deflated several times to clear the artery.

PCI has several obvious advantages over bypass surgery. First, it is performed under a local rather than a general anesthetic and does not involve opening the chest or using a heart-lung machine. It is less expensive, and the patient is usually out of the hospital and recovering in a few days. Still, PCI is not always completely effective, and nearly one-third of patients who have had PCI eventually require bypass surgery or another PCI because the initial procedure is unsuccessful or the blockage recurs.

According to Lloyd-Jones et al., 1.3 million PCI procedures were performed in the United States in 2006. Of these procedures, 65% were performed on men. About 1.3 million angioplasties were performed in 2006.

As technology advances, catheter-based interventions using devices such as fiber optics and laser methods may replace angioplasty as the treatments of choice. Some physicians are also using a tiny cutting blade attached to the end of a fiber-optic tube to remove accumulated plaque, although this method has not yet been proven to be more effective than balloon angioplasty.

Physicians are also placing stents into arteries after angioplasty or PCI to prevent later collapse or restenosis. However, even with stents, arteries renarrow in about a quarter of patients.

In "Effects of Percutaneous Coronary Interventions in Silent Ischemia after Myocardial Infarction" (*Journal of the American Medical Association*, vol. 297, no. 18, May 9, 2007), Paul Erne et al. of Kantonsspital Luzern in Lucerne, Switzerland, report the results of a study following patients who had PCI following a heart attack. The researchers find that PCI and drug therapy reduced the subjects' risk of suffering another major cardiac event. By 2009 PCI was considered the "treatment of choice" for the majority of patients who experience heart attack, as noted by Nevio Taglieri and Carlo Di Mario of the Royal Brompton Hospital and Imperial College, in London, England, in "Percutaneous Coronary Intervention Following Thombolysis: For Whom and When?" (*Acute Cardiac Care*, vol. 11, no. 4, 2009).

HEART TRANSPLANTS. In December 1967 Christiaan Barnard (1922–2001) of South Africa performed the first successful heart transplant. This feat was repeated one month later in the United States by Norman Shumway (1923–2006) at Stanford University Hospital in California. According to the Health Resources and Services Administration (HRSA) Organ Procurement and Transplantation Network (December 26, 2009, http://optn.transplant.hrsa.gov/latestData/rptData.asp), in 2008, 2,163 heart transplants were performed in the United States, and in 2009, 2,212 heart transplants were performed. As of March 2010, 3,147 patients were awaiting heart transplants in the United States.

Risk Factors for Heart Disease

Various risk factors exist for heart disease. Even though some cannot be changed, others can be modified.

UNCHANGEABLE RISK FACTORS. Four risk factors for heart disease that cannot be altered are heredity, race, gender, and increasing age. People whose parents had or have cardiovascular diseases are more likely to develop them. Race is also a significant factor. For example, Lloyd-Jones et al. indicate that African-American adults have the highest rates of high blood pressure in the world (greater than 43%), which increases the risk for heart disease. Men have a greater risk of heart attack than do women. Heart attacks are the leading cause of death among men older than the age of 40, but heart disease is not a major cause of death among women until they reach the age of 60. Heart attacks are also more likely to occur as a person ages. More than half of the Americans who experience heart attacks are aged 65 or older. Of those who die from their attacks, the vast majority are older than age 65.

CHANGEABLE RISK FACTORS. Cigarette smoking doubles the risk of heart attack. A smoker who suffers a heart attack is more likely to die from it and more likely to die suddenly than a nonsmoker. Once people stop smoking, however, regardless of the length of time or the amount they smoked, the risk of heart disease decreases significantly. The prevalence of cigarette smoking declined dramatically from 1965 to 1997 and then slowly decreased to 24% of men and 18% of women in 2007. (See Figure 5.2.) In *Health, United States, 2009* the CDC reports that in 2007, 20% of high school students had smoked cigarettes, 14% of high school students had smoked cigars, and 8% had used smokeless tobacco in the month preceding the survey. Cigarette smoking rates among high school students peaked in 1997 and then decreased and leveled off.

High blood pressure, which usually has no symptoms or warning signs, is called the "silent killer." High blood pressure means that it is more difficult for blood to pump through the arteries, which increases the heart's workload, causing it to weaken and enlarge over time. Generally, blood pressure increases with age. Men have a higher incidence of high blood pressure than women until 45 to 54 years of age, when the risks become equal for both

FIGURE 5.2

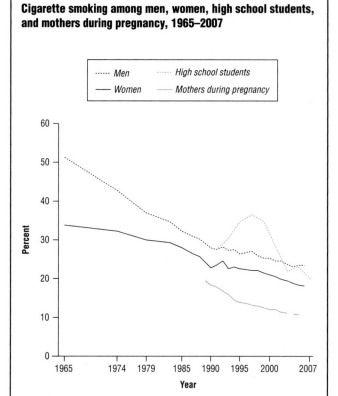

Cigarette smoking among men, women, high school students, and mothers during pregnancy, 1965–2007

Notes: Estimates for men and women are age-adjusted. Cigarette smoking is defined as: (for men and women 18 years and over) at least 100 cigarettes in lifetime and now smoke every day or some days; (for students in grades 9–12) 1 or more cigarettes in the 30 days preceding the survey; and (for mothers with a live birth) during pregnancy. Data for 2004 and 2005 for mothers during pregnancy are based on the 36 states, D.C., and New York City that continued to use the 1989 Revision of the U.S. Certificate of Live Births in 2005.

SOURCE: "Figure 6. Cigarette Smoking among Men, Women, High School Students, and Mothers during Pregnancy: United States, 1965–2007," in *Health, United States, 2008. With Chartbook*, Centers for Disease Control and Prevention, National Center for Health Statistics, 2009, http://www.cdc.gov/nchs/data/hus/hus08.pdf (accessed December 29, 2009)

sexes. The prevalence of high blood pressure increased from 25.5% in 1988–94 to 31.3% in 2003–06. (Table 5.1 defines hypertension as having elevated blood pressure and/or taking antihypertensive medication. Elevated blood pressure is defined as having systolic pressure of at least 140 mm Hg or diastolic pressure of at least 90 mm Hg. Those with elevated blood pressure also may be taking prescribed medicine for high blood pressure. Those taking antihypertensive medication may not have measured elevated blood pressure but are still classified as having hypertension.) In most cases, high blood pressure can be controlled through diet, exercise, and medication.

High serum cholesterol levels increase the risk of coronary heart disease. High serum cholesterol is defined as greater than or equal to 240 mg/dL (6.20 mmol/L). Borderline high serum cholesterol is defined as greater than or equal to 200 mg/dL and less than 240 mg/dL. In 2003–06, 16.3% of adults aged 20 to 74 had high cholesterol levels.

TABLE 5.1

High blood pressure in adults age 20 and older, by selected characteristics, 1988–94, 1999–2002, and 2003–06

[Data are based on interviews and physical examinations of a sample of the civilian noninstitutionalized population]

Sex, age, race and Hispanic origin[a], and percent of poverty level	Hypertension[b, c] (elevated blood pressure and/or taking antihypertensive medication)			Elevated blood pressure[b]		
	1988–1994	1999–2002	2003–2006	1988–1994	1999–2002	2003–2006
20 years and over, age-adjusted[d]			Percent of population			
Both sexes[e]	25.5	30.0	31.3	18.5	19.9	17.9
Male	26.4	28.8	31.8	20.6	19.1	18.2
Female	24.4	30.6	30.3	16.4	20.2	17.3
Not Hispanic or Latino:						
White only, male	25.6	27.6	31.2	19.7	17.6	17.4
White only, female	23.0	28.5	28.3	15.1	18.5	15.9
Black or African American only, male	37.5	40.6	42.2	30.3	28.2	26.5
Black or African American only, female	38.3	43.5	44.1	26.4	28.8	23.9
Mexican male	26.9	26.8	24.8	22.2	21.5	15.3
Mexican female	25.0	27.9	28.6	20.4	21.2	19.2
Percent of poverty level:[f]						
Below 100%	31.7	33.9	35.0	22.5	23.3	22.6
100%–less than 200%	26.6	33.5	34.1	19.3	23.0	21.1
200% or more	23.9	28.2	30.3	17.5	18.2	16.6
20 years and over, crude						
Both sexes[e]	24.1	30.2	32.1	17.6	19.9	18.2
Male	23.8	27.6	31.3	18.7	18.2	17.9
Female	24.4	32.7	32.9	16.5	21.6	18.6
Not Hispanic or Latino:						
White only, male	24.3	28.3	32.4	18.7	17.8	17.9
White only, female	24.6	32.8	33.4	16.4	21.6	18.8
Black or African American only, male	31.1	35.9	38.8	25.5	25.2	24.8
Black or African American only, female	32.5	41.9	42.8	22.2	27.2	22.4
Mexican male	16.4	16.5	16.6	13.9	14.1	10.9
Mexican female	15.9	18.8	20.0	12.7	13.8	13.0
Percent of poverty level:[f]						
Below 100%	25.7	30.3	28.8	18.7	21.1	18.3
100%–less than 200%	26.7	34.8	36.8	19.8	24.1	22.5
200% or more	22.2	28.2	31.1	16.2	17.8	16.8
Male						
20–34 years	7.1	*8.1	9.2	6.6	*7.3	7.6
35–44 years	17.1	17.1	21.1	15.2	12.1	13.2
45–54 years	29.2	31.0	36.2	21.9	20.4	21.0
55–64 years	40.6	45.0	50.2	28.4	24.8	26.4
65–74 years	54.4	59.6	64.1	39.9	34.9	29.2
75 years and over	60.4	69.0	65.0	49.7	50.6	38.2
Female						
20–34 years	2.9	*2.7	*2.2	*2.4	*1.4	*
35–44 years	11.2	15.1	12.6	6.4	8.5	5.8
45–54 years	23.9	31.8	36.2	13.7	19.1	20.0
55–64 years	42.6	53.9	54.4	27.0	31.9	28.6
65–74 years	56.2	72.7	70.8	38.2	53.0	40.8
75 years and over	73.6	83.1	80.2	59.9	64.4	55.4

(See Table 5.2.) A reduction of dietary fat, especially artery-clogging saturated fat, can reduce blood cholesterol levels, as can exercise. Maintaining a healthy weight, eating a proper diet, and exercising can also enhance the effectiveness of cholesterol-lowering drugs.

A lack of physical exercise is also a risk factor for heart disease. According to the CDC in *Health in the United States, 2009*, in 2007 the percentage of Americans engaged in regular leisure-time physical activity declined with increasing age from 37.1% among adults aged 18 to 24 years of age to 30.8% of 45 to 54 year olds to 24.7% among adults aged 65 to 74. For adults aged 18 to 64, in "Physical Activity Guidelines for Americans" (November 4, 2009, http://www.health.gov/paguidelines/), the U.S. Department of Health and Human Services (DHHS) recommends 2 hours and 30 minutes a week of moderate-intensity, or 1 hour and 15 minutes (75 minutes) a week of vigorous-intensity aerobic physical activity, or an equivalent combination of moderate- and vigorous-intensity aerobic physical activity. Aerobic activity should be performed in episodes of at least ten minutes, preferably spread throughout the week. Adults also should engage in muscle-strengthening activities that involve all major muscle groups performed on two or more days per week. The Guidelines assert that additional health benefits are provided by increasing to 5 hours (300 minutes) a week of moderate-intensity aerobic physical activity, or 2 hours and 30 minutes a week of

TABLE 5.1

High blood pressure in adults age 20 and older, by selected characteristics, 1988–94, 1999–2002, and 2003–06 [CONTINUED]

[Data are based on interviews and physical examinations of a sample of the civilian noninstitutionalized population]

*Estimates are considered unreliable.
[a]Persons of Mexican origin may be of any race. Starting with 1999 data, race-specific estimates are tabulated according to the 1997 Revisions to the Standards for the Classification of Federal Data on Race and Ethnicity and are not strictly comparable with estimates for earlier years. The two non-Hispanic race categories shown in the table conform to the 1997 Standards. Starting with 1999 data, race-specific estimates are for persons who reported only one racial group. Prior to data year 1999, estimates were tabulated according to the 1977 Standards. Estimates for single-race categories prior to 1999 included persons who reported one race or, if they reported more than one race, identified one race as best representing their race.
[b]Hypertension is defined as having measured elevated blood pressure and/or taking antihypertensive medication. Elevated blood pressure is defined as having a measured systolic pressure of at least 140 mmHg or diastolic pressure of at least 90 mmHg. Those with elevated blood pressure also may be taking prescribed medicine for high blood pressure. Those taking antihypertensive medication may not have measured elevated blood pressure but are still classified as having hypertension.
[c]Respondents were asked, "Are you now taking prescribed medicine for your high blood pressure?"
[d]Age-adjusted to the 2000 standard population using five age groups: 20–34 years, 35–44 years, 45–54 years, 55–64 years, and 65 years and over (65–74 years for estimates for 20–74 years). Age-adjusted estimates may differ from other age-adjusted estimates based on the same data and presented elsewhere if different age groups are used in the adjustment procedure.
[e]Includes persons of all races and Hispanic origins, not just those shown separately.
[f]Percent of poverty level is based on family income and family size. Persons with unknown percent of poverty level are excluded (5% in 2003–2006).
Notes: Percents are based on the average of blood pressure measurements taken. In 2003–2006, 81% of participants had three blood pressure readings. Excludes pregnant women. Estimates for persons 20 years and over are used for setting and tracking Healthy People 2010 objectives. Data have been revised and differ from previous editions of Health, United States. Data for additional years are available.

SOURCE: Adapted from "Table 68. Hypertension and Elevated Blood Pressure among Persons 20 Years of Age and over, by Selected Characteristics: United States, 1988–1994, 1999–2002, and 2003–2006," in *Health, United States, 2009. With Special Feature on Medical Technology*, Centers for Disease Control and Prevention, National Center for Health Statistics, 2010, http://www.cdc.gov/nchs/data/hus/hus09.pdf (accessed March 12, 2010)

vigorous-intensity physical activity, or an equivalent combination of both.

CONTRIBUTING FACTORS. Diabetes, or elevated blood glucose, affects cholesterol and triglyceride levels. The disease can sharply increase the risk of heart attack, especially when blood glucose is uncontrolled or poorly controlled. According to the National Institute of Diabetes and Digestive and Kidney Diseases (NIDDK), in "National Diabetes Statistics, 2007" (June 2008, http://diabetes.niddk.nih.gov/dm/pubs/statistics/index.htm), about 68% of deaths among people with diabetes result from heart disease and stroke. Adults with diabetes have heart disease death rates that are two to four times higher than adults without diabetes. Table 5.3 shows that more than 10% of adults over age 20 had diabetes in 2005–06.

Obesity is also a factor contributing to heart disease. Research shows that the location of body fat may affect the risk of suffering a heart attack significantly. Men with a waist measurement that exceeds their hip measurement ("pot bellies," or excessive abdominal fat) and women whose waistline measurement is more than 80% of their hip dimension (apple-shaped) are at greater risk. Even though obesity is directly associated with an increased risk for cardiovascular disease, being overweight to any degree strains the heart.

The prevalence of obesity among adults aged 20 and older in the United States has increased from 19.4% in 1997 to 27.6% in 2009. (See Figure 5.3.) The National Center for Health Statistics (NCHS) notes in *Early Release of Selected Estimates Based on Data from the January–June 2009 National Health Interview Survey* (December 2009, http://www.cdc.gov/nchs/data/nhis/earlyrelease/200912_06.pdf) that even though the prevalence of overweight and

obesity has increased in both males and females in all racial and ethnic groups, non-Hispanic white women were less likely to be obese than Hispanic and non-Hispanic African-American women. Obesity was highest among non-Hispanic African-American women (44.1%).

Women and Heart Disease

Until the early 1990s, almost all research on heart disease was carried out on middle-aged men. However, heart disease affects women, too. When a woman enters menopause, she begins to lose the protection provided by the hormones that appear to reduce the risk of heart disease. As a result, the rates of coronary heart disease are two to three times higher among postmenopausal women than among premenopausal women, and 52.1% of deaths attributable to cardiovascular disease are women. More than one out of three women suffers from some form of cardiovascular disease, according to the American Heart Association in "Women and Cardiovascular Diseases—Statistics 2010" (2009, http://www.americanheart.org/downloadable/heart/1260905040318FS10WM10.pdf). In fact, starting at age 75, the prevalence of cardiovascular disease is higher among women than among men of the same age group.

Wayne Rosamond et al. note in "Heart Disease and Stroke Statistics—2008 Update: A Report from the American Heart Association Statistics Committee and Stroke Statistics Subcommittee" (*Circulation*, vol. 117, no. 4, 2008) that of women age 40 or older who have heart attacks, 23% die within the first year, compared with 18% of men. In part because women have heart attacks at older ages than men do, they are more likely to die from one within a few weeks of its occurrence. Within five years of a first heart attack, 43% of women age 40 or older and 33%

TABLE 5.2

High cholesterol levels in adults age 20 and older, by selected characteristics, 1960–62 through 2003–06

[Data are based on interviews and laboratory work of a sample of the civilian noninstitutionalized population]

Sex, age, race and Hispanic origin[a], and percent of poverty level	1960–1962	1971–1974	1976–1980[b]	1988–1994	1999–2002	2003–2006
20–74 years, age-adjusted[c]	Percent of population with high serum total cholesterol (greater than or equal to 240 mg/dL)					
Both sexes[d]	33.3	28.6	27.8	19.7	17.0	16.3
Male	30.6	27.9	26.4	18.8	16.9	15.6
Female	35.6	29.1	28.8	20.5	17.0	16.9
Not Hispanic or Latino:						
White only, male	—	—	26.4	18.7	17.0	16.0
White only, female	—	—	29.6	20.7	17.4	17.9
Black or African American only, male	—	—	25.5	16.4	12.5	11.2
Black or African American only, female	—	—	26.3	19.9	16.6	13.0
Mexican male	—	—	20.3	18.7	17.6	17.7
Mexican female	—	—	20.5	17.7	12.7	13.8
Percent of poverty level:[e]						
Below 100%	—	24.4	23.5	19.3	17.8	18.2
100%–less than 200%	—	28.9	26.5	19.4	18.8	16.5
200% or more	—	28.9	29.0	19.6	16.5	16.2
20 years and over, age-adjusted[c]						
Both sexes[d]	—	—	—	20.8	17.3	16.3
Male	—	—	—	19.0	16.4	15.1
Female	—	—	—	22.0	17.8	17.1
Not Hispanic or Latino:						
White only, male	—	—	—	18.8	16.5	15.5
White only, female	—	—	—	22.2	18.1	18.0
Black or African American only, male	—	—	—	16.9	12.4	10.9
Black or African American only, female	—	—	—	21.4	17.7	13.3
Mexican male	—	—	—	18.5	17.4	17.6
Mexican female	—	—	—	18.7	13.8	14.4
Percent of poverty level:[e]						
Below 100%	—	—	—	20.6	18.3	18.1
100%–less than 200%	—	—	—	20.6	19.1	16.7
200% or more	—	—	—	20.4	16.5	16.0
20 years and over, crude						
Both sexes[d]	—	—	—	19.6	17.3	16.4
Male	—	—	—	17.7	16.6	15.2
Female	—	—	—	21.3	18.0	17.5
Not Hispanic or Latino:						
White only, male	—	—	—	18.0	16.9	15.7
White only, female	—	—	—	22.5	19.1	18.9
Black or African American only, male	—	—	—	14.7	12.2	10.8
Black or African American only, female	—	—	—	18.2	16.1	12.5
Mexican male	—	—	—	15.4	15.0	15.7
Mexican female	—	—	—	14.3	10.7	12.6
Percent of poverty level:[e]						
Below 100%	—	—	—	17.6	16.4	16.8
100%–less than 200%	—	—	—	19.8	18.2	16.0
200% or more	—	—	—	19.5	16.9	16.5
Male						
20–34 years	15.1	12.4	11.9	8.2	9.8	9.5
35–44 years	33.9	31.8	27.9	19.4	19.8	20.5
45–54 years	39.2	37.5	36.9	26.6	23.6	20.8
55–64 years	41.6	36.2	36.8	28.0	19.9	16.0
65–74 years	38.0	34.7	31.7	21.9	13.7	10.9
75 years and over	—	—	—	20.4	10.2	9.6

of men in the same age group will die. Of those who have experienced a heart attack, the percent having another heart attack or fatal coronary heart disease is 22% among women aged 40 to 69 years and 16% of men in the same age group; 12% of women heart attack sufferers aged 40 to 69 will experience heart failure within five years, compared with 7% of men in the same age group. Women heart attack sufferers aged 40 to 69 experience a stroke rate of 6%

within five years of their heart attack, compared with 4% of men in the same age group. Rosamond and his coauthors note that the overall death rate for coronary heart disease in the United States in 2004 was 150.2 deaths per 100,000 population. Higher death rates were experienced by African-American males (223.9 per 100,000) and white males (194.2 per 100,000) than for African-American females (148.7 per 100,000) and white

TABLE 5.2

High cholesterol levels in adults age 20 and older, by selected characteristics, 1960–62 through 2003–06 [CONTINUED]

[Data are based on interviews and laboratory work of a sample of the civilian noninstitutionalized population]

Sex, age, race and Hispanic origin[a], and percent of poverty level	1960–1962	1971–1974	1976–1980[b]	1988–1994	1999–2002	2003–2006
20–74 years, age-adjusted[c]	Percent of population with high serum total cholesterol (greater than or equal to 240 mg/dL)					
Female						
20–34 years	12.4	10.9	9.8	7.3	8.9	10.3
35–44 years	23.1	19.3	20.7	12.3	12.4	12.7
45–54 years	46.9	38.7	40.5	26.7	21.4	19.7
55–64 years	70.1	53.1	52.9	40.9	25.6	30.5
65–74 years	68.5	57.7	51.6	41.3	32.3	24.2
75 years and over	—	—	—	38.2	26.5	18.6

—Data not available.

[a]Persons of Mexican origin may be of any race. Starting with 1999 data, race-specific estimates are tabulated according to the 1997 Revisions to the Standards for the Classification of Federal Data on Race and Ethnicity and are not strictly comparable with estimates for earlier years. The two non-Hispanic race categories shown in the table conform to the 1997 Standards. Starting with 1999 data, race-specific estimates are for persons who reported only one racial group. Prior to data year 1999, estimates were tabulated according to the 1977 Standards. Estimates for single-race categories prior to 1999 included persons who reported one race or, if they reported more than one race, identified one race as best representing their race.

[b]Data for Mexicans are for 1982–1984.

[c]Age-adjusted to the 2000 standard population using five age groups: 20–34 years, 35–44 years, 45–54 years, 55–64 years, and 65 years and over (65–74 years for estimates for 20–74 years). Age-adjusted estimates may differ from other age-adjusted estimates based on the same data and presented elsewhere if different age groups are used in the adjustment procedure.

[d]Includes persons of all races and Hispanic origins, not just those shown separately.

[e]Percent of poverty level is based on family income and family size. Persons with unknown percent of poverty level are excluded (4% in 2003–2006).

Notes: High serum cholesterol is defined as greater than or equal to 240 mg/dL (6.20 mmol/L). Borderline high serum cholesterol is defined as greater than or equal to 200 mg/dL and less than 240 mg/dL. Risk levels have been defined by the Third Report of the National Cholesterol Education Program Expert Panel on Detection, Evaluation, and Treatment of High Blood Cholesterol in Adults. National Heart, Lung, and Blood Institute, National Institutes of Health. September 2002. Individuals who take medicine to lower their serum cholesterol levels and whose measured total serum cholesterol levels are below the cut-offs for high and borderline high cholesterol are notdefined as having high or borderline high cholesterol, respectively. Data for additional years are available.

SOURCE: Adapted from "Table 69. Serum Total Cholesterol Levels among Persons 20 Years of Age and over, by Sex, Age, Race and Hispanic Origin, and Poverty Level: United States, Selected Years 1960–1962 through 2003–2006," in *Health, United States, 2009. With Special Feature on Medical Technology*, Centers for Disease Control and Prevention, National Center for Health Statistics, 2010, http://www.cdc.gov/nchs/data/hus/hus09.pdf (accessed March 12, 2010)

females (114.7 per 100,000). Death rates were even lower for Hispanics (119.2 per 100,000), Native Americans and Alaska Natives (106.5 per 100,000), and Asian/Pacific Islanders (84.1 per 100,000).

Women are more seriously affected by heart disease than men are because women have smaller arteries, they frequently wait longer to get care, and they are generally older (typically by ten years) when heart disease strikes. Another reason could be that women's early symptoms of heart disease often differ from those of the "classic" heart attack. According to Samantha J. Zbierajewski-Eischeid of Geisinger Health System and Susan J. Loeb of Pennsylvania State University in "Myocardial Infarction in Women: Promoting Symptom Recognition, Early Diagnosis, and Risk Assessment" (*Dimensions of Critical Care Nursing*, vol. 28, no. 1, January/February 2009), symptoms that often occur in women before a heart attack are unusual fatigue, sleep disturbance, shortness of breath, indigestion, and anxiety. Although many symptoms that may occur during a heart attack are comparable to the symptoms men experience: shortness of breath, weakness, unusual fatigue, cold sweat, and dizziness, women also may experience nausea—with or without vomiting and back pain. Zbierajewski-Eischeid and Loeb also assert that health professionals may fail to accurately identify MI in women.

Women also undergo fewer cardiac procedures than do men. Furthermore, there has been research demon-strating that anticlotting drugs, which were originally formulated for men, do not offer women comparable benefits. Finally, women may underestimate their vulnerability to heart disease. In "National Study of Women's Awareness, Preventive Action, and Barriers to Cardiovascular Health" (*Circulation*, vol. 113, no. 4, 2006), Lori Mosca of Columbia University Medical Center, New York, et al. note that past AHA surveys revealed that women feared breast cancer more than cardiovascular disease, even though more women die as a result of cardiovascular disease (1 out of 2.5 deaths) than from breast cancer (1 out of 30 deaths).

Stroke

Stroke (cerebrovascular disease) is a cardiovascular disease that affects the blood vessels of the central nervous system. When an artery supplying oxygen and nutrients to the brain bursts or becomes clogged with a blood clot, a part of the brain does not receive the oxygen it needs. Without the necessary oxygen, the affected nerve cells die within moments. The parts of the body controlled by these nerve cells also become dysfunctional. Because dead brain cells cannot be replaced, the damage done by a stroke is often permanent.

Stroke affects people in different ways. The extent of the resulting damage or loss depends on the type of stroke and the area of the brain that has been damaged. Physicians

TABLE 5.3

Selected health conditions and risk factors, 1988–94 through 2005–06

[Data are based on interviews and physical examinations of a sample of the civilian noninstitutionalized population]

Health conditions	1988–1994	1999–2000	2001–2002	2003–2004	2005–2006
Diabetes[a]		Percent of persons 20 years of age and over			
Total, age-adjusted[b]	8.0	8.8	10.0	10.4	10.1
Total, crude	7.8	8.3	9.6	10.3	10.2
High serum total cholesterol[c]					
Total, age-adjusted[d]	20.8	18.3	16.5	16.9	15.6
Total, crude	19.6	17.8	16.4	17.0	15.9
Hypertension[e]					
Total, age-adjusted[d]	25.5	30.0	29.7	32.1	30.5
Total, crude	24.1	28.9	28.9	32.5	31.7
Overweight (includes obesity)[f]					
Total, age-adjusted[d]	56.0	64.0	65.3	66.0	66.6
Total, crude	54.9	63.6	65.2	66.2	67.0
Obesity[g]					
Total, age-adjusted[d]	22.9	30.1	29.9	32.0	33.9
Total, crude	22.3	29.9	30.0	32.0	34.2
Untreated dental caries[h]					
Total, age-adjusted[d]	27.7	24.3	21.3	30.0	—
Total, crude	28.2	25.0	21.6	30.3	—
Overweight[i]		Percent of persons under 20 years of age			
2–5 years	7.2	10.3	10.6	13.9	11.0
6–11 years	11.3	15.1	16.3	18.8	15.1
12–19 years	10.5	14.8	16.7	17.4	17.8
Untreated dental caries[h]					
2–5 years	19.1	23.2	15.8	23.4	—
6–19 years	23.6	22.7	20.6	25.2	—

— Data not available.

[a]Includes physician-diagnosed and undiagnosed diabetes. Physician-diagnosed diabetes was obtained by self-report and excludes women who reported having diabetes only during pregnancy. Undiagnosed diabetes is defined as a fasting blood glucose (FBG) of at least 126 mg/dL and no reported physician diagnosis. In 2005–2006, FBG testing was performed at a different laboratory and using a different instrument than testing in earlier years. NHANES conducted a crossover study to evaluate the impact of these changes on FBG measurements. As a result of that study, NHANES recommended that 2005–2006 data on FBG measurements be adjusted to be compatible with earlier years. Undiagnosed diabetes estimates in *Health, United States* were produced after adjusting the 2005–2006 FGC data as recommended.

[b]Estimates are age-adjusted to the year 2000 standard population using three age groups: 20–39 years, 40–59 years, and 60 years and over. Because of the smaller sample size for fasting tests, age adjustment is to three age groups only. Age-adjusted estimates in this table may differ from other age-adjusted estimates based on the same data and presented elsewhere if different age groups are used in the adjustment procedure.

[c]High serum cholesterol is defined as greater than or equal to 240 mg/dL (6.20 mmol/L). Risk levels have been defined by the Third Report of the National Cholesterol Education Program Expert Panel on Detection, Evaluation, and Treatment of High Blood Cholesterol in Adults. National Heart, Lung, and Blood Institute, National Institutes of Health. September 2002. Individuals who take medicine to lower their serum cholesterol levels and whose measured total serum cholesterol levels are below the cut-offs for high cholesterol are not defined as having high cholesterol.

[d]Age-adjusted to the 2000 standard population using five age groups: 20–34 years, 35–44 years, 45–54 years, 55–64 years, and 65 years and over. Age-adjusted estimates may differ from other age-adjusted estimates based on the same data and presented elsewhere if different age groups are used in the adjustment procedure.

[e]Hypertension is defined as having elevated blood pressure and/or taking antihypertensive medication. Elevated blood pressure is defined as having systolic pressure of at least 140 mmHg or diastolic pressure of at least 90 mmHg. Those with elevated blood pressure may be taking prescribed medicine for high blood pressure. Respondents were asked, "Are you now taking prescribed medicine for your high blood pressure?"

[f]Excludes pregnant women. Overweight is defined as body mass index (BMI) greater than or equal to 25 kilograms/meter^2

[g]Excludes pregnant women. Obesity is defined as body mass index (BMI) greater than or equal to 30 kilograms/meter^2

[h]Untreated dental caries refers to untreated coronal caries, that is, caries on the crown or enamel surface of the tooth. Root tips are classified as coronal caries. Root caries are not included. For children 2–5 years of age, only dental caries in primary teeth was evaluated. Caries in both permanent and primary teeth was evaluated for children 6–11 years of age. For children 12 years and over and for adults, only dental caries in permanent teeth was evaluated. Persons without at least one primary or one permanent tooth or one root tip were classified as edentulous and were excluded from this analysis. The majority of edentulous persons are 65 years of age and over. Estimates of edentulism among persons 65 years of age and over are 33% in 1988–1994 and 27% in 1999–2004.

[i]Overweight is defined as body mass index (BMI) at or above the sex- and age-specific 95th percentile BMI cutoff points from the 2000 CDC Growth Charts: United States. Advance data from vital and health statistics; no 314. Hyattsville, MD: National Center for Health Statistics. 2000. Excludes pregnant girls.

Note: Data have been revised and differ from previous editions of *Health, United States*.

SOURCE: "Table 67. Selected Health Conditions and Risk Factors: United States, 1988–1994 through 2005–2006," in *Health, United States, 2009. With Special Feature on Medical Technology*, Centers for Disease Control and Prevention, National Center for Health Statistics, 2010, http://www.cdc.gov/nchs/data/hus/hus09.pdf (accessed March 12, 2010)

can often identify the location of a stroke in the brain from the symptoms and deficits observed during a neurologic examination, even before an imaging study (computed tomography or magnetic resonance imaging) confirms the region of the brain affected. The senses, speech, the ability to understand speech, behavioral patterns, thought, and memory are affected most frequently. The most common effect is for one side of the body to become paralyzed or severely weakened. A loss of sensation or vision as the result of the stroke can result in a loss of awareness of the affected parts, so many stroke victims may forget or "neglect" the parts of the body that are weakened or

FIGURE 5.3

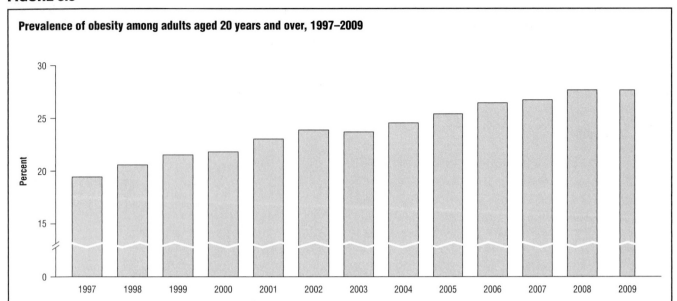

Prevalence of obesity among adults aged 20 years and over, 1997–2009

Notes: Obesity is defined as a body mass index (BMI) of 30 kg/m² or more. The measure is based on self-reported height and weight. Estimates of obesity are restricted to adults aged 20 years and over for consistency with the Healthy People 2010 (3) program. The analyses excluded people with unknown height or weight (about 6% of respondents each year). Beginning with the 2003 data, the National Health Interview Survey (NHIS) transitioned to weights derived from the 2000 census. In this Early Release, estimates for 2000–2002 were recalculated using weights derived from the 2000 census.

SOURCE: "Figure 6.1. Prevalence of Obesity among Adults Aged 20 Years and over: United States, 1997–June 2009," in *Early Release of Selected Estimates Based on Data from the January–June 2009 National Health Interview Survey*, Centers for Disease Control and Prevention, National Center for Health Statistics, December 2009, http://www.cdc.gov/nchs/data/nhis/earlyrelease/200912_06.pdf (accessed December 29, 2009)

paralyzed. Falls, bumping into objects, or dressing only one side of the body tend to result from this sudden lack of awareness.

INCIDENCE OF STROKE DEATHS IS DECLINING. In *Health, United States, 2009*, the NCHS notes that in 2006 stroke was the third-leading cause of death in the United States, following heart disease and cancer, and that 137,119 Americans died of stroke. (See Table 1.9 in Chapter 1.) Lloyd-Jones et al. indicate that each year about 610,000 people suffer a new stroke and 185,000 experience recurrent strokes. The AHA explains in the fact sheet "Older Americans and Cardiovascular Diseases—Statistics" (2010, http://www.americanheart.org/downloadable/heart/1260811877868FS08OLD10.pdf) that 86% of stroke deaths occur in persons age 65 and older.

Lloyd-Jones and his coauthors observe that in 2006, stroke accounted for 1 in every 18 deaths. The death rate for stroke declined by 33.5% between 1996 and 2006, and the actual number of stroke deaths fell by 18.4%. Figure 5.4 shows that the rate of stroke deaths substantially declined from 1950. In *Health, United States, 2009*, the CDC notes that the age-adjusted death rate for stroke declined 76% between 1950 and 2006. In "Women and Cardiovascular Diseases—Statistics" (2010, http://www.americanheart.org/downloadable/heart/1260905040318FS10WM10.pdf), the AHA reports that because women live longer than men, more women die of stroke each year. In 2006 women accounted for 60.2% of stroke deaths in the United States.

The two blood thinners heparin and warfarin are often used to reduce the chance of blood clots and recurrent strokes, even though these drugs pose some risk of bleeding problems. Clinical trials show that the drugs are safe if their use is closely monitored. Another drug, tissue plasminogen activator (tPA), is a "clot-busting drug" approved specifically for fighting strokes. tPA, which became available in 1996, must be administered within three hours after the onset of a stroke. The drug works to stop the swift advance of damage caused by clots shutting off blood flow to the brain, which accounts for four-fifths of strokes. Early detection and immediate treatment are vital for tPA treatment to be optimally effective. Regular, low doses of aspirin have also proved effective in preventing stroke.

REHABILITATION FOR STROKE SURVIVORS. Stroke is a leading cause of serious long-term disability. The AHA asserts that stroke accounts for more than half of all patients hospitalized for acute brain diseases. According to Kate Hardie of the University of Western Australia, Perth, et al. in "Ten-Year Risk of First Recurrent Stroke and Disability after First-Ever Stroke in the Perth Community Stroke Study" (*Stroke*, vol. 35, no. 3, February 5, 2005), the risk of first recurrent stroke is six times greater than the risk of first-ever stroke in the general population of the same age and sex, almost one-half of survivors remain disabled, and one-seventh require institutional care. In "Predicting Recurrent Stroke after Minor Stroke and Transient Ischemic Attack" (*Expert Review of Cardiovascular Therapy*, vol. 7, no. 1, October 2009), Philippe

FIGURE 5.4

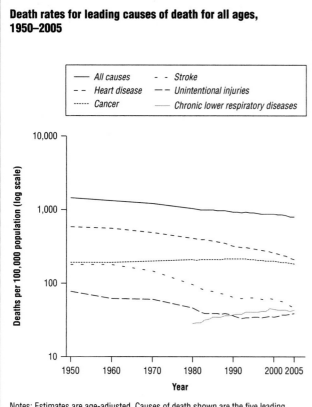

Death rates for leading causes of death for all ages, 1950–2005

Notes: Estimates are age-adjusted. Causes of death shown are the five leading causes of death for all ages in 2005. Starting with 1999 data, causes of death were coded according to International Classification of Diseases (ICD)–10.

SOURCE: "Figure 16. Death Rates for Leading Causes of Death for All Ages: United States, 1950–2005," in *Health, United States, 2008. With Chartbook*, Centers for Disease Control and Prevention, National Center for Health Statistics, 2009, http://www.cdc.gov/nchs/data/hus/hus08.pdf (accessed December 29, 2009)

Couillard et al. of the University of Calgary in Canada explain that the risk of recurrent stroke after even a minor stroke is quite high—10% in the 90 days following the first stroke.

Many survivors lose mental and physical abilities and need expensive, long, and intensive rehabilitation to regain their independence. In some cases independence is not achievable. Stroke can affect most senses and perception, and patients who have had a stroke may find even familiar surroundings incomprehensible. They may be unable to recognize or understand well-known objects or people. The simplest activities become difficult, and depression is a common problem because patients who have had a stroke may feel overwhelmed and develop a sense of despair.

According to Lloyd-Jones et al., the duration of recovery depends on the severity of the stroke. Between 50% and 70% of stroke survivors regain the ability to function independently, whereas 15% to 30% suffer permanent disability. Three months after a stroke, 20% of patients require institutional care. Lloyd-Jones et al.

also note a study of sex differences among first-time stroke patients showed that women suffered more disability than men—33% of women compared with 27% of men had moderate to severe disability when they were discharged from the hospital.

In *Acute Stroke Management* (April 9, 2007, http://www.emedicine.com/neuro/TOPIC9.HTM), Edward C. Jauch of the Medical University of South Carolina et al. explain that according to the Framingham Heart Study (a study of heart health initiated in the town of Framingham, Massachusetts, in 1948 that by 2002 included the grandchildren of the original 5,209 participants), 31% of stroke survivors needed help taking care of themselves, 20% required help walking, and 71% had some type of impaired vocational ability when examined seven years after the occurrence of their strokes. Sixteen percent needed to be institutionalized.

Spontaneous recovery in the initial 30 days after a stroke probably accounts for the highest levels of regained functional ability. However, rehabilitation to reduce dependency and improve physical ability is also vital. The patient's attitude, the skills of the rehabilitation team, and support and understanding from the patient's family all affect the quality of recovery.

High Blood Pressure

Blood pressure is a combination of two forces: the heart pumping blood into the arteries and the resistance of small arteries called arterioles to the flow of blood. The greater the resistance, the greater the pressure needed by the heart to keep the blood moving. The walls of the arterioles are elastic enough to allow for the expansion and contraction caused by the constantly changing rate of blood flow, thus allowing for a steady blood pressure in normal bodies. If the arterioles stay contracted or lose their elasticity as a result of atherosclerosis (commonly known as "hardening of the arteries"), the resistance to blood flow increases and blood pressure rises.

Blood pressure is measured in millimeters of mercury (mm Hg) by an instrument known as a sphygmomanometer. The sphygmomanometer produces two values: the systolic pressure (a measurement of the maximum pressure of the blood flow when the heart contracts or beats) and the diastolic pressure (the minimum pressure of the blood flow between beats). A typical normal range of values may vary, but the more resistance there is to blood flow, the higher the reading. High blood pressure (hypertension) for adults is defined as a systolic pressure equal to or greater than 140 mm Hg and/or a diastolic pressure equal to or greater than 90 mm Hg.

Prehypertension is defined as systolic pressure of 120 mm Hg to 139 mm Hg and diastolic pressure over 80 mm Hg to 89 mm Hg. According to the Agency for Healthcare Research and Quality, in "Prehypertension Accounts for a Substantial Number of Hospitalizations, Nursing Home Admissions, and Premature Deaths" (April 2005, http://www.ahrq.gov/research/apr05/0405RA10.htm), about two-thirds of individuals aged 45 to 64 and 80% of those aged 65 to 74 have prehypertension.

Elevated blood pressure causes the heart to work harder than normal and places the arteries under a strain that might contribute to a heart attack, stroke, or atherosclerosis. When the heart works too hard, it can become enlarged and will eventually be unable to function at maximum pumping capacity.

PREVALENCE OF HYPERTENSION. In "Hypertension Awareness, Treatment, and Control—Continued Disparities in Adults: United States, 2005–2006" (NCHS Data Brief, 2008, http://www.cdc.gov/nchs/data/databriefs/db03 .pdf), Yechiam Ostchega et al. of the CDC's Division of Health and Nutrition Examination Surveys report that in 2005–2006, 29% of all U.S. adults aged 18 years and older were hypertensive (either had blood pressure readings equal to or greater than 140/90 or were taking antihypertensive medication). The prevalence of hypertension was nearly equal between men and women, and an additional 28% of U.S. adults had prehypertension (systolic blood pressure of 120 mm to 139 mm Hg or diastolic blood pressure of 80 mm to 89 mm Hg, and not pharmacologically treated for high blood pressure). More than three-quarters (78%) of hypertensive adults were aware of their condition and more than two-thirds (68%) were taking medication to control it.

Ostchega et al. report that African-Americans were more likely to suffer from hypertension than whites or Mexican Americans in 2005–06. Table 5.1 shows data about hypertension among people 20 years of age and older by race, poverty status, and Hispanic origin. In the period 2003 through 2006 hypertension was more prevalent among African-American males (42.2%) and females (44.1%) than among white males (31.2%) and females (28.3%) or Mexican-American males (24.8%) and females (28.6%).

TREATMENT. In almost all cases, hypertension is treatable. A variety of medications, including diuretics, which rid the body of excess fluid and salt, can lower blood pressure.

Diet and lifestyle changes are also essential to control hypertension. Some people with only mildly elevated blood pressure need only to reduce or eliminate salt in their diet. Blood pressure in overweight or obese people often declines when they lose weight. Heavy drinkers often see improved blood pressure when they abstain from alcohol or drink less. Some people find exercise, stress management techniques, and relaxation therapy helpful. When people are aware of the problem and follow prescribed treatments, hypertension can be controlled and need not be fatal. Patients, however, often stop taking high

blood pressure medication once their hypertension is controlled. This poses a serious danger; it is essential that patients continue to take the medication even if they feel perfectly well.

CANCER

Cancer is a large group of diseases characterized by the uncontrolled growth and spread of abnormal cells. These cells may grow into masses of tissue called tumors. Tumors made up of cells that are not cancerous are called benign tumors. The tumors consisting of cancer cells are called malignant tumors. The dangerous aspect of cancer is that cancer cells invade and destroy normal tissue.

The spread of cancer cells occurs either by a local growth of the tumor or by some of the cells becoming detached and traveling through the blood and lymph systems to start additional tumors in other parts of the body. Metastasis (the spread of cancer cells) may be confined to a region of the body, but if left untreated (and often despite treatment), the cancer cells can spread throughout the entire body, causing death. The rapid, invasive, and destructive nature of cancer makes it, arguably, the most feared of all diseases, even though it is second to heart disease as the leading cause of death in the United States.

What Causes Cancer, Who Gets Cancer, and Who Survives?

Cancer may be caused by both external factors (chemicals, radiation, and viruses) and internal factors (hormones, immune conditions, and inherited mutations). These factors act together or in sequence to begin or promote cancer.

It seems no one is immune to cancer. Because the incidence increases with age, most cases are found among adults in midlife or older. However, in *Health, United States, 2009*, the NCHS reports that in 2006 cancer was the second-leading cause of death in the United States among children aged 5 to 14. (See Table 1.11 in Chapter 1.) The American Cancer Society (ACS) estimates in *Cancer Facts and Figures, 2009* (2009, http://www.cancer.org/downloads/STT/500809web.pdf) that about one out of two men and a little higher than one in three women in the United States will have some type of cancer at some point during their lifetime.

The ACS estimates that in 2009, 1.5 million new cancer cases would be diagnosed and 562,340 people would die of cancer. In the United States cancer causes one out of every four deaths. Although the five-year survival rate for all cancers diagnosed between 1996 and 2004 is 66%, up from 50% in 1975 through 1977, the death rates for many forms of cancer have remained fairly steady since the 1930s. Three exceptions are lung, stomach, and uterine cancer. In the 1930s stomach cancer and uterine cancer had some of the highest death rates, but they have since declined to some of the lowest. Meanwhile, the lung cancer death rate increased dramatically from 1930 up until 1990, especially for men, then began to decline.

The improved rates of survival are largely attributable to earlier diagnosis as well as improved treatment. Just 50 years ago fewer than one out of four patients treated for cancer were still living after five years. Approximately 11.1 million Americans have a history of cancer. Many of these individuals are considered "cured," meaning that there is no evidence of the disease, and survivors have a life expectancy comparable to people who have never had cancer.

Research reveals that long-term survivors of childhood cancers are at an increased risk for subsequent health problems or limitations in physical performance and are likely to have difficulty with certain activities of daily living. In "Limitations on Physical Performance and Daily Activities among Long-Term Survivors of Childhood Cancer" (*Annals of Internal Medicine*, vol. 143, no. 9, November 1, 2005), Kirsten K. Ness of St. Jude Children's Research Hospital et al. analyze data from 11,481 subjects who were diagnosed with cancer before age 21 and survived at least five years. Survivors were 80% more likely than their siblings to report performance limitations and at least four times more likely to describe restricted participation in routine activities including the ability to attend school or work.

The survivors most likely to report performance limitations, restrictions in routine activities, and difficulty attending school or work were those with brain and bone cancers. Not surprisingly, brain cancer survivors were more likely than other survivors to report impairments in performing personal care. Ness et al. observe that even though some treatment for childhood cancers is known to cause functional limitations, the prevalence of these problems and their relationship to cancer type and treatment received remains unclear.

In "Survivors of Childhood Cancer" in the December 2009 issue of *BMJ*, Meriel Jenney of Children's Hospital for Wales, Cardiff, and Gill Levitt of the Great Ormond Street Hospital, London, observe that the numbers of children who survive cancer are increasing but that some may suffer lifelong problems as a result of the disease or its treatment. For example, Jenney and Levitt report that childhood cancer survivors are more likely than their siblings to report heart problems in young adult life.

BEHAVIORAL AND ENVIRONMENTAL RISK FACTORS CONTRIBUTE TO CANCER DEATHS. In "Causes of Cancer in the World: Comparative Risk Assessment of Nine Behavioral and Environmental Risk Factors" (*Lancet*, vol. 366, no. 9,499, November 19, 2005), Goodarz Danaei et al. of the Harvard School of Public Health collaborated with more than 100 scientists around the world in 2001 to estimate mortality for 12 types of cancer linked to certain risk factors. They find that of the 7 million cancer deaths worldwide, 35% were attributable to the nine potentially modifiable behavioral and environmental risk factors: overweight and obesity, low fruit and vegetable intake, physical inactivity, smoking, alcohol use, unsafe sex, urban air pollution, indoor smoke from household use of coal, and contaminated injections in health-care settings.

Worldwide, the nine risk factors caused 1.6 million cancer deaths among men and 830,000 cancer deaths among women. Smoking alone was estimated to have caused 21% of deaths from cancer worldwide. Smoking, which is linked to lung, mouth, stomach, pancreatic, and bladder cancers, is the biggest avoidable risk factor, followed by alcohol and not eating enough fruit and vegetables. In high-income countries these nine risks caused 760,000 cancer deaths; smoking, alcohol, and overweight and obesity were the most important causes of cancer in these nations.

In low- and middle-income regions the nine risks caused nearly 1.7 million cancer deaths; smoking, alcohol consumption, and low fruit and vegetable intake were the leading risk factors for these deaths. The sexual transmission of the human papillomavirus (HPV) is the leading risk factor for cervical cancer in women in low- and middle-income countries, particularly in sub-Saharan Africa and South Asia, mainly because access to cervical cancer screening is limited.

Danaei et al. conclude that "these results clearly show that many globally important types of cancer are preventable by changes in lifestyle behaviors and environmental interventions. To win the war against cancer we must focus not just on advances in biomedical technologies, but also on technologies and policies that change the behaviors and environments that cause those cancers."

In "The Global Burden of Cancer: Priorities for Prevention" (*Carcinogenesis*, November 2009), Michael J. Thun and his colleagues at the ACS observe that despite decreasing cancer death rates in high-resource countries such as the United States, the number of cancer cases and deaths is projected to more than double worldwide during the coming 20 to 40 years. By 2030, it is projected that there will be approximately 26 million new cancer cases and 17 million cancer deaths per year. Thun et al. advocate intensified efforts to control and limit international tobacco use, which is the single largest preventable cause of cancer worldwide and increased availability of vaccines against hepatitis B (HBV) and HPV. (Chronic infection with HPV is associated with cancer of the uterine cervix, the opening of the uterus into the vagina, and chronic infection with HBV is associated with liver cancer.)

The Seven Warning Signs

In "Signs and Symptoms of Cancer" (February 24, 2009, http://www.cancer.org/), the ACS identifies general signs and symptoms that may be associated with cancer, such as fever, unexplained weight loss, fatigue, pain and skin changes such as hyperpigmentation (darker looking skin), jaundice (yellow-tinged eyes and skin), erythema (reddened skin), itching, and excessive hair growth. The ACS also lists the following symptoms or changes as possible signals of cancer and indications to see a physician:

- Change in bowel or bladder habits
- A sore that does not heal
- White patches inside the mouth or white spots on the tongue
- Unusual bleeding or discharge
- Thickening or lump in breast or elsewhere
- Indigestion or difficulty swallowing
- Obvious change in wart or mole
- Persistent cough or hoarseness

Could More Americans Be Saved?

The ACS estimates in "The American Cancer Society Great American Health Check" (2008, http://www.cancer.org/downloads/GAHC/GAHC_Community_Tool_Kit.pdf) that many more lives could be saved with early detection and treatment. Regular screening can detect cancers of the breast, oral cavity, colon, rectum, cervix, prostate, and skin at early stages when treatment is more likely to be successful. Approximately 86% of all patients treated for these kinds of cancers currently survive five years or more. With early detection, the ACS points out that an estimated 95% could survive. For example, protecting skin from sunlight would prevent many of the 1 million skin cancers found annually.

In 2009 the U.S. Preventive Services Task Force (USPSTF) issued new mammogram guidelines for breast cancer screening. The USPSTF calls for screening mammograms every two years beginning at age 50 for women with average risk of breast cancer and advises against teaching women self-examination. The ACS and many other health organizations including the American College of Surgeons (ACoS) and Mayo Clinic continue to recommend an annual screening mammogram beginning at the age of 40. Although there is not yet consensus about when to begin mammography screening or the optimal frequency of screening, there is widespread agreement that mammography screening as well as other cancer screens such as Pap tests to detect changes that could lead to cervical cancer do save lives.

According to Table 5.4, the percent of women aged 40 and older who reported that they had received a mammogram within the past two years rose from 1990 to 2000, then stabilized at about 70% until 2003. In 2005 the percent of women screened for breast cancer dropped to 67%, where it remained through 2008. A higher percentage of women aged 50 to 64 (74.2%) than those aged 40 to 49 (61.5%) reported having had a mammogram within the past two years. Table 5.5 shows that the percentage of women aged 18 and older that reported receiving a Pap (Papanicolaou) test to screen for cervical cancer within the past three years rose until 2000 but by 2008 had fallen slightly to 75.6%.

Cancer among African-Americans

African-Americans are more likely to be diagnosed with cancer and to die from the disease than any other racial or ethnic population. Table 5.6 shows the rate of cancer deaths among African-American males in 2006 was 284.9 per 100,000 compared with 217.9 per 100,000 among white men. According to the ACS, in *Cancer Facts and Figures, 2009*, most of these differences are not likely due to genetics; they are more likely due to social, cultural, behavioral, and environmental factors. Examples of social and economic inequities include a lack of health insurance, transportation, or access to affordable health care that prevents or delays testing and timely treatment.

Gender and Cancer

Men and women are each more prone to certain types of cancer—most obviously, the cancers of the reproductive system, such as ovarian and cervical cancer in women and prostate or testicular cancer in men. Breast cancer also occurs mainly in women, although some men do die from this disease.

Similarly, cancer claims more males than females. In 2006 there were 220.1 cancer deaths per 100,000 males, compared with 153.6 per 100,000 females. (See Table 5.6.) The cancer death rates were higher among males of all ages.

Lung Cancer

The ACS estimates in *Cancer Facts and Figures, 2009* that 219,440 new cases of lung cancer would be diagnosed in 2009. The incidence of lung cancer increased until 1991, after which it declined slightly. The incidence of new cases of lung cancer in men declined from a high of 102.1 per 100,000 in 1984 to 73.2 per 100,000 in 2005.

Lung cancer was estimated to claim 159,390 lives in 2009, accounting for 28% of all cancer deaths. Each year since 1987 more women have died of lung cancer than breast cancer, which had been the leading cause of cancer deaths for women for more than 40 years. For men, lung cancer is also the leading cause of cancer-related deaths.

TABLE 5.4

Use of mammography by selected age groups, selected years 1987–2008

[Data are based on household interviews of a sample of the civilian noninstitutionalized population]

Characteristic	1987	1990	1991	1993	1994	1998	1999	2000	2003	2005	2008
	Percent of women having a mammogram within the past 2 years[a]										
40 years and over, age-adjusted[b,c]	29.0	51.7	54.7	59.7	61.0	67.0	70.3	70.4	69.5	66.6	67.1
40 years and over, crude[b]	28.7	51.4	54.6	59.7	60.9	66.9	70.3	70.4	69.7	66.8	67.6
50 years and over, age-adjusted[b,c]	27.3	49.8	54.3	59.7	60.9	69.0	72.1	73.7	72.4	68.2	70.3
50 years and over, crude[b]	27.4	49.7	54.1	59.7	60.6	68.9	71.9	73.6	72.4	68.4	70.5
Age											
40–49 years	31.9	55.1	55.6	59.9	61.3	63.4	67.2	64.3	64.4	63.5	61.5
50–64 years	31.7	56.0	60.3	65.1	66.5	73.7	76.5	78.7	76.2	71.8	74.2
65 years and over	22.8	43.4	48.1	54.2	55.0	63.8	66.8	67.9	67.7	63.8	65.4
65–74 years	26.6	48.7	55.7	64.2	63.0	69.4	73.9	74.0	74.6	72.5	72.6
75 years and over	17.3	35.8	37.8	41.0	44.6	57.2	58.9	61.3	60.6	54.7	57.9

*Estimates are considered unreliable.
—Data not available.
[a]Questions concerning use of mammography differed slightly on the National Health Interview Survey across the years for which data are shown.
[b]Includes all other races not shown separately, unknown poverty level in 1987, unknown health insurance status, and unknown education level.
[c]Estimates for women 40 years and over are age-adjusted to the year 2000 standard population using four age groups: 40–49 years, 50–64 years, 65–74 years, and 75 years and over. Estimates for women 50 years and over are age-adjusted using three age groups.
[d]The race groups, white, black, American Indian or Alaska Native, Asian, Native Hawaiian or Other Pacific Islander, and 2 or more races, include persons of Hispanic and non-Hispanic origin. Persons of Hispanic origin may be of any race. Starting with 1999 data, race-specific estimates are tabulated according to the 1997 Revisions to the Standards for the Classification of Federal Data on Race and Ethnicity and are not strictly comparable with estimates for earlier years. The five single-race categories plus multiple-race categories shown in the table conform to the 1997 Standards. Starting with 1999 data, race-specific estimates are for persons who reported only one racial group, the category 2 or more races includes persons who reported more than one racial group. Prior to 1999, data were tabulated according to the 1977 Standards with four racial groups and the Asian only category included Native Hawaiian or Other Pacific Islander. Estimates for single-race categories prior to 1999 included persons who reported one race or, if they reported more than one race, identified one race as best representing their race. Starting with 2003 data, race responses of other race and unspecified multiple race were treated as missing, and then race was imputed if these were the only race responses. Almost all persons with a race response of other race were of Hispanic origin.
[e]Percent of poverty level is based on family income and family size and composition using U.S. Census Bureau poverty thresholds. Poverty level was unknown for 11% of women 40 years of age and over in 1987. Missing family income data were imputed for 19%–23% of women 40 years of age and over in 1990–1994 and 34%–38% in 1998–2005.
[f]Health insurance categories are mutually exclusive. Persons who reported both Medicaid and private coverage are classified as having private coverage. Starting with 1997 data, state-sponsored health plan coverage is included as Medicaid coverage. Starting with 1999 data, coverage by the State Children's Health Insurance Program (SCHIP) is included as Medicaid coverage. In addition to private and Medicaid, the insured category also includes military plans, other government-sponsored health plans, and Medicare, not shown separately. Persons not covered by private insurance, Medicaid, SCHIP, public assistance (through 1996), state-sponsored or other government-sponsored health plans (starting in 1997), Medicare, or military plans are considered to have no health insurance coverage. Persons with only Indian Health Service coverage are considered to have no health insurance coverage.
[g]Education categories shown are for 1998 and subsequent years. GED stands for General Educational Development high school equivalency diploma. In years prior to 1998 the following categories based on number of years of school completed were used: less than 12 years, 12 years, 13 years or more.
Notes: Data starting in 1997 are not strictly comparable with data for earlier years due to the 1997 questionnaire redesign.

SOURCE: Adapted from "Table 89. Use of Mammography among Women 40 Years of Age and over, by Selected Characteristics: United States, Selected Years 1987–2008," in *Health, United States, 2008. With Chartbook*, Centers for Disease Control and Prevention, National Center for Health Statistics, 2009, http://www.cdc.gov/nchs/data/hus/hus08.pdf (accessed December 29, 2009)

The main risk factor for lung cancer is cigarette smoking, especially a long history of smoking (20 years or more). In addition, exposure to certain industrial substances, such as asbestos, organic chemicals, and radon, can increase the risk of developing the disease.

Passive, or involuntary or secondhand smoking (inhaling other people's smoke), also increases the risk for nonsmokers. Research shows that the risk to a nonsmoking woman who is married to a smoker is 30% greater than for a woman with a nonsmoking spouse. In "Health Effects of Exposure to Secondhand Smoke" (February 29, 2008, http://www.epa.gov/smokefree/healtheffects.html), the Environmental Protection Agency claims that an estimated 3,000 nonsmokers die each year from secondhand-smoke-induced lung cancer. The agency added secondhand smoke to its list of known carcinogens in 1993.

Early diagnosis of lung cancer is difficult. By the time a tumor is visible on x-rays, it is often in the advanced stages. However, if an individual stops smoking before cellular changes occur, damaged tissues often return to normal. New diagnostic tests such as low-dose helical computed tomography scans, which provide detailed three-dimensional images of the lungs, and laboratory procedures that can detect cancer cells in sputum have demonstrated an ability to diagnose lung cancer earlier than conventional tests, and research to evaluate their effects on survival rates is under way. As of 2010, efforts to detect lung cancer earlier had not yet demonstrated the capacity to reduce mortality from the disease. The treatment options for lung cancer include surgery, radiation therapy, and chemotherapy (anticancer drugs).

Colon and Rectal Cancer

The ACS reports in *Cancer Facts and Figures, 2009* that in 2009 an estimated 106,100 cases of colon cancer and 40,870 cases of rectal cancer would be diagnosed and that an estimated 49,920 people would die of the diseases. The incidence of colorectal cancer has been decreasing since the mid-1980s, from 66.3 cases per 100,000 population in 1985 to 46.4 in 2005.

TABLE 5.5

Use of Pap smears by selected age groups, selected years 1987–2008

[Data are based on household interviews of a sample of the civilian noninstitutionalized population]

Characteristic	1987	1993	1994	1998	1999	2000	2003	2005	2008
	Percent of women having a Pap smear within the past 3 years[a]								
18 years and over, age-adjusted[b, c]	74.1	77.7	76.8	79.3	80.8	81.3	79.2	77.9	75.6
18 years and over, crude[b]	74.4	77.7	76.8	79.1	80.8	81.2	79.0	77.7	75.1
18–44 years	83.3	84.6	82.8	86.8	84.9	83.9	83.6	81.8	—
18–24 years	74.8	78.8	76.6	76.8	73.5	75.1	74.5	70.7	—
25–44 years	86.3	86.3	84.6	89.9	88.5	86.8	86.8	85.7	—
45–64 years	70.5	77.2	77.4	81.7	84.6	81.3	80.6	78.8	—
45–54 years	75.7	82.1	81.9	83.8	86.3	83.6	83.4	81.0	—
55–64 years	65.2	70.6	71.0	78.4	82.0	77.8	76.8	76.0	—
65 years and over	50.8	57.6	57.3	61.0	64.5	60.8	54.9	50.0	—
65–74 years	57.9	64.7	64.9	70.0	71.6	70.1	66.3	61.6	—
75 years and over	40.4	48.0	47.3	50.8	56.7	51.1	42.7	37.5	—

*Estimates are considered unreliable.
—Data not available.
[a]Questions concerning use of Pap smears differed slightly on the National Health Interview Survey across the years for which data are shown.
[b]Includes all other races not shown separately, unknown poverty level in 1987, unknown health insurance status, and unknown education level.
[c]Estimates are age-adjusted to the year 2000 standard population using five age groups: 18–44 years, 45–54 years, 55–64 years, 65–74 years, and 75 years and over. Age-adjusted estimates in this table may differ from other age-adjusted estimates based on the same data and presented elsewhere if different age groups are used in the adjustment procedure.
Notes: Data starting in 1997 are not strictly comparable with data for earlier years due to the 1997 questionnaire redesign.

SOURCE: Adapted from "Table 87. Use of Pap Smears among Women 18 Years of Age and over, by Selected Characteristics: United States, Selected Years 1987–2008," in *Health, United States, 2009. With Special Feature on Medical Technology,* Centers for Disease Control and Prevention, National Center for Health Statistics, 2010, http://www.cdc.gov/nchs/data/hus/hus09.pdf (accessed March 27, 2010)

When colon and rectal cancers are detected early, the ACS indicates that the five-year survival rates are 90%. However, only 40% of such cancers are found at this stage. If the malignancy has spread regionally, the five-year survival rate drops to 64%.

Colon cancer occurs most often in people without any known risk factors. However, people with a family history of polyps in the colon or rectum and people who have suffered from ulcerative colitis and other diseases of the bowel are considered to be at a greater risk for developing the disease. Other significant risk factors may be physical inactivity, obesity, diabetes, smoking, heavy alcohol consumption, and a diet high in fat and low in fiber.

The ACS recommends a variety of screening tests to detect bowel cancer in its early stages. A digital rectal examination, performed by a physician during a routine office visit, is recommended annually for those older than 40 years of age. For people older than age 50, an annual stool test for fecal occult blood (hidden blood) is recommended, along with flexible sigmoidoscopy (examination of the lower colon and rectum using a hollow, lighted tube) every five years or as often as recommended by the physician. The ACS also recommends an imaging procedure called a double-contrast barium enema, which provides a complete radiologic examination of the colon, every five years for people older than 50 and a screening colonoscopy (examination of the entire colon) every ten years or as often as recommended by the physician. Although it is a more costly screening test, some people prefer a virtual colonoscopy, which uses x-rays and computers to produce images of the entire length of the colon.

Despite overwhelming evidence that screening and early detection save lives, many adults do not receive even the simplest of the colon cancer screening tests. The CDC asserts in "Colorectal Cancer Control Program (CRCCP)" (January 28, 2010, http://www.cdc.gov/cancer/colorectal/statistics/screening_rates.htm) that if everyone aged 50 or older had regular screening tests and all precancerous polyps were removed, as many as 60% of deaths from colorectal cancer could be prevented.

The most common treatment for cancer of the bowel is surgery to remove the diseased area, in combination with radiation. A colostomy (an opening in the abdomen to allow for waste elimination) is seldom necessary for patients with colon cancer but may be required for patients with rectal cancer. The ACS reports that few patients with rectal cancer require a permanent colostomy if the cancer is detected in the early stages. Of those who do require a permanent colostomy, most go on to lead normal, active lives. Chemotherapeutic agents used to treat metastatic (spreading) colon and rectal cancer include the drugs oxaliplatin with 5-fluorouracil followed by leucovorin as well as bevacizumab, which blocks the growth of blood vessels to the tumor, and cetuximab and panitumumab, both of which block the effects of hormone-like factors that promote cancer cell growth.

Breast Cancer

Breast cancer is the most common form of cancer among women. According the ACS, in *Cancer Facts and Figures, 2009,* an estimated 192,370 new cases of invasive breast cancer in women and 62,280 new cases of in

TABLE 5.6

Death rates for cancer by sex, age, ethnicity and race, selected years 1950–2006

[Data are based on death certificates]

Sex, race, Hispanic origin, and age	1950[a,b]	1960[a,b]	1970[b]	1980[b]	1990[b]	2000[c]	2001[c]	2002[c]	2003[c]	2004[c]	2005[c]	2006[c]
						Deaths per 100,000 resident population						
All persons												
All ages, age-adjusted[d]	193.9	193.9	198.6	207.9	216.0	199.6	196.0	193.5	190.1	185.8	183.8	180.7
All ages, crude	139.8	149.2	162.8	183.9	203.2	196.5	194.4	193.2	191.5	188.6	188.7	187.0
Under 1 year	8.7	7.2	4.7	3.2	2.3	2.4	1.6	1.8	1.9	1.8	1.8	1.8
1–4 years	11.7	10.9	7.5	4.5	3.5	2.7	2.7	2.6	2.5	2.5	2.3	2.3
5–14 years	6.7	6.8	6.0	4.3	3.1	2.5	2.5	2.6	2.6	2.5	2.5	2.2
15–24 years	8.6	8.3	8.3	6.3	4.9	4.4	4.3	4.3	4.0	4.1	4.1	3.9
25–34 years	20.0	19.5	16.5	13.7	12.6	9.8	10.1	9.7	9.4	9.1	9.0	9.0
35–44 years	62.7	59.7	59.5	48.6	43.3	36.6	36.8	35.8	35.0	33.4	33.2	31.9
45–54 years	175.1	177.0	182.5	180.0	158.9	127.5	126.5	123.8	122.2	119.0	118.6	116.3
55–64 years	390.7	396.8	423.0	436.1	449.6	366.7	356.5	351.1	343.0	333.4	326.9	321.2
65–74 years	698.8	713.9	754.2	817.9	872.3	816.3	802.8	792.1	770.3	755.1	742.7	727.2
75–84 years	1,153.3	1,127.4	1,169.2	1,232.3	1,348.5	1,335.6	1,315.8	1,311.9	1,302.5	1,280.4	1,274.8	1,263.8
85 years and over	1,451.0	1,450.0	1,320.7	1,594.6	1,752.9	1,819.4	1,765.6	1,723.9	1,698.2	1,653.3	1,637.7	1,606.1
Male												
All ages, age-adjusted[d]	208.1	225.1	247.6	271.2	280.4	248.9	243.7	238.9	233.3	227.7	225.1	220.1
All ages, crude	142.9	162.5	182.1	205.3	221.3	207.2	205.3	203.8	201.3	198.4	198.9	196.6
Under 1 year	9.7	7.7	4.4	3.7	2.4	2.6	1.5	2.0	1.7	1.8	2.1	1.8
1–4 years	12.5	12.4	8.3	5.2	3.7	3.0	2.9	2.7	2.8	2.6	2.6	2.5
5–14 years	7.4	7.6	6.7	4.9	3.5	2.7	2.5	2.9	2.8	2.7	2.7	2.5
15–24 years	9.7	10.2	10.4	7.8	5.7	5.1	5.0	4.9	4.6	4.8	4.8	4.6
25–34 years	17.7	18.8	16.3	13.4	12.6	9.2	9.3	9.2	8.9	8.6	8.8	8.6
35–44 years	45.6	48.9	53.0	44.0	38.5	32.7	32.6	31.5	30.8	29.1	28.9	27.4
45–54 years	156.2	170.8	183.5	188.7	162.5	130.9	130.3	128.0	127.4	124.3	121.6	119.0
55–64 years	413.1	459.9	511.8	520.8	532.9	415.8	405.2	399.8	386.8	376.7	369.5	363.6
65–74 years	791.5	890.5	1,006.8	1,093.2	1,122.2	1,001.9	984.6	964.8	931.7	907.6	899.1	870.4
75–84 years	1,332.6	1,389.4	1,588.3	1,790.5	1,914.4	1,760.6	1,727.1	1,711.3	1,695.4	1,662.1	1,649.7	1,631.3
85 years and over	1,668.3	1,741.2	1,720.8	2,369.5	2,739.9	2,710.7	2,613.6	2,491.1	2,413.8	2,349.5	2,319.3	2,248.7
Female												
All ages, age-adjusted[d]	182.3	168.7	163.2	166.7	175.7	167.6	164.7	163.1	160.9	157.4	155.6	153.6
All ages, crude	136.8	136.4	144.4	163.6	186.0	186.2	183.9	183.0	182.0	179.1	178.8	177.6
Under 1 year	7.6	6.8	5.0	2.7	2.2	2.3	1.8	1.6	2.1	1.9	1.5	1.8
1–4 years	10.8	9.3	6.7	3.7	3.2	2.5	2.5	2.4	2.1	2.4	2.0	2.1
5–14 years	6.0	6.0	5.2	3.6	2.8	2.2	2.4	2.4	2.4	2.2	2.2	2.0
15–24 years	7.6	6.5	6.2	4.8	4.1	3.6	3.5	3.6	3.4	3.4	3.3	3.1
25–34 years	22.2	20.1	16.7	14.0	12.6	10.4	10.9	10.2	9.9	9.6	9.1	9.5
35–44 years	79.3	70.0	65.6	53.1	48.1	40.4	41.0	40.0	39.1	37.7	37.5	36.4
45–54 years	194.0	183.0	181.5	171.8	155.5	124.2	122.7	119.8	117.1	113.8	115.8	113.7
55–64 years	368.2	337.7	343.2	361.7	375.2	321.3	311.5	306.0	302.3	293.2	287.4	281.8
65–74 years	612.3	560.2	557.9	607.1	677.4	663.6	652.2	648.5	635.3	627.1	610.9	605.9
75–84 years	1,000.7	924.1	891.9	903.1	1,010.3	1,058.5	1,045.4	1,046.7	1,040.1	1,023.5	1,020.3	1,012.5
85 years and over	1,299.7	1,263.9	1,096.7	1,255.7	1,372.1	1,456.4	1,410.7	1,391.1	1,381.9	1,340.1	1,324.6	1,305.5

TABLE 5.6

Death rates for cancer by sex, age, ethnicity and race, selected years 1950–2006 [CONTINUED]

[Data are based on death certificates]

Sex, race, Hispanic origin, and age	1950[a,b]	1960[a,b]	1970[b]	1980[b]	1990[b]	2000[c]	2001[c]	2002[c]	2003[c]	2004[c]	2005[c]	2006[c]
						Deaths per 100,000 resident population						
White male[e]												
All ages, age-adjusted[d]	210.0	224.7	244.8	265.1	272.2	243.9	239.2	235.2	230.1	224.4	222.3	217.9
All ages, crude	147.2	166.1	185.1	208.7	227.7	218.1	216.4	215.5	213.1	209.9	210.6	208.7
25–34 years	17.7	18.8	16.2	13.6	12.3	9.2	9.3	9.1	8.9	8.6	8.5	8.6
35–44 years	44.5	46.3	50.1	41.1	35.8	30.9	31.3	30.5	29.9	28.2	28.4	26.7
45–54 years	150.8	164.1	172.0	175.4	149.9	123.5	123.6	121.8	119.9	117.5	115.7	113.6
55–64 years	409.4	450.9	498.1	497.4	508.2	401.9	392.1	386.0	375.6	364.9	356.5	352.9
65–74 years	798.7	887.3	997.0	1,070.7	1,090.7	984.3	969.4	954.8	922.7	896.3	889.9	862.0
75–84 years	1,367.6	1,413.7	1,592.7	1,779.7	1,883.2	1,736.0	1,704.6	1,695.3	1,683.6	1,652.7	1,646.2	1,631.3
85 years and over	1,732.7	1,791.4	1,772.2	2,375.6	2,715.1	2,693.7	2,597.6	2,486.8	2,412.1	2,348.9	2,322.7	2,258.3
Black or African American male[e]												
All ages, age-adjusted[d]	178.9	227.6	291.9	353.4	397.9	340.3	330.9	319.6	308.8	301.2	293.7	284.9
All ages, crude	106.6	136.7	171.6	205.5	221.9	188.5	184.5	181.5	178.3	176.2	175.4	172.3
25–34 years	18.0	18.4	18.8	14.1	15.7	10.1	10.5	11.2	10.3	10.0	11.9	10.0
35–44 years	55.7	72.9	81.3	73.8	64.3	48.4	44.6	43.0	41.7	38.4	36.2	36.5
45–54 years	211.7	244.7	311.2	333.0	302.6	214.2	204.8	197.3	207.0	197.0	186.1	182.2
55–64 years	490.8	579.7	689.2	812.5	859.2	626.4	604.2	610.3	583.8	569.2	568.3	542.9
65–74 years	636.5	938.5	1,168.9	1,417.2	1,613.9	1,363.8	1,335.3	1,274.7	1,221.5	1,209.7	1,183.8	1,156.5
75–84 years[f]	853.5	1,053.3	1,624.8	2,029.6	2,478.3	2,351.8	2,290.0	2,223.0	2,144.2	2,087.2	2,017.5	1,979.1
85 years and over	—	1,155.2	1,387.0	2,393.9	3,238.3	3,264.8	3,209.9	2,976.1	2,825.5	2,748.8	2,683.7	2,543.3
American Indian or Alaska Native male[e]												
All ages, age-adjusted[d]	—	—	—	140.5	145.8	155.8	155.3	141.9	139.9	147.1	147.6	135.5
All ages, crude	—	—	—	58.1	61.4	67.0	72.4	70.4	70.3	78.9	82.2	76.1
25–34 years	—	—	—	*	*	*	*	*	*	*	*	*
35–44 years	—	—	—	*	22.8	21.4	22.9	18.9	19.0	18.1	26.9	15.1
45–54 years	—	—	—	86.9	86.9	70.3	77.1	76.1	81.9	86.3	81.7	74.5
55–64 years	—	—	—	213.4	246.2	255.6	256.0	261.4	222.7	268.6	269.1	222.8
65–74 years	—	—	—	613.0	530.6	648.0	673.9	604.9	565.4	642.0	622.2	583.5
75–84 years	—	—	—	936.4	1,038.4	1,152.5	1,093.0	1,069.3	995.2	1,060.0	1,020.7	1,016.8
85 years and over	—	—	—	1,471.2	1,654.4	1,584.2	1,487.5	1,036.3	1,459.1	1,134.1	1,302.6	1,161.0
Asian or Pacific Islander male[e]												
All ages, age-adjusted[d]	—	—	—	165.2	172.5	150.8	147.0	137.9	137.2	136.3	133.0	126.7
All ages, crude	—	—	—	81.9	82.7	85.2	87.0	84.0	84.2	85.9	86.7	84.5
25–34 years	—	—	—	6.3	9.2	7.4	7.1	7.9	7.6	5.9	7.2	6.9
35–44 years	—	—	—	29.4	27.7	26.1	24.8	22.7	21.7	23.6	20.0	19.6
45–54 years	—	—	—	108.2	92.6	78.5	83.9	82.8	77.0	77.2	75.9	70.2
55–64 years	—	—	—	298.5	274.6	229.2	234.8	224.7	196.1	198.7	199.4	197.2
65–74 years	—	—	—	581.2	687.2	559.4	515.1	481.7	498.1	496.8	492.2	459.9
75–84 years	—	—	—	1,147.6	1,229.9	1,086.1	1,095.9	1,012.7	1,056.9	1,021.6	991.4	942.3
85 years and over	—	—	—	1,798.7	1,837.0	1,823.2	1,676.4	1,544.3	1,545.6	1,552.4	1,488.6	1,439.0

TABLE 5.6

Death rates for cancer by sex, age, ethnicity and race, selected years 1950–2006 [CONTINUED]

[Data are based on death certificates]

Sex, race, Hispanic origin, and age	1950 a,b	1960 a,b	1970 b	1980 b	1990 b	2000 c	2001 c	2002 c	2003 c	2004 c	2005 c	2006 c
						Deaths per 100,000 resident population						
Hispanic or Latino male e,g												
All ages, age-adjusted d	—	—	—	—	174.7	171.7	168.2	161.4	156.5	151.2	152.7	143.4
All ages, crude	—	—	—	—	65.5	61.3	62.2	61.2	61.5	60.9	63.0	60.4
25–34 years	—	—	—	—	8.0	6.9	6.3	6.3	6.8	6.4	6.5	6.1
35–44 years	—	—	—	—	22.5	20.1	21.7	18.4	18.2	18.6	17.8	16.0
45–54 years	—	—	—	—	96.6	79.4	81.5	78.4	81.1	77.4	75.9	71.4
55–64 years	—	—	—	—	294.0	253.1	253.5	254.3	246.5	239.0	236.9	224.8
65–74 years	—	—	—	—	655.5	651.2	642.8	622.3	617.6	585.8	603.5	574.8
75–84 years	—	—	—	—	1,233.4	1,306.4	1,258.3	1,190.8	1,163.9	1,174.2	1,161.8	1,098.4
85 years and over	—	—	—	—	2,019.4	2,049.7	1,967.4	1,869.0	1,668.6	1,508.8	1,601.5	1,440.1
White, not Hispanic or Latino male g												
All ages, age-adjusted d	—	—	—	—	276.7	247.7	243.1	239.6	234.6	229.2	227.3	223.4
All ages, crude	—	—	—	—	246.2	244.4	243.4	243.8	241.8	239.2	240.7	239.9
25–34 years	—	—	—	—	12.8	9.7	10.0	9.8	9.4	9.3	9.0	9.3
35–44 years	—	—	—	—	36.8	32.3	32.6	32.5	31.9	29.9	30.5	28.9
45–54 years	—	—	—	—	153.9	127.2	127.3	125.9	123.8	121.9	120.3	118.7
55–64 years	—	—	—	—	520.6	412.0	401.7	395.5	384.8	374.6	366.1	363.4
65–74 years	—	—	—	—	1,109.0	1,002.1	988.2	975.3	942.0	917.5	910.4	883.0
75–84 years	—	—	—	—	1,906.6	1,750.2	1,721.8	1,716.5	1,707.8	1,677.3	1,673.7	1,662.9
85 years and over	—	—	—	—	2,744.4	2,714.1	2,676.8	2,507.7	2,441.7	2,387.1	2,358.3	2,300.2
White female e												
All ages, age-adjusted d	182.0	167.7	162.5	165.2	174.0	166.9	163.9	162.4	160.2	157.0	155.2	153.6
All ages, crude	139.9	139.8	149.4	170.3	196.1	199.4	196.7	195.8	194.6	191.7	191.1	190.1
25–34 years	20.9	18.8	16.3	13.5	11.9	10.1	10.4	9.9	9.4	9.0	8.6	9.1
35–44 years	74.5	66.6	62.4	50.9	46.2	38.2	39.3	38.5	37.3	35.8	36.0	34.9
45–54 years	185.8	175.7	177.3	166.4	150.9	120.1	118.9	115.3	112.1	109.2	110.7	109.5
55–64 years	362.5	329.0	338.6	355.5	368.5	319.7	303.6	303.1	299.8	290.8	284.0	279.1
65–74 years	616.5	562.1	554.7	605.2	675.1	665.6	652.9	650.4	638.9	630.8	616.2	611.5
75–84 years	1,026.6	939.3	903.5	905.4	1,011.8	1,063.4	1,043.8	1,053.1	1,046.3	1,033.1	1,030.5	1,023.0
85 years and over	1,348.3	1,304.9	1,126.6	1,266.8	1,372.3	1,459.1	1,416.7	1,395.1	1,386.5	1,348.9	1,333.6	1,317.5
Black or African American female e												
All ages, age-adjusted d	174.1	174.3	173.4	189.5	205.9	193.8	193.3	190.3	187.7	182.5	179.6	176.1
All ages, crude	111.8	113.8	117.3	136.5	156.1	151.8	152.3	151.7	151.4	148.9	149.1	147.7
25–34 years	34.3	31.0	20.9	18.3	18.7	13.5	13.0	13.3	13.9	13.9	12.6	12.5
35–44 years	119.8	102.4	94.6	73.5	67.4	58.9	57.3	56.2	55.4	54.2	52.5	50.8
45–54 years	277.0	254.8	228.6	230.2	209.9	173.9	168.8	168.2	167.2	160.9	166.3	158.7
55–64 years	484.6	442.7	404.8	450.4	482.4	391.0	390.9	385.4	380.4	369.4	365.4	356.9
65–74 years	477.3	541.6	615.8	662.4	773.2	753.1	748.4	741.1	714.6	706.2	679.6	672.9
75–84 years f	605.3	696.3	763.3	923.9	1,059.9	1,124.0	1,125.0	1,123.1	1,116.9	1,083.6	1,071.9	1,065.3
85 years and over	—	728.9	791.5	1,159.9	1,431.3	1,527.7	1,457.5	1,468.0	1,475.3	1,387.7	1,365.8	1,324.4

TABLE 5.6

Death rates for cancer by sex, age, ethnicity and race, selected years 1950–2006 [CONTINUED]

[Data are based on death certificates]

Sex, race, Hispanic origin, and age	1950[a,b]	1960[a,b]	1970[b]	1980[b]	1990[b]	2000[c]	2001[c]	2002[c]	2003[c]	2004[c]	2005[c]	2006[c]
						Deaths per 100,000 resident population						
American Indian or Alaska Native female[e]												
All ages, age-adjusted[d]	—	—	—	94.0	106.9	108.3	114.1	112.9	105.6	108.6	105.9	108.3
All ages, crude	—	—	—	50.4	62.1	61.3	68.8	71.0	68.2	73.0	73.8	76.8
25–34 years	—	—	—	*		*	*	9.4	*	*	*	*
35–44 years	—	—	—	36.9	31.0	23.7	25.7	23.6	24.3	27.4	23.5	25.4
45–54 years	—	—	—	96.9	104.5	59.7	79.4	80.6	75.7	72.0	85.5	72.8
55–64 years	—	—	—	198.4	213.3	200.9	221.7	202.5	195.8	211.8	201.5	193.8
65–74 years	—	—	—	350.8	438.9	458.3	463.8	473.2	411.2	480.7	475.8	469.8
75–84 years	—	—	—	446.4	554.3	714.0	752.7	703.9	784.4	707.3	701.5	756.8
85 years and over	—	—	—	786.5	843.7	983.2	905.2	1,001.2	686.0	724.6	581.0	684.8
Asian or Pacific Islander female[e]												
All ages, age-adjusted[d]	—	—	—	93.0	103.0	100.7	99.3	95.9	96.7	92.0	94.5	92.2
All ages, crude	—	—	—	54.1	60.5	72.1	74.0	72.6	75.6	73.8	78.1	77.8
25–34 years	—	—	—	9.5	7.3	8.1	8.0	6.4	7.2	6.6	7.7	7.3
35–44 years	—	—	—	38.7	29.8	28.9	25.6	23.6	25.8	24.2	25.1	24.7
45–54 years	—	—	—	99.8	93.9	78.2	82.5	78.5	77.6	77.0	75.4	73.5
55–64 years	—	—	—	174.7	196.2	176.5	167.7	171.2	166.7	159.1	171.3	160.2
65–74 years	—	—	—	301.9	346.2	357.4	373.3	358.1	361.5	344.2	328.1	330.9
75–84 years	—	—	—	522.1	641.4	650.1	633.1	606.4	616.9	578.4	606.8	602.4
85 years and over	—	—	—	800.0	971.7	988.5	929.2	910.1	907.9	872.9	942.0	878.4
Hispanic or Latina female[e, g]												
All ages, age-adjusted[d]	—	—	—	—	111.9	110.8	108.6	106.1	105.9	101.4	101.9	100.4
All ages, crude	—	—	—	—	60.7	58.5	58.7	58.1	59.1	57.7	59.5	59.7
25–34 years	—	—	—	—	9.7	7.8	8.3	7.5	7.4	7.5	7.1	8.5
35–44 years	—	—	—	—	34.8	30.7	29.8	28.4	28.0	25.4	27.0	27.9
45–54 years	—	—	—	—	100.5	84.7	84.2	78.0	80.2	73.5	79.9	78.1
55–64 years	—	—	—	—	205.4	192.5	196.7	179.8	185.9	183.0	172.5	174.4
65–74 years	—	—	—	—	404.8	410.0	394.5	395.6	379.7	380.7	382.5	370.2
75–84 years	—	—	—	—	663.0	716.5	681.2	692.2	702.1	663.6	688.5	665.9
85 years and over	—	—	—	—	1,022.7	1,056.5	1,068.6	1,031.2	1,014.8	937.0	880.4	884.9

TABLE 5.6

Death rates for cancer by sex, age, ethnicity and race, selected years 1950–2006 [CONTINUED]

[Data are based on death certificates]

Sex, race, Hispanic origin, and age	1950[a, b]	1960[a, b]	1970[b]	1980[b]	1990[b]	2000[c]	2001[c]	2002[c]	2003[c]	2004[c]	2005[c]	2006[c]
White, not Hispanic or Latina female[g]						Deaths per 100,000 resident population						
All ages, age-adjusted[d]	—	—	—	—	177.5	170.0	167.2	165.9	163.8	160.9	159.1	157.6
All ages, crude	—	—	—	—	210.6	220.6	218.4	218.5	217.6	215.3	215.1	214.7
25–34 years	—	—	—	—	11.9	10.5	10.7	10.3	9.8	9.3	8.9	9.2
35–44 years	—	—	—	—	47.0	38.9	40.4	39.9	38.6	37.5	37.5	35.9
45–54 years	—	—	—	—	154.9	123.0	121.9	118.7	115.1	112.9	113.9	113.0
55–64 years	—	—	—	—	379.5	328.9	317.3	312.8	308.9	299.8	293.6	288.5
65–74 years	—	—	—	—	688.5	681.0	660.7	667.7	657.6	649.8	634.4	631.3
75–84 years	—	—	—	—	1,027.2	1,075.3	1,064.4	1,068.3	1,062.4	1,052.0	1,049.5	1,044.4
85 years and over	—	—	—	—	1,385.7	1,468.7	1,425.1	1,405.4	1,399.1	1,364.5	1,353.2	1,336.7

—Data not available.

*Rates based on fewer than 20 deaths are considered unreliable and are not shown.

[a]Includes deaths of persons who were not residents of the 50 states and the District of Columbia (D.C.).

[b]Underlying cause of death was coded according to the Sixth Revision of the International Classification of Diseases (ICD) in 1950, Seventh Revision in 1960, Eighth Revision in 1970, and Ninth Revision in 1980–1998.

[c]Starting with 1999 data, cause of death is coded according to ICD-10.

[d]Age-adjusted rates are calculated using the year 2000 standard population. Prior to 2003, age-adjusted rates were calculated using standard million proportions based on rounded population numbers. Starting with 2003 data, unrounded population numbers are used to calculate age-adjusted rates.

[e]The race groups, white, black, Asian or Pacific Islander, and American Indian or Alaska Native, include persons of Hispanic and non-Hispanic origin. Persons of Hispanic origin may be of any race. Death rates for the American Indian or Alaska Native and Asian or Pacific Islander populations are known to be underestimated.

[f]In 1950, rate is for the age group 75 years and over.

[g]Prior to 1997, excludes data from states lacking an Hispanic-origin item on the death certificate.

Notes: Starting with Health, United States, 2003, rates for 1991–1999 were revised based on 2000 census counts. Rates for 2001 and later years were computed using 2000-based postcensal estimates. Age groups were selected to minimize the presentation of unstable age-specific death rates based on small numbers of deaths and for consistency among comparison groups. In 2003, seven states reported multiple-race data. In 2004, 15 states reported multiple-race data. In 2005, 21 states and D.C. reported multiple-race data. In 2006, 25 states and D.C. reported multiple-race data. The multiple-race data for these states were bridged to the single-race categories of the 1977 Office of Management and Budget standards for comparability with other states.

SOURCE: Adapted from "Table 37. Death Rates for Malignant Neoplasms, by Sex, Race, Hispanic Origin, and Age: United States, Selected Years 1950–2006," in Health, United States, 2008. With Chartbook, Centers for Disease Control and Prevention, National Center for Health Statistics, 2009, http://www.cdc.gov/nchs/data/hus/hus08.pdf (accessed December 29, 2009)

situ breast cancer as well as 1,910 new cases of breast cancer in men would be diagnosed in 2009. (In situ, or noninvasive, breast cancer is confined to the milk-ducts or glands, whereas invasive forms of breast cancer spread to surrounding breast tissue.) An estimated 40,610 people were expected to die from breast cancer in 2009. The disease ranks second in terms of cancer deaths in women, after lung cancer.

Both the incidence of breast cancer and deaths from the disease have been declining since 2000. According to the ACS, the declining incidence is due to earlier detection and improved treatment; however, the decline also may in part be attributed to the sharply decreased use of hormone replacement therapy, which has been linked to increased breast cancer risk.

The five-year survival rates for cancers of the breast are encouraging. The ACS reports that if the cancer is localized, the survival rate is 98%—up from 80% in the 1950s. If the cancer is undetected and has spread regionally, however, the survival rate decreases to 84%, and for women whose cancer has spread to distant parts of the body, the survival rate is only 27%.

The precise causes of breast cancer are still unknown. The disease is most common in women older than age 50, and the risks are higher among women with a family history of breast cancer, those who have never had children, and women who gave birth to their first baby after age 30. Other factors that may contribute to increased risk for breast cancer include having a longer-than-average menstrual history (menstruation beginning at an early age and ending late in life), being obese after menopause, consuming alcohol, and eating a high-fat diet.

CHOICES OF TREATMENT. Breast cancer treatment remains a subject of continuing medical debate. If a breast contains cancerous tissue, the patient and her physician have four standard treatment options: surgery, radiation therapy, chemotherapy, or hormone therapy. Treatment choices depend on the location and size of the tumor, the stage of the cancer (whether the cancer has spread within the breast or to other parts of the body affects staging), and the size of the breast. A small, contained tumor can be removed in a procedure commonly called a lumpectomy (removal of the tumor, or "lump") and lymph node dissection (microscopic examination of lymph nodes to detect cancer cells), followed by radiation therapy to the whole breast. If the cancer is more advanced and invasive, removing the breast (mastectomy) and usually the adjoining lymph nodes, combined with chemotherapy or hormone therapy, may be the most effective treatment.

Favorable outcomes for women with early stage breast cancer who undergo breast conserving therapy (lumpectomy, usually with radiation therapy) have been confirmed in many studies. For example, in "Long-Term Outcomes after Breast Conservation Therapy for Early Stage Breast Cancer in a Community Setting" (*Breast Journal*, vol. 12, no. 2, March 2006), Susan A. McClosky et al. of Valley Radiotherapy Associates Medical Group in El Segundo, California, compared cancer survival and recurrence rates of 744 breast cancer patients over the course of eight years and concluded that breast conserving therapy in place of mastectomy was "an accepted option for patients with early stage breast cancer." In *Cancer Facts and Figures, 2009* the ACS confirms that numerous studies have shown that long-term survival rates after lumpectomy plus radiation therapy are similar to survival rates after mastectomy for women whose cancer has not spread.

Some treatments are standard (the treatment used currently), and some treatments are being tested in clinical trials. A clinical trial is a research study designed to help improve already-existing treatments or obtain information about the safety and efficacy of new treatments for patients with cancer. If a clinical trial shows that a new treatment is better than the standard treatment, the new treatment then may become the standard treatment.

Sentinel lymph node (SLN) biopsy is a form of treatment that was tested in two large clinical trials that compared SLN biopsy with conventional axillary lymph node dissection. The trials were conducted by the National Surgical Adjuvant Breast and Bowel Project and the American College of Surgeons Oncology Group—which are networks of institutions and physicians across the country that jointly conduct trials under the sponsorship of the National Cancer Institute. SLN biopsy is a surgical procedure involving the removal of the sentinel lymph node (the first lymph node the cancer is likely to spread to from the tumor) during surgery. Either a radioactive substance or a blue dye (in some cases both) is injected near the tumor. This flows through the lymph ducts to the lymph nodes. The first lymph node to receive the substance or dye is removed for biopsy. If cancer cells are not found, no more lymph nodes may need to be removed. After the SLN biopsy, the surgeon performs a lumpectomy or mastectomy to remove the tumor.

Peer and professionally facilitated support groups are available to help patients deal with the emotional consequences and physical side effects of breast cancer treatment. Significant advances and techniques have made breast reconstruction possible—frequently during or immediately following surgery.

GENETIC RESEARCH. Physicians have known for some time that a predisposition to some forms of breast cancer is inherited. For this reason, physicians have been searching for the gene or genes responsible so that they can test patients and provide more careful monitoring for those at risk. In 1994 doctors identified the BRCA1 gene, and in late 1995 they also isolated the BRCA2 gene.

In the fact sheet "Oophorectomy for Breast Cancer Prevention in Women with BRCA1 or BRCA2 Mutations" (*Future Medicine*, vol. 5, no. 1, January 2009), Kelly A. Metcalfe of the University of Toronto explains that if a woman with a family history of breast cancer inherits a defective form of either BRCA1 or BRCA2, she has an estimated 80% to 90% risk of developing breast cancer. Researchers also think that the two genes are linked to ovarian, prostate, and colon cancer, and BRCA2 likely plays some role in breast cancer in men. Scientists suspect that the two genes may also participate in some way in the development of breast cancer in women with no family history of the disease. In *Cancer Facts and Figures, 2009*, the ACS reports that only 5% to 10% of all cases of breast cancer are attributable to defects in BRCA1 and BRCA2. Variations of other genes also are associated with an increased risk for breast cancer.

According to the Mayo Clinic in "Herceptin: Novel Therapy Targets HER2-Positive Breast Cancer" (October 6, 2007, http://www.riversideonline.com/health_reference/Breast-Cancer/BR00012.cfm), another form of breast cancer, driven by multiple copies of a gene called HER2, causes an estimated 30% of the new cases of the disease in the United States each year. HER2/neu is an aggressive form of cancer that can cause death more quickly than other breast cancers, often within 10 to 18 months after the cancer spreads. The HER2 gene produces a protein on the surface of cells that serves as a receiving point for growth-stimulating hormones.

Trastuzumab, a genetically engineered antibody drug that became available in 1998, increases the benefits of chemotherapy by shrinking tumors and slowing the progression of HER2/neu. By 2010 promising therapies included treatment with the anti-HER2/neu antibody trastuzumab (for patients with high levels of the HER2 protein) and aromatase inhibitors. Clinical trials of trastuzumab in combination with other chemotherapeutic agents were underway in 2009 and 2010. One such study was conducted by Andrew M. Wardley et al. of the Cancer Research UK Department of Medical Oncology at The Christie in Manchester, England. In "Randomized Phase II Trial of First-Line Trastuzumab Plus Docetaxel and Capecitabine Compared with Trastuzumab Plus Docetaxel in HER2-Positive Metastatic Breast Cancer" (*Journal of Clinical Oncology*, December 28, 2009), Wardley and his collaborators find the combination of trastuzumab and docetaxel with or without capecitabine effective therapy for HER2-positive locally advanced or metastatic breast cancer. Many breast tumors are "estrogen sensitive," meaning the hormone estrogen helps them to grow. Aromatase inhibitors help block the growth of these tumors by lowering the amount of estrogen in the body. In 2010 there were three aromatase inhibitors approved by the FDA: anastrozole, exemestane, and letrozole.

Skin Cancer

According to the ACS in *Cancer Facts and Figures, 2009*, more than 1 million unreported cases of basal cell or squamous cell cancers occur annually. The majority will be nonmelanoma types—basal or squamous cell cancers that can be easily cured. The ACS estimates that 68,720 new cases of malignant melanoma, a far more serious form of skin cancer, would be diagnosed in 2009. In *Cancer Incidence and Mortality Rates—United States, 2004* (November 7, 2007, http://progressreport.cancer.gov/appendices_incidence-mortality.asp), the NCI notes that among whites, melanoma more than tripled in incidence from 8.7 per 100,000 in 1975 to 28.1 per 100,000 in 2005.

The ACS reports an estimated 11,590 deaths from skin cancer (8,650 from malignant melanoma) in 2009. Melanoma can spread to other parts of the body quickly, but if it is detected early and properly treated, it is highly curable. The five-year survival rate for a localized malignant melanoma is 99%.

Simple precautions can prevent most skin cancers. According to the ACS, avoiding the sun between 10 a.m. and 4 p.m. (when the ultraviolet rays are the strongest), using sunscreens, and wearing protective clothing decrease the risk of skin cancer considerably.

Prostate Cancer

According to the ACS in *Cancer Facts and Figures, 2009*, an estimated 192,280 American men would be diagnosed with prostate cancer in 2009. Approximately 27,360 men would die from the disease, making it the second-leading cause of cancer death in men, exceeded only by lung cancer. The probability of developing prostate cancer increases with advancing age.

During the late 1980s prostate-specific antigen (PSA) screening became available to test for the disease. This is a blood test that measures a protein made by prostate cells. PSA blood tests are reported in nanograms per milliliter (ng/mL). Results are considered normal if the reading is under 4 ng/mL; borderline results are between 4 and 10 ng/mL; and any reading of more than 10 ng/mL is high. The higher the reading, the more likely prostate cancer is present. However, normal levels increase with age, and older men with higher readings are frequently found to have no prostate cancer. For example, PSA levels greater than or equal to 2.5 ng/mL are considered abnormally high for men younger than age 49, whereas PSA levels greater than or equal to 4.5 are considered abnormally high for men between the ages of 60 and 69 years.

To help detect prostate cancer early, at a stage when it is most likely to be successfully treated, a PSA blood test and a digital rectal examination should be offered once a year to men aged 50 and older with a life expectancy of at least 10 years. African-American men and men who have a first-degree relative who had prostate cancer should begin receiving these tests at age 40 to 45 because they are at a higher risk of developing the disease. The ACS reports that in 2009, two large clinical trials intended to help determine the efficacy of PSA testing were underway.

Prostate cancer may be treated in several ways, depending on the age of the patient, the severity of the cancer, and any other medical conditions the patient may have. Radiation and surgery may be used if the disease is in an early stage. Hormone therapy (which shrinks the tumor, thus relieving pain and other symptoms for a long period), chemotherapy, and radiation may be used alone or in combination if the cancer has spread, and these methods may be effective as supplements to treatments during early stages. "Watchful waiting" (close observation with no treatment) may also be appropriate in patients who are older or who have less aggressive tumors.

A radical prostatectomy is the removal of the prostate and some of the tissue surrounding the gland. This is done when the cancer has not spread outside the gland. Radiation therapy kills cancer cells and shrinks tumors and may be used before or after prostate surgery. Impotence (erectile dysfunction) and urinary incontinence occur slightly more often when radiation is used following surgery. Radiation therapy can also cause damage to the rectum.

Therapy to reduce hormone (testosterone) levels may be prescribed to limit prostate cancer cell growth. Patients may be given drugs such as luteinizing hormone-releasing hormone agonists, which decrease the amount of testosterone in the body, or antiandrogens, which block the activity of testosterone. These cause cancer cells to shrink because testosterone promotes the growth of prostate cancer cells.

Transurethral resection relieves the blockage of urinary flow caused by cancer of the prostate gland. This procedure is often performed to relieve symptoms of urinary obstruction caused by the tumor. Chemotherapy is used to treat prostate cancer if it returns after being treated with other types of treatment. For men who have less aggressive tumors, are older than 70 years of age, or have coexisting illnesses, many physicians will use a watch-and-wait approach before suggesting active treatment.

Because more than 90% of all prostate cancers are detected in the local and regional stages, five-year relative survival rate for patients whose tumors are diagnosed at these stages approaches 100%. The ACS reports that since the mid-1980s, the five-year survival rate for all stages combined has increased from 69% to almost 99%.

RESPIRATORY DISEASES AND LUNG HEALTH

The lungs are especially vulnerable to airborne particles, such as viruses, bacteria, tobacco smoke, pollen, fungi, and air pollution. Workers exposed to certain air-borne hazards—cotton fibers, asbestos, and coal, metal, and silica dust—can also develop serious lung diseases. Pneumoconiosis is the general term for occupationally induced lung diseases.

Asthma

According to the CDC (May 15, 2009, http://www.cdc.gov/nchs/fastats/asthma.htm), in 2006 an estimated 16.4 million American adults had asthma. In *Summary Health Statistics for U.S. Children: National Health Interview Survey, 2008* (August 2009, http://www.cdc.gov/nchs/data/series/sr_10/sr10_244.pdf), the NCHS indicates that asthma is the most common chronic illness among children. In 2008 an estimated 10 million children younger than 18 years of age had ever been diagnosed with asthma and nearly 7 million still had asthma.

People with asthma experience acute attacks of wheezing and shortness of breath. This difficulty in breathing is caused by a sudden narrowing of the bronchial tubes. Usually, it is not life threatening, but asthma often limits activities and can be extremely serious for the very young and the very old.

The incidence of asthma has increased dramatically since the 1980s in the United States and in other industrialized nations as a result of lifestyle changes and living conditions in modern society. Exposure to air pollutants including tobacco smoke, ozone, and diesel exhaust may be contributing to this increased incidence. Indoor exposures to allergens may also contribute to the increase in asthma because many indoor environments have been made more air tight to improve energy efficiency. Other factors implicated in the rise in asthma include the increased incidence of obesity, decreased physical activity, change in diet, decreased exposure to microbes during early life, and increased viral respiratory infections such as those contracted by children in daycare settings. Even though children appear to be the population most at risk, new cases are also occurring in adults, particularly older adults.

RACIAL, AGE, AND GENDER DISPARITIES. The CDC explains in "Healthy Youth! Health Topics: Asthma" (August 14, 2009, http://www.cdc.gov/HealthyYouth/asthma/index.htm) that Puerto Ricans and African-Americans had higher rates of asthma and asthma-related problems than white children in the United States. In 2009 the asthma prevalence rates continued to be highest among African-Americans under 15 years old. (See Figure 5.5.)

Asthma was more prevalent in all children under age 15, and boys were more likely to have asthma than girls. (See Figure 5.6.) However, in all other age groups, the prevalence was higher among females than among males.

CAUSES OF ASTHMA ATTACKS. Even though the specific cause of asthma is not known, the disease appears to be associated with allergic reactions, heredity, and environment.

FIGURE 5.5

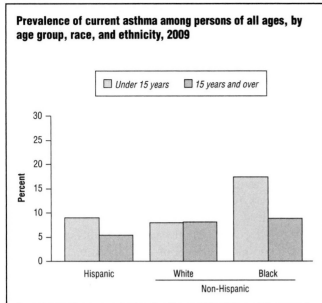

Prevalence of current asthma among persons of all ages, by age group, race, and ethnicity, 2009

Notes: Information on current asthma is self-reported by adults aged 18 years and over. For children under age 18, the information is collected from an adult family member, usually a parent, who is knowledgeable about the child's health. The analyses excluded 20 persons (0.1%) with unknown current asthma status.

SOURCE: "Figure 15.6. Sex-Adjusted Prevalence of Current Asthma among Persons of All Ages, by Age Group and Race/Ethnicity: United States, January–June 2009," in *Early Release of Selected Estimates Based on Data from the January–June 2009 National Health Interview Survey*, Centers for Disease Control and Prevention, National Center for Health Statistics, December 2009, http://www.cdc.gov/nchs/data/nhis/earlyrelease/200912_15.pdf (accessed December 29, 2009)

FIGURE 5.6

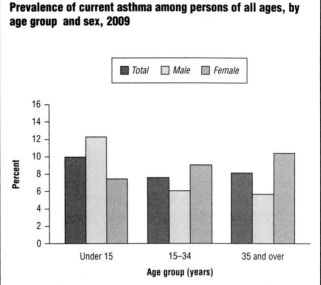

Prevalence of current asthma among persons of all ages, by age group and sex, 2009

Notes: Information on current asthma is self-reported by adults aged 18 years and over. For children under age 18, the information is collected from an adult family member, usually a parent, who is knowledgeable about the child's health. The analyses excluded 20 persons (0.1%) with unknown current asthma status.

SOURCE: "Figure 15.5. Prevalence of Current Asthma among Persons of All Ages, by Age Group and Sex: United States, January–June 2009," in *Early Release of Selected Estimates Based on Data from the January–June 2009 National Health Interview Survey*, Centers for Disease Control and Prevention, National Center for Health Statistics, December 2009, http://www.cdc.gov/nchs/data/nhis/earlyrelease/200912_15.pdf (accessed December 29, 2009)

Many environmental factors can trigger an asthma attack in susceptible individuals. Indoor and outdoor pollution do not cause the disease, but pollutants such as ozone, sulfur dioxide, nitrogen dioxide, and tobacco smoke can trigger an episode of asthma. Allergens such as pollen and dust mites can also provoke asthma attacks.

MANY PATIENTS AND THEIR PHYSICIANS DO MANAGE ASTHMA SYMPTOMS. In "Managing Asthma in Primary Care: Putting New Guideline Recommendations into Context" (*Mayo Clinic Proceedings*, vol. 84, no. 8, August 2009), Michael E. Wechsler of Harvard Medical School notes that many people with asthma are unable to effectively manage their symptoms. Wechsler avers that "many patients overestimate their level of disease control, often tolerating substantial asthma symptoms and having low expectations about the degree of control that is possible." Patients may mistakenly assume that symptoms and resulting reduced activity or disability are the natural and unavoidable consequences of the disease. Wechsler contends that patients and physicians must learn to recognize exactly what constitutes good control of asthma symptoms and advises physicians to adhere to treatment guidelines issued in 2007 by the National Asthma Education and Prevention Program, which emphasize how to manage asthma more effectively with an increased focus on achieving and maintaining good asthma control over time.

Chronic Obstructive Pulmonary Disease

Chronic obstructive pulmonary diseases (COPD; also referred to as chronic lower respiratory diseases), which include emphysema and chronic bronchitis, are progressive diseases that cause obstruction of airflow. The ALA estimates in "Understanding COPD" (2009, http://www.lungusa.org/lung-disease/copd/about-copd/understanding-copd.html) that between 12 and 24 million people suffer from COPD. The National Heart Lung and Blood Institute (NHLBI) reports that in 2006 COPD was the fourth leading cause of death in the United States. (See Figure 5.1.) In *Health, United States, 2009*, the NCHS states that deaths attributable to COPD have increased sharply. In 1980, 56,050 people died from COPD; by 2006 the number had more than doubled to 124,583. (See Table 1.9 in Chapter 1.)

CHRONIC BRONCHITIS. Bronchitis is an inflammation of the lining of the bronchi, tubes that connect the trachea (windpipe) to the lungs. When the bronchi are inflamed and infected, less air is able to flow to and from the lungs, and mucus forms and is coughed up. Acute bronchitis is usually brief in duration and follows the flu or a cold. Chronic bronchitis, however, lingers for months or even years and is characterized by a persistent mucus-producing cough. It is a long-term disease characterized by breathlessness and wheezing.

In 2007, 7.6 million adults over age 18 had chronic bronchitis. (See Table 5.7.) In all age, sex, and race categories, people who smoke cigarettes are far more likely to develop chronic bronchitis than nonsmokers. Workers whose jobs involve inhaling large amounts of dust and irritating fumes are also more likely to get the disease. When air pollution becomes excessive, symptoms intensify.

Antibiotics and bronchodilator drugs are useful treatments, but even more important is the need to eliminate the sources of respiratory irritation. This could mean quitting smoking or avoiding polluted air, fumes, and dust. Chronic bronchitis is often the forerunner of emphysema.

EMPHYSEMA. Emphysema is a severe disease of the lungs that usually develops gradually. The air sacs on the walls of the lungs slowly lose their elasticity, and stale air becomes trapped in the lungs, which become overly inflated. This interferes with the normal exchange of oxygen and carbon dioxide. People with emphysema often feel as if they are drowning in a sea of air. In its late stage, emphysema also affects the heart, because the flow of blood from the lungs is disrupted by changes caused by emphysema. The heart has to pump harder to compensate for the disease and may become enlarged. Death often results from heart failure.

About 3.7 million Americans had emphysema in 2007. (See Table 5.7.) Of these, 2 million were males and 1.7 million were females.

DIABETES

Diabetes is a disease that affects the body's use of food, causing levels of blood glucose (sugar in the blood) to become too high. Normally, the body converts sugars, starches, and proteins into a form of sugar called glucose. The blood then carries glucose to all cells throughout the body. In the cells, with the help of the hormone insulin, the glucose is either converted into energy for use immediately or stored for the future. Beta cells of the pancreas, a small organ located behind the stomach, manufacture insulin. The process of turning food into energy via glucose is important because the body depends on glucose for every function.

Because diabetes deprives body cells of the glucose needed to function properly, several complications can develop to threaten the lives of diabetics further. The healing process of the body is slowed or impaired, and the risk of infection increases. Complications of diabetes include higher risk and rates of heart disease; circulatory problems, especially in the legs, which often are severe enough to require surgery or even amputation; diabetic retinopathy, a condition that can cause blindness; kidney disease that may require dialysis; dental problems; and

problems with pregnancy. Close attention to preventive health care such as regular eye, dental, and foot examinations and tight control of blood sugar levels have been shown to prevent some of the consequences of diabetes. The types of diabetes, populations at risk of developing the disease, complications of diabetes, and measures to prevent the development of diabetes and its complications are described in Chapter 2.

Warning Signs of Prediabetes and Diabetes

To determine whether someone has prediabetes or diabetes, a fasting plasma glucose test or an oral glucose tolerance test (OGTT) is done in the doctor's office. A fasting blood glucose level between 100 and 125 milligrams per deciliter (mg/dL) signals prediabetes, and a fasting blood glucose level of 126 mg/dL or higher signals diabetes. With the OGTT test, a patient fasts overnight, then drinks a solution rich in glucose. The patient's blood glucose level is then measured at one-hour intervals, commonly over two to five hours, to determine the rate at which the glucose is consumed. A diagnosis of prediabetes is made when the two-hour blood glucose level is between 140 and 199 mg/dL, and diabetes is diagnosed when the level is 200 mg/dL or higher.

The symptoms of Type 1 diabetes usually occur suddenly. These include excessive thirst, frequent urination, weight loss, weakness and fatigue, nausea and vomiting, and irritability. The symptoms of Type 2 diabetes generally appear gradually. These may include any of the symptoms seen in Type 1 diabetes, plus recurring infections that are slow to heal, drowsiness, blurred vision, numbness in the hands or feet, and itching.

Prevalence of Diabetes

From 1997 through 2009 there was an increase in diagnosed diabetes among U.S. adults. (See Figure 5.7.) In 2009, 9.3% of the U.S adult population aged 18 and older had been diagnosed with diabetes by a physician or other health professional. The prevalence of diabetes increases with age among men and women, with the highest rates among older adults—people aged 65 and older. In all age categories except for ages 55 to 64, the prevalence of diagnosed diabetes in 2009 was higher in men than in women. (See Figure 5.8.) The prevalence of diagnosed diabetes was higher among non-Hispanic African-Americans (13.5%) and Hispanics (13.1%) than among non-Hispanic whites (7.6%). (See Figure 5.9.)

People who are older than age 40, overweight, have a family history of diabetes, and are physically inactive are at greater risk of developing Type 2 diabetes. There is an increased prevalence of diabetes with age. The percentage of people diagnosed with diabetes over age 65 (20%) is more than six times as high as for people aged 18 to 44 (3%). (See Figure 5.8.)

TABLE 5.7

Frequency of selected respiratory diseases among persons 18 and older, by selected characteristics, 2007

Selected characteristic	All persons 18 years of age and over	Emphysema	Asthma		Hay fever	Sinusitis	Chronic bronchitis
			Ever had	Still has			
			Number in thousands[b]				
Total[c]	223,181	3,736	24,402	16,177	16,882	25,953	7,604
Sex							
Male	107,750	2,018	10,383	5,825	7,120	9,748	2,559
Female	115,431	1,718	14,020	10,351	9,763	16,205	5,045
Age							
18–44 years	110,890	226	12,996	7,996	7,420	10,261	2,515
45–64 years	76,136	1,765	7,895	5,476	7,210	11,154	3,226
65–74 years	19,258	861	2,030	1,591	1,302	2,589	1,050
75 years and over	16,897	884	1,481	1,113	950	1,949	813
Race							
1 race[d]	220,175	3,612	23,824	15,781	16,589	25,555	7,367
White	180,815	3,341	19,997	13,229	14,265	21,990	6,356
Black or African American	26,366	210	2,699	2,025	1,489	2,872	825
American Indian or Alaska Native	2,222	†	*241	*146	*159	186	*58
Asian	10,437	*21	842	357	675	502	121
Native Hawaiian or Other Pacific Islander	335	—	†	†	—	†	†
2 or more races[e]	3,006	*124	579	396	293	398	237
Black or African American, white	378	—	*55	†	†	†	†
American Indian or Alaska Native, white	1,578	*105	247	165	168	271	161
Hispanic or Latino origin[f] and race							
Hispanic or Latino	29,857	262	2,687	1,664	1,471	2,053	503
Mexican or Mexican American	18,309	97	1,331	784	862	1,161	206
Not Hispanic or Latino	193,324	3,474	21,715	14,512	15,411	23,900	7,101
White, single race	153,359	3,093	17,615	11,743	12,933	20,080	5,914
Black or African American, single race	25,574	199	2,585	1,963	1,447	2,817	805
Education[g]							
Less than a high school diploma	29,790	1,288	3,011	2,329	1,876	3,329	1,520
High school diploma or GED[h]	55,363	1,310	5,068	3,560	3,156	6,841	2,353
Some college	50,281	831	5,936	4,168	4,675	7,028	2,042
Bachelor's degree or higher	56,971	268	6,174	3,683	5,883	7,146	1,076
Family income[i]							
Less than $35,000	69,738	2,158	9,084	6,503	4,445	8,488	3,882
$35,000 or more	130,163	1,366	13,457	8,502	11,099	14,967	3,139
$35,000–$49,999	30,247	514	3,062	2,037	2,081	3,104	818
$50,000–$74,999	37,717	531	4,285	2,849	3,021	4,467	992
$75,000–$99,999	24,193	*203	2,167	1,384	2,080	3,055	707
$100,000 or more	38,006	*118	3,943	2,233	3,917	4,340	621
Poverty status[i]							
Poor	23,083	596	3,315	2,454	1,312	2,552	1,244
Near poor	31,110	937	3,853	2,649	2,186	3,491	1,584
Not poor	139,879	1,725	14,644	9,290	11,903	17,229	3,865
Health insurance coverage[k]							
Under age 65 years:							
Private	127,870	777	13,770	8,637	10,814	15,530	2,892
Medicaid	14,440	409	2,497	1,979	1,184	1,834	1,023
Other	6,933	448	927	618	585	1,085	576
Uninsured	36,974	348	3,591	2,212	2,036	2,912	1,226
Age 65 years and over:							
Private	20,872	904	2,044	1,516	1,409	2,496	1,004
Medicaid and Medicare	2,238	178	343	305	152	346	226
Medicare only	10,166	431	798	647	521	1,269	420
Other	2,612	210	312	228	153	404	209
Uninsured	223	†	†	†	†	†	†
Marital status							
Married	124,214	1,870	11,691	7,900	10,319	15,850	3,783
Widowed	14,080	747	1,563	1,243	896	1,870	900
Divorced or separated	24,008	648	3,198	2,224	1,864	3,501	1,177
Never married	45,472	219	5,651	3,236	2,556	3,455	1,057
Living with a partner	14,619	246	2,226	1,524	1,225	1,218	663

Causes of Diabetes

The causes of both Type 1 and Type 2 diabetes are unknown, but a family history of diabetes increases the risk for both types, strongly suggesting a genetic component in the genesis of the disease. Some scientists believe that a flaw in the body's immune system may be a factor

TABLE 5.7

Frequency of selected respiratory diseases among persons 18 and older, by selected characteristics, 2007 [CONTINUED]

Selected characteristic	All persons 18 years of age and over	Selected respiratory conditions[a]					
		Emphysema	Asthma		Hay fever	Sinusitis	Chronic bronchitis
			Ever had	Still has			
		Number in thousands[b]					
Place of residence[l]							
Large MSA	111,359	1,237	11,683	7,474	8,597	11,700	3,031
Small MSA	73,818	1,455	8,724	5,769	5,521	8,903	2,774
Not in MSA	38,004	1,044	3,995	2,934	2,764	5,350	1,799
Region							
Northeast	38,209	456	4,460	2,932	3,163	3,950	1,085
Midwest	53,802	983	6,141	4,245	3,387	6,096	1,733
South	81,850	1,527	8,131	5,464	5,850	11,604	3,346
West	49,320	770	5,670	3,535	4,483	4,303	1,440
Sex and ethnicity							
Hispanic or Latino, male	15,375	90	1,137	515	646	918	190
Hispanic or Latina, female	14,482	172	1,550	1,149	825	1,135	313
Not Hispanic or Latino:							
White, single race, male	73,878	1,703	7,658	4,397	5,521	7,690	1,989
White, single race, female	79,480	1,390	9,956	7,346	7,412	12,390	3,925
Black or African American, single race, male	11,482	102	904	589	514	750	227
Black or African American, single race, female	14,092	*96	1,681	1,373	933	2,067	578

†Estimates with a relative standard error of greater than 50% are replaced with a dagger and are not shown.

*Estimates preceded by an asterisk have a relative standard error of greater than 30% and less than or equal to 50% and should be used with caution as they do not meet the standard of reliability or precision.

—Quantity zero.

[a]Respondents were asked in two separate questions if they had ever been told by a doctor or other health professional that they had emphysema or asthma. Respondents who had been told they had asthma were asked if they still had asthma. Respondents were asked in three separate questions if they had been told by a doctor or other health professional in the past 12 months that they had hay fever, sinusitis, or bronchitis. A person may be represented in more than one column.

[b]Unknowns for the columns are not included in the frequencies, but they are included in the "All persons 18 years of age and over" column. The numbers in this table are rounded.

[c]Total includes other races not shown separately and persons with unknown education, family income, poverty status, health insurance, and marital status characteristics.

[d]In accordance with the 1997 standards for federal data on race and Hispanic or Latino origin, the category "1 race" refers to persons who indicated only a single race group. Persons who indicated a single race other than the groups shown are included in the total for "1 race," but not shown separately due to small sample sizes. Therefore, the frequencies for the category "1 race" will be greater than the sum of the frequencies for the specific groups shown separately. Persons of Hispanic or Latino origin may be of any race or combination of races. This table uses the complete new Office of Management and Budget race and Hispanic origin terms.

[e]The category "2 or more races" refers to all persons who indicated more than one race group. Only two combinations of multiple race groups are shown due to small sample sizes for other combinations. Therefore, the frequencies for the category "2 or more races" will be greater than the sum of the frequencies for the specific combinations shown separately. Persons of Hispanic or Latino origin may be of any race or combination of races.

[f]Persons of Hispanic or Latino origin may be of any race or combination of races. Similarly, the category "not Hispanic or Latino" refers to all persons who are not of Hispanic or Latino origin, regardless of race.

[g]Education is shown only for persons aged 25 years and over.

[h]GED is General Educational Development high school equivalency diploma.

[i]The categories "Less than $35,000" and "$35,000 or more" include both persons reporting dollar amounts and persons reporting only that their incomes were within one of these two categories. The indented categories include only those persons who reported dollar amounts. Because of the different income questions used in 2007, income estimates may not be comparable with those from earlier years.

[j]Poverty status is based on family income and family size using the U.S. Census Bureau's poverty thresholds for the previous calendar year. "Poor" persons are defined as below the poverty threshold. "Near poor" persons have incomes of 100% to less than 200% of the poverty threshold. "Not poor" persons have incomes that are 200% of the poverty threshold or greater. Because of the different income questions used in 2007, poverty ratio estimates may not be comparable with those from earlier years.

[k]Classification of health insurance coverage is based on a hierarchy of mutually exclusive categories. Persons with more than one type of health insurance were assigned to the first appropriate category in the hierarchy. Persons under age 65 years and those age 65 years and over were classified separately due to the prominence of Medicare coverage in the older population. The category "Private" includes persons who had any type of private coverage either alone or in combination with other coverage. For example, for persons age 65 years and over, "Private" includes persons with only private or private in combination with Medicare. The category "Uninsured" includes persons who had no coverage as well as those who had only Indian Health Service coverage or had only a private plan that paid for one type of service such as accidents or dental care.

[l]MSA is metropolitan statistical area. Large MSAs have a population size of 1,000,000 or more; small MSAs have a population size of less than 1,000,000. "Not in MSA" consists of persons not living in a metropolitan statistical area.

SOURCE: J. R. Pleis and J. W. Lucas, "Table 3. Frequencies of Selected Respiratory Diseases among Persons 18 Years of Age and over, by Selected Characteristics: United States, 2007," in "Summary Health Statistics for U.S. Adults: National Health Interview Survey, 2007," *Vital and Health Statistics*, series 10, no. 240, May 2009, http://www.cdc.gov/nchs/data/series/sr_10/sr10_240.pdf (December 30, 2009)

in Type 1 diabetes. Other researchers believe that physical inactivity and the resulting poor cardiovascular fitness is a risk factor for developing diabetes.

In Type 2 diabetes heredity may be a factor, but because the pancreas continues to produce insulin, the disease is considered more of a problem of insulin resistance, in which the body is not using the hormone efficiently. In people prone to Type 2 diabetes, being overweight can set off the disease because excess fat prevents insulin from working correctly. Maintaining a healthy weight and keeping physically fit can usually prevent Type 2 diabetes. To date, Type 1 diabetes cannot be prevented.

"Diabesity" and "Double Diabetes"

The recognition of obesity-dependent diabetes prompted scientists and physicians to coin a new term to describe this condition: diabesity. The term was first used in the 1990s and has gained widespread acceptance. Even though diabesity is attributed to the same causes as

FIGURE 5.7

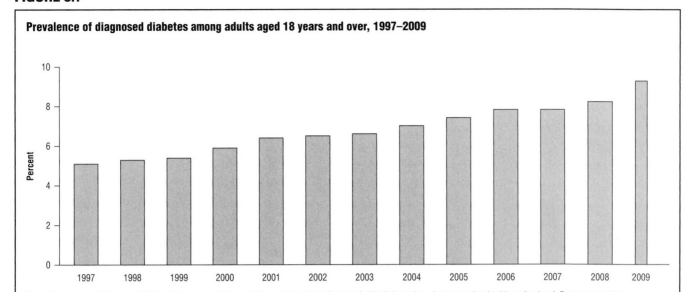

Prevalence of diagnosed diabetes among adults aged 18 years and over, 1997–2009

Notes: Prevalence of diagnosed diabetes is based on self-report of ever having been diagnosed with diabetes by a doctor or other health professional. Persons reporting "borderline" diabetes status and women reporting diabetes only during pregnancy were not coded as having diabetes in the analyses. The analyses excluded persons with unknown diabetes status (about 0.1% of respondents each year). Beginning with the 2003 data, the National Health Interview Survey transitioned to weights derived from the 2000 census. In this early release, estimates for 2000–2002 were recalculated using weights derived from the 2000 census.

SOURCE: "Figure 14.1. Prevalence of Diagnosed Diabetes among Adults Aged 18 Years and over: United States, 1997–June 2009," in *Early Release of Selected Estimates Based on Data from the January–June 2009 National Health Interview Survey*, Centers for Disease Control and Prevention, National Center for Health Statistics, December 2009, http://www.cdc.gov/nchs/data/nhis/earlyrelease/200912_14.pdf (accessed December 29, 2009)

Type 2 diabetes—insulin resistance and pancreatic cell dysfunction—researchers are beginning to link the inflammation associated with obesity to the development of diabetes and cardiovascular disease.

In *Diabesity: The Obesity-Diabetes Epidemic That Threatens America—And What We Must Do to Stop It* (2005), Francine R. Kaufman, director of the Center for Endocrinology, Diabetes and Metabolism at Children's Hospital in Los Angeles, asserts that the diabesity epidemic "imperils human existence as we now know it." Kaufman predicts that based on current trends, more than one-third of American children born in 2000 will develop diabetes in their lifetime. She cautions that unless drastic measures are taken to reverse or slow this trend, by 2020 there will be a 72% increase in the number of diabetics in the United States.

In "Projecting the Future Diabetes Population Size and Related Costs for the U.S." (*Diabetes Care*, vol. 32, no. 12, December 2009), Elbert S. Huang of the University of Chicago et al. predict that between 2009 and 2034, the number of Americans with diagnosed and undiagnosed diabetes will nearly double from 23.7 million to 44.1 million. Huang and his colleagues caution that, "Without significant changes in public or private strategies, this population and cost growth are expected to add a significant strain to an overburdened health care system."

Another recently recognized and increasingly prevalent problem is posed by patients diagnosed with both Type 1 and Type 2 diabetes simultaneously. Called "dou-

ble diabetes," it has been diagnosed in both children and adults. It occurs when children with Type 1 diabetes who rely on insulin injections to control their diabetes gain weight and develop the insulin resistance that is the hallmark of Type 2 diabetes. Among adults who have been diagnosed with Type 2 diabetes, those who fail to respond to conventional treatment have been found to also suffer from the Type 1, insulin-dependent form of the disease.

Even though there are not yet reliable statistics about the prevalence of double diabetes, Dorothy Becker, a pediatric endocrinologist and leading double-diabetes researcher at Children's Hospital of Pittsburgh, estimates in an interview with Lauran Neergaard in "'Double Diabetes' Harder to Detect, Treat" (Associated Press, July 19, 2005), that 25% of children with Type 1 diabetes who are overweight also have symptoms of Type 2 diabetes. Becker posits that overweight people require more insulin to process glucose regardless of whether they are insulin resistant. It may be that obesity overworks the pancreas until it wears out. It is also possible that obesity triggers or hastens the autoimmune destruction, which implies that individuals genetically predisposed to Type 1 diabetes might not develop the disease if they maintained a healthy weight.

In "Double Diabetes: A Mixture of Type 1 and Type 2 Diabetes in Youth" (*Endocrine Involvement in Developmental Syndromes*, vol. 14, 2009), Paolo Pozzilli and Chiara Guglielmi of the University Campus Bio-Medico

FIGURE 5.8

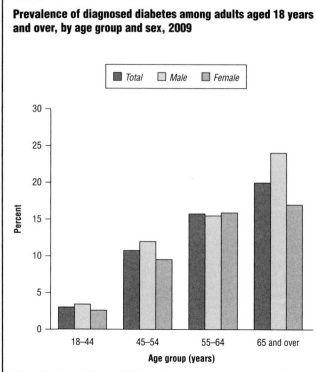

Prevalence of diagnosed diabetes among adults aged 18 years and over, by age group and sex, 2009

Notes: Prevalence of diagnosed diabetes is based on self-report of ever having been diagnosed with diabetes by a doctor or other health professional. Persons reporting "borderline" diabetes status and women reporting diabetes only during pregnancy were not coded as having diabetes in the analyses. The analyses excluded 6 persons (0.1%) with unknown diabetes status.

SOURCE: "Figure 14.2. Prevalence of Diagnosed Diabetes among Adults Aged 18 Years and over, by Age Group and Sex: United States, 2009," in *Early Release of Selected Estimates Based on Data from the January–June 2009 National Health Interview Survey*, Centers for Disease Control and Prevention, National Center for Health Statistics, December 2009, http://www.cdc.gov/nchs/data/nhis/earlyrelease/200912_14.pdf (accessed December 29, 2009)

FIGURE 5.9

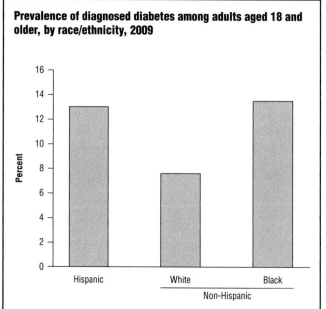

Prevalence of diagnosed diabetes among adults aged 18 and older, by race/ethnicity, 2009

Notes: Prevalence of diagnosed diabetes is based on self-report of ever having been diagnosed with diabetes by a doctor or other health professional. Persons reporting "borderline" diabetes status and women reporting diabetes only during pregnancy were not coded as having diabetes in the analyses. The analyses excluded 6 persons (0.1%) with unknown diabetes status. Estimates are age-sex adjusted using the projected 2000 U.S. population as the standard population and using four age groups: 18–44 years, 45–54 years, 55–64 years, and 65 years and over.

SOURCE: "Figure 14.3. Age-Sex-Adjusted Prevalence of Diagnosed Diabetes among Adults Aged 18 Years and over, by Race/Ethnicity: United States, January–June 2009," in *Early Release of Selected Estimates Based on Data from the January–June 2009 National Health Interview Survey*, Centers for Disease Control and Prevention, National Center for Health Statistics, December 2009, http://www.cdc.gov/nchs/data/nhis/earlyrelease/200912_14.pdf (accessed December 29, 2009)

in Rome, Italy, observe that there was an increase in Type 1 diabetes, especially in children younger than five years old, during the previous decade that may be attributed to changes in environmental factors, rather than to genetic factors. They assert that marked increase in the incidence of Type 2 diabetes in children and adolescents is very likely the result of the increase in obesity and sedentary lifestyle occurring in developed countries. Pozzilli and Guglielmi opine that the "current classification of diabetes should be revised taking into account this new form of diabetes which [is] called double diabetes or hybrid diabetes."

Deaths Resulting from Diabetes

The risk of death among people with diabetes is about twice that of their age peers without diabetes. In 2006 diabetes was the seventh leading cause of death in the United States. (See Figure 5.1.) The NCHS notes in *Health, United States, 2009* that 72,449 people died from it in 2006. (See Table 1.9 in Chapter 1.) In "National Diabetes Statistics, 2007" (June 2008, http://diabetes.niddk

.nih.gov/dm/pubs/statistics/index.htm) the NIDDK asserts that diabetes is likely to be underreported as a cause of death. The institute notes that only about 35% to 40% of the deceased with diabetes had diabetes listed on their death certificates, and just 10% to 15% had it listed as the underlying cause of death.

CHRONIC CONDITIONS LIMIT ACTIVITY

Besides the personal suffering associated with chronic conditions, these diseases generate an enormous financial burden on families of affected individuals and the nation in terms of medical care costs and lost productivity. The NCHS reports in *Health, United States, 2008* (2009, http://www.cdc.gov/nchs/data/hus/hus08.pdf) that in 2005–06 just 3 out of 1,000 adults aged 18 to 44 said their activity was limited by diabetes, compared with 31 out of 1,000 adults aged 55 to 64. Chronic conditions endanger health and compromise wellness, or quality of life. Figure 5.10 shows that among working-age adults, arthritis and musculoskeletal disorders were the activity-limiting chronic conditions named most frequently in 2005–06. Among adults aged 45 to 54, heart and circulatory problems were the second-most common cause of activity

FIGURE 5.10

FIGURE 5.11

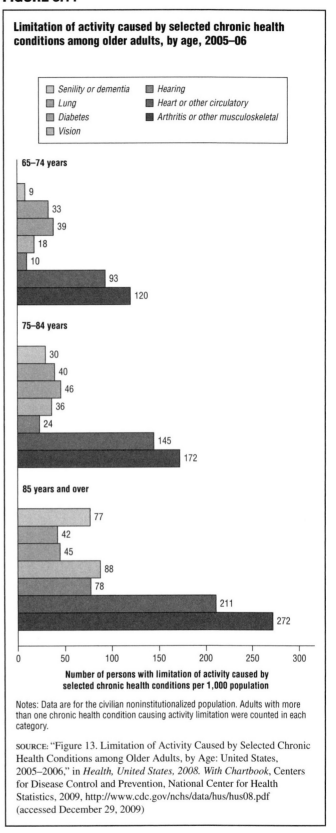

FIGURE 5.10

Limitation of activity caused by selected chronic health conditions among working-age adults, by age, 2005–06

Legend: Mental illness; Fractures or joint injury; Lung; Diabetes; Heart or other circulatory; Arthritis or other musculoskeletal; Mental retardation

18–44 years
13, 5, 4, 3, 6, 18, 6

45–54 years
23, 13, 11, 14, 26, 56, 3

55–64 years
25, 19, 21, 31, 63, 99, 3

Number of persons with limitation of activity caused by selected chronic health conditions per 1,000 population

Notes: Data are for the civilian noninstitutionalized population. Adults with more than one chronic health condition causing activity limitation were counted in each category.

SOURCE: "Figure 12. Limitation of Activity Caused by Selected Chronic Health Conditions among Working-Age Adults, by Age: United States, 2005–2006," in *Health, United States, 2008. With Chartbook*, Centers for Disease Control and Prevention, National Center for Health Statistics, 2009, http://www.cdc.gov/nchs/data/hus/hus08.pdf (accessed December 29, 2009)

FIGURE 5.11

Limitation of activity caused by selected chronic health conditions among older adults, by age, 2005–06

Legend: Senility or dementia; Lung; Diabetes; Vision; Hearing; Heart or other circulatory; Arthritis or other musculoskeletal

65–74 years
9, 33, 39, 18, 10, 93, 120

75–84 years
30, 40, 46, 36, 24, 145, 172

85 years and over
77, 42, 45, 88, 78, 211, 272

Number of persons with limitation of activity caused by selected chronic health conditions per 1,000 population

Notes: Data are for the civilian noninstitutionalized population. Adults with more than one chronic health condition causing activity limitation were counted in each category.

SOURCE: "Figure 13. Limitation of Activity Caused by Selected Chronic Health Conditions among Older Adults, by Age: United States, 2005–2006," in *Health, United States, 2008. With Chartbook*, Centers for Disease Control and Prevention, National Center for Health Statistics, 2009, http://www.cdc.gov/nchs/data/hus/hus08.pdf (accessed December 29, 2009)

limitation. Mental illness also contributed to activity limitation. Not surprisingly, the rate per 1,000 adults with activity limitation resulting from chronic conditions increases with advancing age. (See Figure 5.11.) The NCHS reports in *Health, United States, 2009* that these rates remained steady in 2006–07.

CHAPTER 6
DEGENERATIVE DISEASES

Degenerative diseases are noninfectious disorders characterized by progressive disability. Patients can often live for years with their diseases. Even though they may not die from degenerative diseases, patients' symptoms usually grow more disabling, and they often succumb to complications of their disorders.

ARTHRITIS

The word *arthritis* literally means joint inflammation, and it is applied to more than 100 related diseases known as rheumatic diseases. When a joint (the point where two bones meet) becomes inflamed, swelling, redness, pain, and loss of motion occur. In the most serious forms of the disease, the loss of motion can be physically disabling.

Normally, inflammation is the body's response to an injury or a disease. It causes pain, redness, swelling, and warmth in the inflamed body part. Once the injury is healed or the disease is cured, the inflammation stops. In arthritis, however, the inflammation does not subside. Instead, it becomes part of the problem, damaging healthy tissues. This generates more inflammation and more damage, and the painful cycle continues. The damage can change the shape of bones and other tissues of the joints, making movement difficult and painful.

Types of Arthritis

More than 100 types of arthritis have been identified, but 4 major types affect large numbers of Americans:

- Osteoarthritis—The most common type of arthritis, osteoarthritis generally affects people as they grow older. Sometimes called degenerative arthritis, it causes the breakdown of bones and cartilage (connective tissue attached to bones) and usually causes pain and stiffness in the fingers, knees, feet, hips, and back. The Arthritis Foundation (2010, http://www.arthritis.org/disease-center .php?disease_id=32) notes that osteoarthritis affects about 27 million Americans.

- Fibromyalgia—Fibromyalgia affects the muscles and connective tissues and causes widespread pain, fatigue, sleep problems, and stiffness. Fibromyalgia also causes "tender points" that are more sensitive to pain than other areas of the body. According to the National Fibromyalgia Association (2009, http://www.fmaware.org/site/Page Server?pagename=fibromyalgia_affected), 10 million Americans, mostly women, have this condition.

- Rheumatoid arthritis—Rheumatoid arthritis is caused by a flaw in the body's immune system that results in inflammation and swelling in joint linings, followed by damage to bone and cartilage in the hands, wrists, feet, knees, ankles, shoulders, or elbows. The Arthritis Foundation (2010, http://www.arthritis.org/disease-center.php?disease_id=31) reports that 1.3 million Americans, mostly women, have this form of arthritis.

- Gout—Gout is an inflammation of a joint caused by an accumulation of uric acid (a natural substance) in the joint, usually the big toe, knee, or wrist. The uric acid forms crystals in the affected joint, causing severe pain and swelling. According to the Arthritis Foundation (2010, http://www.arthritis.org/disease-center.php?disease _id=42&df=whos_at_risk), gout affects more men than women and occurs in about 2.1 million Americans.

Other Inflammatory and Autoimmune Disorders

Another less common, but potentially life-threatening, form of rheumatic disease is systemic lupus erythematosus (SLE; also called lupus), an inflammatory autoimmune disease (the immune system mistakenly attacks the body's own tissues) that attacks skin, joints, blood, and the kidneys. The Centers for Disease Control and Prevention (CDC) reports in the fact sheet "Eliminate Disparities in Lupus" (May 14, 2008, http://www.cdc.gov/omhd/AMH/ factsheets/lupus.htm) that SLE occurs more frequently among women than men (9 out of 10 people diagnosed with lupus are women) and that death rates from SLE were

3 times higher for African-Americans than for whites. U.S. prevalence estimates vary from about 322,000 to more than 1.5 million. Generally diagnosed in women of child-bearing age, the symptoms of SLE include:

- Painful or swollen joints, muscle pain, and fatigue

- Fever, weight loss, hair loss, and skin rashes

- Cold, pale, or blue fingers, also known as Raynaud's phenomenon

- Swollen legs or glands

- Nephritis (inflammation of the kidneys)

- Pleuritis (inflammation of the lungs) that may produce chest pain or increase the risk of developing pneumonia

- Myocarditis, endocarditis, or pericarditis (inflammation of the heart valves and the membrane around the heart, respectively) and vasculitis (inflammation of blood vessels)

As with other inflammatory and autoimmune disorders, each patient experiences the disease differently. SLE symptoms ranging from mild to severe flare up and subside throughout the course of the illness. Some patients with SLE also experience headaches, vision disturbances, strokes, or behavior changes as a result of the effects of the disease on the central nervous system.

No cure exists for SLE, and treatment aims to relieve symptoms and reduce the potential for organ damage and complications. Most patients receive corticosteroid hormones, such as prednisone and dexamethasone, which rapidly reduce inflammation. Patients with SLE are also treated with nonsteroidal anti-inflammatory drugs (NSAIDs) such as ibuprofen, naproxen, and indomethacin along with other drugs to combat pain, swelling, and fever. Drugs originally used to treat malaria are also used to treat the fatigue, joint pain, rashes, and pleuritis resulting from SLE.

Many chronic degenerative diseases, especially autoimmune diseases, are thought to occur when a genetically susceptible individual encounters an environmental trigger. For example, some researchers believe viruses may be the environmental triggers for diseases such as SLE and scleroderma, an illness in which skin and internal organs thicken and harden.

Prevalence of Arthritis

Arthritis is a common problem. In "Arthritis Related Statistics" (August 1, 2009, http://www.cdc.gov/arthritis/data_statistics/arthritis_related_stats.htm), the CDC's National Center for Chronic Disease Prevention and Health Promotion reports an estimated 46 million U.S. adults had been diagnosed with arthritis. By 2030 the total number in the United States is expected to increase to 67 million adults suffering from some form of arthritis. (See Table 6.1.)

TABLE 6.1

Projected prevalence of physician-diagnosed arthritis among adults aged 18 and older, selected years 2010–30

Year	Estimated number of adults with doctor-diagnosed arthritis (in 1,000s)		
	Men	Women	Total
2010	20,178	31,701	51,879
2015	21,732	33,993	55,725
2020	23,164	36,244	59,409
2025	24,622	38,587	63,209
2030	26,053	40,915	66,969

SOURCE: Adapted from "Projected Prevalence of Doctor-Diagnosed Arthritis, US Adults Aged 18+ Years, 2005–2030," in *NHIS Arthritis Surveillance—Text Description*, Centers for Disease Control and Prevention, Division of Adult and Community Health, National Center for Chronic Disease Prevention and Health Promotion, October 28, 2009, http://www.cdc.gov/arthritis/data_statistics/national_nhis_text.htm#1 (accessed January 4, 2010)

In *Arthritis: Meeting the Challenge—At a Glance 2009* (2009, http://www.cdc.gov/nccdphp/publications/AAG/pdf/arthritis.pdf), the CDC indicates that arthritis is the leading cause of disability among Americans. Nearly 19 million adults report activity limitations because of arthritis each year. Among all adults aged 18 to 64, about 1 in 20 say they have arthritis that limits their ability to work, and among the 23 million adults in this age group who have arthritis, 1 in 3 experiences work limitations attributable to arthritis. In *Health, United States, 2009* (2010, http://www.cdc.gov/nchs/data/hus/hus09.pdf), the National Center for Health Statistics (NCHS) notes that arthritis and other musculoskeletal diseases account for the greatest proportion of activity limitation among adults of all ages. The Arthritis Foundation observes in "Arthritis Prevalence: A Nation in Pain" (2008, http://www.arthritis.org/media/newsroom/media-kits/Arthritis_Prevalence.pdf) that arthritis is a more frequent cause of activity limitation than heart disease, cancer, or diabetes.

About half of all people older than age 65 will experience some form of arthritis in their lifetime. Even though some think of it as only an older person's disease, it also can affect children. The Arthritis Foundation (2010, http://www.arthritis.org/ja-fact-sheet.php) indicates that arthritis is one of the most common childhood diseases in the United States. About 294,000 children and teenagers suffer from arthritis.

Developments in Arthritis Research

As researchers learn more about inflammation and the body's immune system, they come closer to finding new drugs designed to relieve the pain of arthritis and to block the degenerative process of these diseases. Researchers are investigating ways to improve treatment with the body's own biologic response modifiers (products that modify immune responses). They expect that these substances can be used to control the destructive processes of autoimmune diseases without weakening the whole immune system.

In "Rejuvenating the Immune System in Rheumatoid Arthritis" (*Nature Reviews Rheumatology*, no. 5, October 2009), Cornelia M. Weyand of Emory University et al. explain that in rheumatoid arthritis, the aging process of the immune system is accelerated. This was thought to be a consequence of chronic inflammatory activity. However, recent research indicates that impaired ability to repair damaged DNA may be involved. This finding suggests pursuing treatments aimed at resetting the immune systems of patients with rheumatoid arthritis to help restore their ability to repair broken or defective DNA.

Medications used to help relieve the symptoms of joint pain, stiffness, and swelling include NSAIDs, aspirin, analgesics, and corticosteroids. These drugs may be used in combination. Among recent advances are more effective pain-relief drugs with fewer adverse side effects than those already on the market. One of the problems with NSAIDs, the most widely used class of drugs for osteoarthritis, is the potential to irritate the stomach and cause ulcers.

Disease-modifying antirheumatic drugs (DMARDs) help reduce joint inflammation. They are generally effective but take as long as three to four months to produce benefits, so they must be started as early as possible to help prevent joint deformities and disability later in life. Doctors often prescribe an additional medication, such as a corticosteroid or an NSAID, to help control pain and inflammation while the DMARD starts to work.

DMARDs include low doses of methotrexate, leflunomide, penicillamine, sulfasalazine, auranofin (also known as oral gold), gold sodium thiomalate (also known as injectable gold), minocycline, azathioprine, hydroxychloroquine sulfate (and other antimalarials), cyclosporine, and biologic agents. DMARDs are used most often for rheumatoid arthritis, but some DMARDs can also be used for juvenile rheumatoid arthritis, ankylosing spondylitis, psoriatic arthritis, and SLE.

Other therapies are also available. For instance, patients with moderate to severe rheumatoid arthritis who have not responded well to DMARDs may try Prosorba therapy. This involves drawing blood, separating plasma from red blood cells, and treating plasma through a Prosorba column (a cylinder the size of a soup can that holds a sandlike substance coated with protein A, a molecule that binds antibodies). Treated plasma is then rejoined with red blood cells and returned to the body. Treatments are given in 12 weekly sessions that last about two and a half hours each. The therapy works in much the same way that dialysis does. It cleans and filters the blood, removing the autoantibodies (self-attacking) that may contribute to causing painful, swollen joints. It

may take as long as 16 weeks for patients to feel the benefits of the therapy.

Patients with osteoarthritis of the knee may be treated with joint fluid therapy, called viscosupplements, which act to lubricate the knee joint to relieve pain and ease motion. Along with medical therapies, regular exercise, weight control, and other self-care measures considerably reduce the incidence and effects of the disease.

Setbacks in Arthritis Drug Treatment

In 1999 two new drugs, celecoxib and rofecoxib, were marketed to physicians and directly to consumers as potent painkillers for arthritis sufferers. Celecoxib was marketed as Celebrex and rofecoxib as Vioxx, among other names. The drugs, called COX-2 inhibitors, are NSAIDs and were heralded as superior to conventional NSAIDs because they provided the same pain-relieving effects as aspirin and NSAIDs but with less chance of causing ulcers and intestinal bleeding. Almost immediately after their introduction, the drugs joined the ranks of the nation's best-selling prescription pharmaceuticals.

However, in November 2002, the first reports of increased heart disease among patients taking rofecoxib were issued, and in April 2002 the U.S. Food and Drug Administration (FDA) required Merck, the pharmaceutical company that makes rofecoxib, to inform the public about the potential for increased risk of heart attack and stroke. That same year, a third COX-2 inhibitor, called valdecoxib, was introduced as Bextra.

When the study "Risk of Acute Myocardial Infarction and Sudden Cardiac Death in Patients Treated with COX-2 Selective and Non-selective NSAIDs" (http://www.fda.gov/cder/drug/infopage/vioxx/vioxxgraham.pdf) by David J. Graham of the FDA et al. was released on September 30, 2004, it revealed that patients taking rofecoxib were twice as likely to suffer from stroke and heart attack as nonusers, and Merck withdrew the product from the market. Less than three months later the FDA asked Pfizer to add a "black-box" warning to the valdecoxib label alerting doctors and consumers to the increased risk of heart attack and stroke. (A black-box warning is the strongest form of warning the FDA can request.) One week later, on December 17, 2004, the National Cancer Institute terminated a colon polyp study because of an increased cardiovascular risk in celecoxib users, and the National Institutes of Health (NIH) halted a study of Alzheimer's disease because it suggested that the NSAID naproxen also increased the risk for heart attack or stroke. At the close of 2004 the FDA formally exhorted limited and cautious use of COX-2 inhibitors and traditional NSAIDs.

In February 2005 the FDA reversed its determination about naproxen, stating that it was not associated with increased cardiovascular risk and recommended that COX-2 drugs remain on the market. By April 2005 the FDA asked Pfizer to take valdecoxib off the market, and manufacturers of over-the-counter (nonprescription) and prescription NSAIDs, as well as celecoxib, were asked to change their labels to reflect the increased risk.

Following its withdrawal from the market, more than 20,000 rofecoxib-related lawsuits were filed against Merck by former rofecoxib users or their survivors, alleging harm from the widely marketed drug. CNN/Money correspondent Aaron Smith reports in "Big Win for Merck in Vioxx 2" (November 3, 2005, http://money.cnn.com/2005/11/03/news/fortune500/merck_humeston/index.htm) that Merck lost its first lawsuit—a product liability case—in Texas in the summer of 2005. Merck, however, won its second case in New Jersey. The jury found that Merck did not fail to warn consumers about the safety of rofecoxib, was not guilty of fraud, did not misrepresent the risks of heart attack and stroke when marketing it to physicians, and did not conceal information about the drug.

However, according to the article "Vioxx Trial Loss Raises Merck Strategy Questions" (Associated Press, April 6, 2006), in 2006 a New Jersey jury found Merck liable for two rofecoxib users' heart attacks and awarded one $3 million and the other $1.5 million in damages. Even though the jury asserted that Merck did not adequately warn the users about heart health risks, it also observed that the drug was not the sole factor responsible for the users' heart attacks. In November 2006 a federal judge denied class action status for the 24,000 patient and survivor lawsuits pending against Merck in relation to Vioxx because of the wide variation among the plaintiffs of relative healthiness before taking the drug and of the length of time they took Vioxx (November 22, 2006, http://money.cnn.com/2006/11/22/news/companies/vioxx/index.htm).

Merck also faced legal action from its investors, who accused the company of misleading them about the risks associated with the use of Vioxx. In November 2009 lawyers representing Merck addressed the Supreme Court in an effort to overturn a decision by the 3rd U.S. Circuit Court of Appeals to allow a class-action securities lawsuit brought by the shareholders who lost value after Merck withdrew Vioxx from the market (November 30, 2009, http://www.nj.com/business/index.ssf/2009/11/supreme_court_hears_merck_over.html). Merck's representatives contended that information was made public beginning as early as 2001 that risks associated with Vioxx were becoming evident.

OSTEOPOROSIS

Osteoporosis is a skeletal disorder characterized by compromised bone strength, which predisposes affected individuals to increased risk of fracture. The National Osteoporosis Foundation (NOF; 2008, http://www.nof.org/news/pressroom.htm) defines osteoporosis as about 25% bone loss compared to a healthy young adult, or, on a bone density test, 2.5 standard deviations below normal. Even though some bone loss occurs naturally with advancing age, the stooped posture (kyphosis) and loss of height (greater than one to two inches) experienced by many older adults result from vertebral fractures caused by osteoporosis.

Bone density builds during childhood growth and reaches its peak in early adulthood. From then on, bone loss gradually increases, outpacing the body's natural ability to replace bone. The denser bones are during the growth years, the less likely they will be to develop osteoporosis. Proper diet, especially eating foods rich in calcium and vitamin D long before the visible symptoms of osteoporosis appear, is vitally important.

Osteoporosis worsens with age, leaving its sufferers at risk of broken hips or other bones, curvature of the spine, and other disabilities. According to the NOF in "Fast Facts on Osteoporosis" (2008, http://www.nof.org/osteoporosis/diseasefacts.htm), an estimated 8 million women (non-Hispanic white women are disproportionately affected) and 2 million men have the disease. In severe cases the disease may cause patients to experience spontaneous (without external causes) fractures, generally in the vertebrae of the spine.

The National Institute of Arthritis and Musculoskeletal and Skin Diseases (NIAMS) reports that in addition to the 10 million Americans that have osteoporosis, another 34 million are considered at risk of developing the condition. Like other chronic conditions that disproportionately affect older adults, the prevalence of bone disease and fractures is projected to increase markedly as the population ages. In *Osteoporosis Overview* (May 2009, http://www.niams.nih.gov/Health_Info/Bone/Osteoporosis/default.asp), the NIAMS finds that each year about 1.5 million people suffer an osteoporotic-related fracture, which often leads to a downward spiral in physical and mental health. For example, of the 80,000 men who suffer a hip fracture each year, one-third will die within 12 months of their injury.

The NIAMS notes that one out of every two women over age 50 will have an osteoporosis-related fracture in her lifetime, with the risk of fracture increasing with age. The aging of the population combined with the historic lack of focus on bone health may together cause the number of hip fractures in the United States to double or even triple by 2025.

The 1994 discovery of a gene linked to bone density was hailed as the most important finding in osteoporosis research in a decade. Two forms of the gene, B and b, exist. People with two b genes, one from each parent, have the highest bone density and are the least likely to develop osteoporosis, whereas those with one of each, the Bb genotype, have intermediate bone density. People with two B genes have the lowest bone density and the highest risk of osteoporosis. Women with the BB genotype may be four times as likely to experience hip fractures as those with the bb genotype.

The article "The Latest Osteoporosis Research" (*Arthritis Today*, June 11, 2007) notes that researchers in Iceland identified the bone morphogenetic protein-2 gene in 2003 and that researchers were actively formulating a simple test to identify children at risk for osteoporosis in later life. The test would allow doctors to prescribe an increased intake of calcium, vitamin D, and protein during the growth years for these children, thus preventing or delaying the onset of osteoporosis. Although by early 2010 this specific genetic test was not yet available commercially, it and others continued to be developed and refined. It also is hoped that tests such as these will pave the way for effective gene therapy to prevent osteoporosis.

In December 2009 Interleukin Genetics announced that it is marketing a Bone Health Genetic Test that detects genetic patterns associated with the development of osteoporosis (December 17, 2009, http://www.ilgenetics .com/content/news-events/newsDetail.jsp/q/news-id/209). The test analyzes gene variations that are associated with increased risk for spinal fracture and low bone mineral density.

Table 6.2 summarizes the factors that predispose a person to osteoporosis and fractures. Apart from genetics,

TABLE 6.2

Causes of bone loss and fractures in osteoporosis

Failure to develop a strong skeleton

Genetics—limited growth or abnormal bone composition
Nutrition—calcium, phosphorous and vitamin D deficiency, poor general nutrition
Lifestyle—lack of weight-bearing exercise, smoking

Loss of bone due to excessive breakdown (resorption)

Decreased sex hormone production
Calcium and vitamin D deficiency, increased parathyroid hormone
Excess production of local resorbing factors

Failure to replace lost bone due to impaired formation

Loss of ability to replenish bone cells with age
Decreased production of systemic growth factors
Loss of local growth factors

Increased tendency to fall

Loss of muscle strength
Slow reflexes and poor vision
Drugs that impair balance

SOURCE: "Table 2-2. Causes of Bone Loss and Fractures in Osteoporosis," in *Bone Health and Osteoporosis: A Report of the Surgeon General 2004*, U.S. Department of Health and Human Services, Public Health Service, Office of the Surgeon General, 2004, http://www.surgeongeneral.gov/library/ bonehealth/chapter_2.html (accessed January 5, 2010)

the risk factors—nutrition, physical activity (especially weight-bearing exercise), and choosing not to smoke— are all modifiable.

Treatment of Osteoporosis

The primary goal of therapy is to prevent fractures. Nonpharmacologic (without medicine) preventive measures to help prevent osteoporosis include diet modification (an increase in the intake of calcium and vitamin D), exercise programs, and fall-prevention strategies. These may include such subtle lifestyle changes as wearing rubber-soled shoes for better traction, installing grab bars in bathtubs and showers, and keeping floors clear of clutter. Current pharmacologic (medication) therapies improve bone mass and reduce fracture risk.

At the turn of the 21st century, the typical treatment for postmenopausal women with osteoporosis, or those at risk for the disease, was hormone replacement therapy (HRT), often combined with daily doses of calcium and regular weight-bearing exercise, such as walking and exercising with weights. This treatment slows the advance of the disease and helps prevent fractures and disability. However, serious side effects of HRT were recognized in 2002, including documented increased risks of cardiovascular disease and certain types of cancer, and many women discontinued HRT treatment. For some women at heightened risk for osteoporosis who also have fewer risk factors for cardiovascular disease, HRT remains a treatment option.

One of the goals of osteoporosis treatment is to maintain bone health by preventing bone loss and by building new bone. Another is to minimize the risk and impact of falls because they can cause fractures. Figure 6.1 shows the pyramid of prevention and treatment of osteoporosis. At its base is nutrition, with adequate intake of calcium, vitamin D, and other minerals; physical exercise; and preventive measures to reduce the risk of falls. The second layer of the pyramid involves identifying and treating diseases that can cause osteoporosis, such as thyroid disease. The peak of the pyramid involves drug therapy for osteoporosis.

There are two primary types of drugs used to treat osteoporosis. Antiresorptive agents act to reduce bone loss, and anabolic agents are drugs that build bone. Antiresorptive therapies include use of bisphosphonates, estrogen, selective estrogen receptor modulators, and calcitonin. Antiresorptive therapies reduce bone loss, stabilize the architecture of the bone, and decrease bone turnover. In 2005 the FDA approved two bisphosphonates (alendronate and risedronate) for the prevention or treatment of osteoporosis and one anabolic agent (a synthetic form of parathyroid hormone known as teriparatide that is administered by injection).

FIGURE 6.1

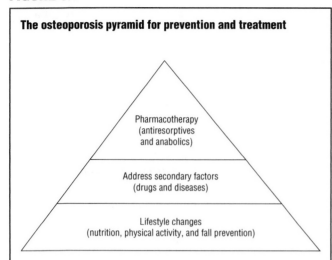

The osteoporosis pyramid for prevention and treatment

Pharmacotherapy
(antiresorptives
and anabolics)

Address secondary factors
(drugs and diseases)

Lifestyle changes
(nutrition, physical activity, and fall prevention)

Note: **The base of the pyramid:** The first step in the prevention and treatment of osteoporosis and the prevention of fractures is to build a foundation of nutrition and lifestyle measures that maximize bone health. The diet should not only be adequate in calcium and vitamin D, but should have a healthy balance of other nutrients. A weight-bearing exercise program should be developed. Cigarette smoking and excessive alcohol use must be avoided. In the older individual, at high risk for fractures, the changes in lifestyle would include a plan not only to maximize physical activity, but also to minimize the risk of falls. The use of hip protectors can be considered in some high-risk patients. Diseases that increase the risk of falls by causing visual impairment, postural hypotension (a drop in blood pressure on standing, which leads to dizziness), or poor balance should be treated. Drugs that cause bone loss or increase the risk of falls should be avoided or given at the lowest effective dose.
The second level of the pyramid: The next step is to identify and treat diseases that produce secondary osteoporosis or aggravate primary osteoporosis. These measures are the foundation upon which specific pharmacotherapy is built and should never be forgotten.
The third level of the pyramid: If there is sufficiently high risk of fracture to warrant pharmacotherapy, the patient is usually started on antiresorptives. Anabolic agents are used in individuals in whom antiresorptive therapy is not adequate to prevent bone loss or fractures.

SOURCE: "Figure 9-1. The Osteoporosis Pyramid for Prevention and Treatment," in *Bone Health and Osteoporosis: A Report of the Surgeon General 2004*, U.S. Department of Health and Human Services, Public Health Service, Office of the Surgeon General, 2004, http://www.surgeongeneral.gov/library/bonehealth/chapter_9.html (accessed January 5, 2010)

EXERCISE IMPROVES BONE HEALTH IN OLDER ADULTS. In "Exercise Effects on Bone Mineral Density: Relationships to Change in Fitness and Fatness" (*American Journal of Preventive Medicine*, vol. 28, no. 5, 2005), Kerry J. Stewart et al. of Johns Hopkins School of Medicine followed 104 older men and women and found that six months of aerobic exercise using a bicycle, treadmill, or stepper, combined with weightlifting, resulted in improved overall fitness and fat loss without significant change (loss) in bone mineral density. Furthermore, the study participants who exercised the hardest and had the greatest increases in aerobic fitness, muscle strength, and muscle tissue showed bone mass increases of 1% to 2%.

Evidence that exercise has measurable positive effects on bone structure continues to mount. In "Short-term Adapted Physical Activity Program Improves Bone Quality in Osteopenic/Osteoporotic Postmenopausal Women" (*Journal of Physical Activity and Health*, vol. 5, no. 6,

November 2008), S. Tolomio et al. of the University of Padova, Italy, found that bone structure in postmenopausal women diagnosed with bone loss was improved by an exercise program that included aerobic, balance, and strength training. Comparing a group of patients who participated in a 20-week supervised exercise program with a control group who did not perform the activities, the researchers found the exercises improved both limb strength and bone density, two factors that contribute to the ability to prevent falls and fractures.

MULTIPLE SCLEROSIS

Multiple sclerosis (MS) is a chronic, degenerative, and often intermittent disease of the central nervous system. It eventually destroys the myelin protein sheaths that surround and insulate nerve fibers in the brain and spinal cord. Myelin is a fatty substance that aids the flow of electrical impulses from the brain through the spinal cord. These nerve impulses control all conscious and unconscious movements. In MS the myelin sheath disintegrates and is replaced by hard sclerotic plaques (scar tissue) that distort or prevent the flow of electrical impulses along the nerves to various parts of the body.

MS usually appears in young adulthood and is common enough to have earned the title "the great crippler of young adults." Many problems and symptoms are associated with the disease, but the major problem is lost mobility. Symptoms can range from mild problems, such as numbness and muscle weakness, to uncontrollable tremors, slurred speech, loss of bowel and bladder control, memory lapses, and paralysis. Even though almost all parts of the nervous system may become involved, the spinal cord is the most vulnerable. Wild mood swings, from euphoria to depression, are another manifestation of the disease. The disease is not fatal in itself, but it weakens its victims and makes them far more susceptible to infection.

The disease is called "multiple" because it usually affects many parts of the nervous system and is often characterized by relapses followed by periods of partial and sometimes complete recovery. Therefore, it is multiple both in how it affects the body and in how often it strikes.

Prevalence

In "Who Gets MS" (2010, http://www.nationalmssociety.org/about-multiple-sclerosis/what-we-know-about-ms/who-gets-ms/index.aspx), the National Multiple Sclerosis Society estimates that 400,000 people in the United States have been diagnosed with MS and that every week approximately 200 people are newly diagnosed with the disease. The disease is most often diagnosed in patients between the ages of 20 and 50 years old. A possible clue to the cause of MS is that it is more common in cold, damp climates. In Europe it is found most often in the Scandinavian countries, the Baltic region, northern Germany, and Great Britain. It is rare in the Mediterranean countries, China, and Japan, and among Native Americans. It is also rare among African-Americans. White females are affected twice as often as males. In the United States most cases are found in the northern areas, and it is more common in Canada than in the southern United States.

Diagnosing MS

The diagnosis of MS is generally made after a thorough history and physical examination and the results of diagnostic tests are evaluated. Among the tests are magnetic resonance imaging (MRI, which provides a detailed view of the brain), spinal tap (to examine spinal fluid for signs of the disease), and evoked potentials (which measure how quickly and accurately a person's nervous system responds to certain stimulation). No single test can detect MS; several must be done and compared.

The neurologic examination for MS focuses on detecting hyperactive (as opposed to normal) reflexes and balance and gait disturbances. An eye examination evaluates damage to the optic nerve. Even though some cases of MS are readily diagnosed by the physician based on the history and physical examination, most physicians confirm the diagnosis using an imaging study to document evidence of plaques in at least two locations of the central nervous system.

Causes of MS

The exact cause of MS is unknown. Many theories about its cause have been proposed—genetics, gender, or exposure to environmental triggers such as viruses, trauma, or heavy metals—but none have been proven. The most widely accepted theory is that damage to myelin results from an abnormal response by the body's immune system. Normally, the immune system defends the body against foreign invaders such as viruses or bacteria. However, in an autoimmune disease the body attacks its own tissue. Some believe that MS is an autoimmune disease in which myelin is attacked.

The National Multiple Sclerosis Society explains in "What Causes MS?" (2010, http://www.nationalmssociety .org/about-multiple-sclerosis/what-we-know-about-ms/what-causes-ms/index.aspx) that like other diseases, genetic factors, in a complex interplay with environmental influences such as exposure to viruses, very likely play a significant role in determining who develops MS. Close relatives of people with MS—such as children, siblings, or a nonidentical twin—have a higher chance of developing the disease than do people without relatives with MS, and an identical twin of someone with MS has a one in four chance of developing the disease. If genes were the sole determinant, an identical twin of someone with MS would have a 100% chance of devel-

oping the disease. Given that the risk is only one out of four reveals that other factors, such as geography, ethnicity, and viral infection, are probably necessary to trigger the development of the disease. Because MS is two to three times more common in women than in men, it is also possible that hormones play a role in determining susceptibility to MS.

Treatment of MS

No known specific treatment halts the disease process. Once nerve fibers have been destroyed, they cannot recover their function. Current methods of treatment include powerful immune-suppressant drugs that often leave patients vulnerable to secondary infections. The best treatment seems to be to build general resistance and avoid fatigue and exposure to extremes in temperature. Physical therapy and psychotherapy are useful in helping patients and their families cope with the limitations caused by MS.

The National Multiple Sclerosis Society recommends that people diagnosed with the disease should start drug treatment immediately, before symptoms worsen. The society recommends prompt treatment with medication, because it appears that patients who receive early treatment will probably have fewer disabling symptoms than those who do not. There are five disease-modifying drugs on the market that slow the progression of the disease.

The drugs to treat MS are beta-interferon products that act by reducing the inflammation of MS lesions and reducing the accumulation of the lesions. All have demonstrated effectiveness in reducing the number and severity of relapses. Two other medications, glatiramer acetate and mitoxantrone, are also used to treat MS. Glatiramer acetate is believed to work by suppressing the immune system's attacks on myelin. Mitoxantrone reduces the activity of white blood cells that attack myelin and is generally prescribed for patients with worsening MS.

Exacerbations, or flare-ups, of the disease, which may last from a few days to several months, are commonly treated with high doses of corticosteroids—drugs used to reduce inflammation. Rehabilitation programs help people with MS maintain fitness and pace themselves to conserve their energy during their daily activities. Other therapy programs provide strategies to maintain independence, to use assistive technologies in the workplace, and to adjust to changes in speech, swallowing, and cognitive abilities.

PARKINSON'S DISEASE

Parkinsonism refers not to a particular disease but to a condition marked by a characteristic set of symptoms affecting more than 1 million people in the United States in 2010, according to the National Parkinson Foundation (2010, http://www.parkinson.org/Parkinson-s-Disease.aspx).

Both men and women are affected, and the probability of developing Parkinson's disease (PD) increases with advancing age. PD usually strikes people older than age 62, but an estimated 10% of patients are 40 years old or younger.

PD is caused by the progressive deterioration of about half a million brain cells in the portion of the brain that controls certain types of muscle movement. These cells secrete dopamine, a neurotransmitter (chemical messenger). Dopamine's function is to allow nerve impulses to move smoothly from one nerve cell to another. These nerve cells, in turn, transmit messages to the muscles of the body to begin movement. When the normal supply of dopamine is reduced, the messages are not correctly sent, and the symptoms of PD appear.

The four early warning signs of PD are tremors, muscle stiffness, unusual slowness, and a stooped posture. Medications can control initial symptoms, but as time goes on they become less effective. As the disease worsens, patients develop tremors, causing them to fall or jerk uncontrollably. (The jerky body movements that patients with PD experience are known as dyskinesias.) At other times rigidity sets in, rendering patients unable to move. About one-third of patients also develop dementia, an impairment of cognition (thought processes).

Treatment of PD

The management of PD is individualized and includes drug therapy and a program that stresses daily exercise. Exercise can often reduce the rigidity of muscles, prevent weakness, and improve the ability to walk.

The main goal of drug treatment is to restore the chemical balance between dopamine and another neurotransmitter, acetylcholine. The standard treatment for most patients is levodopa (L-dopa), which was first approved for use in 1970. L-dopa is a compound that the body converts into dopamine to replace it in the body and help alleviate symptoms. (Without dopamine, signals from the brain cannot "transmit" properly to the body, and movement is impaired.) However, treatment with L-dopa does not slow the progressive course of the disease or even delay the changes in the brain that PD produces, and it may produce some unpleasant side effects because of its change to dopamine before reaching the brain. Simultaneously administering substances that inhibit this change allows a higher concentration of levodopa to reach the brain and considerably decreases the side effects.

Along with L-dopa and other drugs called dopamine agonists, which mimic the action of dopamine, four other classes of drugs are used to treat the symptoms of PD, including anticholinergics, COMT inhibitors, MAO-B inhibitors, and amantadine, which was initially developed as an antiviral drug. Anticholinergics work to relieve tremor and rigidity. COMT inhibitors act by prolonging the effectiveness of a dose of levodopa by preventing its breakdown. MAO-B inhibitors slow the breakdown of dopamine in the brain. Amantadine has demonstrated effectiveness in reducing dyskinesias.

Genetic Link to PD

Two studies, "LRRK2 G2019S as a Cause of Parkinson's Disease in North African Arabs" by Suzanne Lesage of Université Pierre et Marie Curie/INSERM et al. and "LRRK2 G2019S as a Cause of Parkinson's Disease in Ashkenazi Jews" by Laurie J. Ozelius of Mount Sinai Medical School et al. (both published in *New England Journal of Medicine*, vol. 354, no. 4, January 26, 2006), describe the discovery of a single genetic mutation on a gene called leucine-rich repeat kinase 2 (LRRK2) that accounts for as many as 30% of all cases of PD in Arabs, North Africans, and Jews. People with the mutation make an abnormal version of a protein called dardarin (a form of the Basque word for tremor) in which a single amino acid—number 2019—is glycine instead of serine. This finding may help direct the development of a drug to modify the impact of this mutation to prevent or substantially delay onset of the disease.

Subsequent studies, such as "Genomewide Association Study for Onset Age in Parkinson Disease" by Jeanne C. Latourelle of Boston University et al. (*BMC Medical Genetics*, September 22, 2009) have found that in addition to identification of five single genes associated with PD, there are multiple genes and gene interactions that increase susceptibility to PD. The researchers found that the age at which PD begins also is a highly heritable trait. The latter finding is especially important because by identifying genes related to the age of onset, it may be possible to identify ways to delay the onset of PD symptoms. Effectively postponing disease onset could reduce the prevalence of PD.

Experimental Therapies

GENE THERAPY. As of 2010 the use of gene therapy for PD patients remained highly experimental. The therapy entails inserting a beneficial gene into brain cells using technology developed by RheoGene, a University of Pittsburgh Medical Center affiliate, that allows investigators to turn the gene on or off as needed, which is an important safety feature if the proteins it produces have some unanticipated, harmful effect. It also permits investigators to custom-tailor the activity of the gene based on the individual needs of each patient.

One of the genes that is inserted produces glial cell line–derived neurotrophic factor (GDNF), a protein that appears to strengthen brain cells and helps prevent the death of sick cells. In animal studies GDNF has been shown to stop the progression of the disease and perhaps even reverse it. The challenge has been to find a way to deliver the growth factor.

C. W. Christine et al. of the University of California, San Francisco, report in "Safety and Tolerability of Putaminal AADC Gene Therapy for Parkinson's Disease" (*Neurology*, vol. 73, no. 20, October 14, 2009) the promising results of a small (12 patient) clinical trial of gene therapy for PD that proved to be safe, well tolerated, and effective. The therapy subdued overactive circuitry in the brain by stimulating increased production of GABA, an amino acid that acts as an inhibitory neurotransmitter (neurochemical that transmits nerve impulses), without the untoward side effects associated with L-dopa treatment. However, the method of administration was problematical and in some patients produced the undesirable side effect of bleeding in the brain.

ELECTRODE IMPLANTS. Another procedure being tested is the use of electrical implants. Electrodes are surgically implanted in the brain and connected to a battery-operated device, which is also implanted in the body. The device allows patients to "turn off" the tremors that prevent them from performing the activities of daily living such as pouring a glass of milk and feeding themselves. One drawback is that the device's batteries must be surgically replaced every three to five years.

STEM CELL RESEARCH. In August 2001 researchers and patients hoping to benefit from treatment based on this promising area of scientific study were partially relieved when then U.S. President George W. Bush (1946–) announced that federal funds could be used to conduct stem cell research on existing stem cell lines. His decision banned the creation or use of new embryos for federally funded experimental purposes. This meant that federal funds were available to researchers in this field, but it placed significant limits on the scope of research eligible for federal support.

Junying Yu of the Genome Center of Wisconsin/ University of Wisconsin—Madison et al. report in "Induced Pluripotent Stem Cell Lines Derived from Human Somatic Cells" (*Science*, vol. 318, no. 5,858, December 21, 2007) that they created stem cells without using embryos by turning human skin cells into stem cells capable of growing into any of the 220 types of tissue in the body. This accomplishment was seen as not only effectively overcoming any ethical and legal arguments about stem cell research but also improving the odds of clinical efficacy because immune rejection is unlikely to pose a problem using stem cells made this way.

On March 9, 2009, President Barack Obama (1961–) relaxed limitations on stem cell research through an executive order that allowed support for "responsible, scientifically worthy human stem cell research, including human embryonic stem cell research" (August 25, 2009, http://stemcells.nih.gov/policy/2009guidelines.htm). By March 2010, Francis S. Collins, director of the National Institutes of Health, noted in the *Washington Post* that the number of cell lines available for research studies had doubled to 44 and that more than 100 additional lines had been submitted to the NIH for approval (March 20, 2010, http://www.washingtonpost.com/wp-dyn/content/article/2010/03/19/AR2010031904625.html). According to Collins, the new policy "allows for a continually growing number of stem cell lines to be considered and ensures that research will be conducted ethically and responsibly."

The excitement and optimism about human embryonic stem cells centers on the capacity of these cells to renew themselves and develop into specialized cell types. Unlike other cells that have predetermined roles and functions, such as heart or brain cells, stem cells can develop into nearly all the specialized cells of the body—with the potential to replace cells for the nervous system, heart, pancreas, kidneys, skin, bone, or blood.

Research is under way that uses stem cells to treat neurologic disorders by replacing diseased or malfunctioning cells in the brain and spinal cord. The results of this research could have life-changing consequences for people suffering from PD, MS, Alzheimer's disease, and spinal cord injuries. Other research focuses on developing organs and tissues for transplantation, because there is an urgent need for donor organs. Still other investigators are looking at ways to induce stem cells to become insulin-producing cells of the pancreas to treat diabetes.

ALZHEIMER'S DISEASE

Alzheimer's disease (AD) is a progressive, degenerative disease that affects the brain and results in severely impaired memory, thinking, and behavior. The NCHS notes in *Deaths: Final Data for 2006* (April 17, 2009, http://www.cdc.gov/NCHS/data/nvsr/nvsr57/nvsr57_14.pdf) that in 2006 it was the seventh leading cause of death. By 2007, it had outpaced diabetes and had risen to the sixth leading cause of death among American adults. In *2009 Alzheimer's Disease Facts and Figures* (2009, http://www.alz.org/national/documents/report_alzfactsfigures2009.pdf), the Alzheimer's Association, reports that approximately 5.3 million Americans were afflicted with AD in 2009. The overwhelming majority of AD sufferers (5.1 million) were aged 65 and older. The CDC notes that AD usually begins after age 60, and risk goes up with age. About 5% of men and women aged 65 to 74 have Alzheimer's disease, and nearly half of those age 85 and older may have the disease. The number of people with the disease doubles every five years beyond age 65. Women have a higher lifetime risk of developing the disease because, on average, they live longer than men.

The German physician Alois Alzheimer (1864–1915) first described the disease in 1907, after he had cared for a patient with an unusual mental illness. Alzheimer observed anatomic changes in his patient's brain and described them as abnormal clumps and tangled bundles of fibers. Nearly a century later these abnormal findings, now described as amyloid plaques and neurofibrillary tangles, along with abnormal clusters of proteins in the brain, are recognized as the characteristic markers of AD.

Suspected Causes

AD is not a normal consequence of healthy aging, and researchers continue to seek its cause. Like most other chronic, progressive diseases, it is believed to be influenced by some combination of genetic and nongenetic factors.

Researchers have identified different patterns of inheritance, ages of onset (when symptoms begin), genes, chromosomes, and proteins linked to the development of AD. Mutations in at least four genes, situated on chromosomes 1, 14, 19, and 21, and possibly as many as seven genes, are thought to be involved in the disease.

The first genetic breakthrough—the discovery that a mutation in a single gene could cause this progressive neurological illness—was reported in 1991 by Alison Goate et al. of St. Mary's Hospital Medical School, London, in "Segregation of a Missense Mutation in the Amyloid Precursor Protein Gene with Familial Alzheimer's Disease" (*Nature*, vol. 349, no. 6,311, February 21, 1991). The researchers identified the defect in the gene that directs cells to produce a substance called amyloid protein. Goate et al. found that low levels of the brain chemical acetylcholine contribute to the formation of plaques, the hard deposits of amyloid protein that accumulate in the brain tissue of AD patients. In healthy people, these protein fragments are broken down and excreted. Because amyloid protein is found in cells throughout the body, the question is: Why and how does it become a deadly substance in the brain cells of some people and not others?

In 1995 three more genes linked to AD were identified. One gene is linked to a rare, devastating form of early-onset AD, which occurs as early as the third decade of life. When defective, this gene may prevent brain cells from correctly processing a substance called beta amyloid precursor protein. The second gene, which is also involved in the production of beta amyloid, is associated with another early-onset form of AD that strikes people younger than age 65.

According to the National Center for Biotechnology Information (2010, http://www.ncbi.nlm.nih.gov/entrez/dispomim.cgi?id=107741), the third gene, known as apolipoprotein E (apoE), was initially linked to AD in 1993, but its role in the body was not immediately identified. Researchers have since discovered that the gene regulates lipid metabolism within the organs and helps redistribute cholesterol. In the brain, apoE plays a key role in repairing nerve tissue that has been injured. There are three forms (alleles) of the gene: apoE-2, apoE-3, and apoE-4. Between one-half and one-third of all AD patients have at least one apoE-4 gene, whereas only 15.5% of the general population carries an apoE-4 gene. In 1998 Marion R. Meyer of Johns Hopkins University et al. noted in "APOE Genotype Predicts When—Not Whether—One Is Predisposed to Develop Alzheimer Disease" (*Nature Genetics*, vol. 19, no. 4, August 1998) that the apoE-4 gene does not determine whether an individual will develop the disease; instead, it appears to affect when AD will strike—the age when AD symptoms are likely to begin. The National Institute on Aging confirms that while this gene occurs in 40% of people who develop late-onset AD, one-third of people with AD do not have the form of apoE-4 gene associated with AD (2010, http://www.nia.nih.gov/Alzheimers/Alzheimers Information/Causes/).

Also in 1998, Deborah Blacker of Harvard Medical School et al. found in "Alpha-2 Macroglobulin Is Genetically Associated with Alzheimer Disease" (*Nature Genetics*, vol. 19, no. 4, August 1998) that A2M-2, another gene variant, appears to affect whether a person will develop AD. An estimated one-third of Americans may carry this gene, potentially tripling their risk of developing late-onset AD, compared to their siblings with the normal version of the A2M gene. Science writer Misia Landau of Harvard Medical School reports in "Late-Onset Alzheimer's Gene Suggests Interplay of Genes Determines Timing and Risk of Disease" (*Focus*, August 14, 1998) that the discovery of A2M-2 suggests that developing a drug that mimics the A2M gene's normal function might help prevent the development of some cases of AD in genetically susceptible people.

Additional genes related to AD risk may be identified by a genome-wide association study, which rapidly scans markers across the genomes (complete sets of deoxyribonucleic acid [DNA]) of many people to detect genetic variations associated with a particular disease.

Symptoms of AD

AD begins slowly. The symptoms include difficulty with memory and a loss of cognition. The patient with AD may also experience confusion; language problems, such as trouble finding words; impaired judgment; disorientation in place and time; and changes in mood, behavior, and personality. How quickly these changes occur varies from person to person, but eventually the disease leaves its victims unable to care for themselves. In their terminal stages, patients with AD require care 24 hours a day. They no longer recognize family members or themselves, and they need help with daily activities such as eating, dressing, bathing, and using the toilet. Eventually, they may become incontinent, blind, and unable to communicate. Finally, their bodies may "forget" how to breathe or make the heart beat. Many patients die from pneumonia.

Testing for AD

A complete physical, psychiatric, and neurologic evaluation can usually produce a diagnosis of AD that is about 90% accurate. For many years the only sure way to diagnose the disease was to examine brain tissue under a microscope, which was not possible while the AD victim was still alive. An autopsy of someone who has died of AD reveals a characteristic pattern that is the hallmark of the disease: tangles of fibers (neurofibrillary tangles) and clusters of degenerated nerve endings (neuritic plaques) in areas of the brain that are crucial for memory and intellect. Also, the cortex of the brain is shrunken.

In October 2000 John C. Mazziotta of the UCLA School of Medicine reported in "Window on the Brain" (*Archives of Neurology*, vol. 57, no. 10) that the use of MRI techniques could measure the volume of brain tissue in areas of the brain used for memory, organizational ability, and planning. In addition, the use of these measurements could accurately identify people with AD and predict which people would develop AD. That same year, in "Using Serial Registered Brain Magnetic Resonance Imaging to Measure Disease Progression in Alzheimer Disease" (*Archives of Neurology*, vol. 57, no. 3, March 2000), Nick C. Fox et al. of the Institute of Neurology, London, reported using MRI to identify parts of the brain affected by AD before symptoms appear and measure brain atrophy to monitor the progression of AD.

In 2005 Dimitra G. Georganopoulou et al. of Northwestern University announced in "Nanoparticle-Based Detection in Cerebral Spinal Fluid of a Soluble Pathogenic Biomarker for Alzheimer's Disease" (*Proceedings of the National Academy of Sciences*, vol. 102, no. 7, February 15, 2005) the development of yet another diagnostic test that detects small amounts of protein in spinal fluid. Called a bio-barcode assay, the test is as much as a million times more sensitive than other tests. Originally used to identify a marker for prostate cancer, the test is used to detect a protein in the brain called amyloid-beta-derived diffusible ligand (ADDL). ADDLs are small soluble proteins. To detect them the researchers used nanoscale particles that had antibodies specific to ADDL.

In "Finding Alzheimer's before a Mind Fails" (*New York Times*, December 26, 2007), Denise Grady reports on a test that uses a special type of dye called Pittsburgh Compound B that enables positron emission tomography scans (imaging studies) to identify amyloid deposits in the brain. Such testing can help establish the diagnosis by distinguishing Alzheimer's from other kinds of dementia and can help physicians monitor the progress of the disease and the effects of drug treatment.

In 2009 a new test debuted that accurately detects AD in its earliest stages, before the onset of memory problems and other symptoms of cognitive impairment.

In "Cerebrospinal Fluid Biomarker Signature in Alzheimer's Disease Neuroimaging Initiative Subjects" (*Annals of Neurology*, vol. 65, no. 4, April 2009), Leslie M. Shaw et al. of the University of Pennsylvania School of Medicine explain that the test measures the concentration of specific biomarkers, in this case proteins (tau protein and amyloid beta42 polypeptide) in spinal fluid that can indicate AD. Shaw and his coauthors report that subjects with low concentrations of amyloid beta42 and high levels of tau in their spinal fluid were more likely to develop AD. The test had an 87% accuracy rate when predicting which subjects would be diagnosed with AD.

The results of research published in "Pittsburgh Compound B Imaging and Prediction of Progression from Cognitive Normality to Symptomatic Alzheimer's Disease" (*Archives of Neurology*, vol. 66, no. 12, December 14, 2009) suggest that people with no symptoms of dementia may be at risk for developing AD if they have abnormal levels of beta-amyloid. A study conducted by John C. Morris et al. of the Alzheimer's Disease Research Center in St. Louis, Missouri, used imaging studies including PET scans and MRI to detect levels of beta-amyloid protein in the living brain and measure brain volume. Morris and his collaborators find that the level of beta-amyloid is associated with shrinkage in many parts of the brain and over time, with declining ability to perform well on memory and thinking tests.

Investigators continue to look at other biological markers, such as blood tests, and at neuropsychological tests, which measure memory, orientation, judgment, and problem solving, to see if they can accurately predict whether healthy, unaffected older adults will develop AD or whether those with mild cognitive impairment will go on to develop AD. However, the availability of tests raises ethical and practical questions about patients' desires or needs to know their risk of developing AD. Is it helpful or useful to predict a condition that is not yet considered preventable or curable?

Treatments for AD

As of 2010 there was still no cure or prevention for AD, and treatment has focused on managing symptoms. Medication can reduce some of the symptoms, such as agitation, anxiety, unpredictable behavior, and depression. Physical exercise and good nutrition are important, as is a calm and highly structured environment. The object is to help the patient with AD maintain as much comfort, normalcy, and dignity as possible.

In 2010 there were five FDA-approved prescription drugs for the treatment of AD. The first four drugs to be approved were cholinesterase inhibitors, which are drugs designed to prevent the breakdown of acetylcholine.

Cholinesterase inhibitors keep levels of the chemical messenger high, even while the cells that produce the messenger continue to become damaged or die. About half of the people who take cholinesterase inhibitors see modest improvement in cognitive symptoms. Until 1997 tacrine was the nation's only AD medication, but tacrine is rarely prescribed today because of associated side effects, including possible liver damage. However, there are three other cholinesterase inhibitors currently used that produce some delay in the deterioration of memory and other cognitive skills: donepezil, approved in 1996; rivastigmine, approved in 2000; and galantamine, approved in 2001.

Memantine was approved by the FDA in 2003 for the treatment of moderate to severe AD. It is classified as an uncompetitive low-to-moderate affinity N-methyl-D-aspartate (NMDA) receptor antagonist, and it is the first Alzheimer drug of this type approved in the United States. According to the Alzheimer's Association, it acts by regulating the activity of glutamate, one of the brain's specialized messenger chemicals involved in information processing, storage, and retrieval.

Investigational drug research underway in 2010 involved the use of drugs and vaccines to block the production of beta amyloid, which is thought to be the source of the problem, or help rid the body of it quickly. Researchers are also looking at antiamyloid antibodies, proteins made by the immune system that counter the effects of beta amyloid, as a way to halt the progress of the disease early in its course. All the drugs being tested were intended to decrease the frequency or severity of the symptoms of AD and slow its progression, but none were expected to cure AD. The investigational drugs aim to address three aspects of AD: improve cognitive function in people with early AD; slow or postpone the progression of the disease; and control behavioral problems such as wandering, aggression, and agitation of patients with AD.

Investigational drug research targeting two enzymes—beta-secretase and gamma-secretase—involved in plaque formation also may benefit people suffering from AD. In "Modeling an Anti-Amyloid Combination Therapy for Alzheimer's Disease" (*Science Translational Research*, vol. 2, no. 13, January 6, 2010), Vivian W. Chow et al. of Johns Hopkins University School of Medicine report that reduction of these two enzymes reduces the formation of amyloid beta protein or amyloid plaque in the brain.

It also appears that a combination of vitamin E and anti-inflammatory drugs play a role in slowing the progress of AD. According to Valory N. Pavlik et al. of Baylor College of Medicine in "Vitamin E Use Is Associated with Improved Survival in an Alzheimer's Disease Cohort" (*Dementia and Geriatric Cognitive Disorders*, vol. 28, no. 6, December 2009), vitamin E at a dose of 2,000 IU

(international units) per day has been shown to delay AD progression. However, researchers question the safety of this high dose. Pavlik et al. not only found no safety risk associated with the dose but also report that vitamin E use actually improved survival rates among AD patients. In a letter to the editor in the *Journal of Clinical Psychopharmacology* (vol. 29, no. 5, October 2009), Daniel M. Bittner of Otto von Guericke University in Magdeburg, Germany, reports that a small study revealed some evidence that the combination of vitamin E and a cholinesterase inhibitor appear to act synergistically (the combined action is greater than the sum total of each acting separately) to address symptoms of AD.

THE IMPACT OF AD ON CAREGIVERS' HEALTH AND WELL-BEING. The suffering of a patient with AD is only part of the devastating emotional, physical, and financial trauma of AD. People who care for loved ones with AD are considered "second victims" of the disease. Caregivers often neglect their own needs, including their health and social lives, and the needs of other family members. As a result, they may develop more stress-related illnesses and are at a greater risk for depression.

In "Canadian Alzheimer's Disease Caregiver Survey: Baby-Boomer Caregivers and Burden of Care" (*International Journal of Geriatric Psychiatry*, December 22, 2009) Sandra E. Black et al. of Sunnybrook Health Sciences Centre, Toronto, report key findings about the relationship between caregiving and compromised health, including:

- Caregivers reported significant negative effects on emotional health such as increased depression, more stress, and greater fatigue.

- The financial costs associated with caregiving and the impact on their own work situations were significant sources of stress. Caregivers reported retiring early, reducing work hours, or foregoing a promotion in order to provide care.

- There was a significantly greater burden placed on live-in caregivers compared with caregivers who did not reside with the AD patients who were the recipients of care.

Research also demonstrates that caregivers are more likely than their peers who do not provide care for persons suffering from AD or other forms of dementia to suffer from mood and sleep disorders such as insomnia at least in part because they are awakened by their care-recipients at night. In "Insomnia in Caregivers of Persons with Dementia: Who Is at Risk and What Can Be Done about It?" (*Sleep Medicine Clinics*, vol. 4, no. 4, December 2009), Susan M. McCurry et al. of the University of Washington, Seattle, describe sleep as the "new vital sign," because of mounting evidence of its crucial role in maintaining health. AD caregivers, who also may be considered patients because of their increased risk for physical and mental health problems, may be at greater risk of suffering negative consequences from chronic sleep loss in combination with the stress involved in caregiving. Health professionals assert that in view of caregivers' risks of developing health problems, there is an urgent need to exhort family caregivers to engage in such activities as regular exercise and preventive medical care that will benefit their own health, well-being, and longevity.

CHAPTER 7
INFECTIOUS DISEASES

Pursue him to his house, and pluck him thence;

Lest his infection, being of a catching nature,

Spread further.

—William Shakespeare, *Coriolanus* (1607–1608)

Infectious (contagious) diseases are caused by microorganisms—viruses, bacteria, parasites, or fungi—transmitted from one person to another through casual contact, such as influenza; through bodily fluids, such as the human immunodeficiency virus (HIV); or via contaminated air, food, or water supplies. Infectious diseases may also spread by vectors of disease such as insects or arthropods that carry the infectious agent.

According to the World Health Organization (WHO), infectious diseases are a leading cause of death worldwide. Not long ago, the U.S. government and medical experts believed that widespread use of vaccines, antibiotics, and public health measures had effectively eliminated the public health threat of infectious diseases. Throughout the world, however, new and rare diseases are emerging, and old diseases are resurfacing. Some of these infections reflect changes associated with increasing population, growing poverty, urban migration, drug-resistant microbes, and expanding international travel.

The mistaken belief that infectious diseases were problems of the past prompted the governments of many countries, including the United States, to neglect public health programs aimed at preventing and treating infectious disease. By the close of the 20th century, however, enough troubling new diseases had arisen and old ones recurred that the United States resurrected and intensified efforts to respond to and contain infections.

The National Electronic Telecommunications System for Surveillance (NETSS) is a computerized public health surveillance information system that provides the Centers for Disease Control and Prevention (CDC) with weekly data to track certain infectious diseases (notifiable dis-

eases). The CDC (January 25, 2010, http://www.cdc.gov/ncphi/disss/nndss/netss.htm) defines a notifiable disease as "one for which regular, frequent, timely information on individual cases is considered necessary to prevent and control that disease." The list of nationally notifiable diseases is revised periodically. For example, a disease might be added to the list as a new pathogen (an organism that causes disease) emerges, or a disease might be deleted as its incidence declines. Physicians, clinics, and hospitals must report any occurrences of these diseases to the CDC each week. Table 7.1 shows the nationally notifiable infectious diseases tracked in 2010.

MOST FREQUENTLY REPORTED DISEASES

Among the CDC's notifiable diseases, the three most frequently reported infectious diseases in the United States in 2007 were chlamydia (1,108,374 cases—the highest it has been since voluntary reporting began in the mid-1980s), gonorrhea (355,991 cases), and acquired immunodeficiency syndrome (AIDS; 37,503 cases)—all sexually transmitted diseases (STDs). (See Table 7.2.) The remaining notifiable infectious diseases in the top 10 were:

- Salmonellosis (47,995 cases)—a food-borne disease causing fever and intestinal disorders

- Syphilis, all stages (40,920 cases)—an STD that occurs in three stages; it can also be congenital (an infant can be born with the disease)

- Varicella (chicken pox; 40,146 cases)—a disease (usually of childhood) marked by a vesicular (small, blister-like elevations on the skin with fluid in them) rash on the face and body caused by the herpes varicella zoster virus

- Lyme disease (27,444 cases)—a disease spread by ticks

- Shigellosis (19,758 cases)—food-borne and water-borne dysentery

TABLE 7.1

Nationally notifiable infectious diseases, 2010

Anthrax
Arboviral neuroinvasive and non-neuroinvasive diseases
    California serogroup virus disease
    Eastern equine encephalitis virus disease
    Powassan virus disease
    St. Louis encephalitis virus disease
    West Nile virus disease
    Western equine encephalitis virus disease
Botulism
    Botulism, foodborne
    Botulism, infant
    Botulism, other (wound & unspecified)
Brucellosis
Chancroid
Chlamydia trachomatis infection
Cholera
Cryptosporidiosis
Cyclosporiasis
Dengue
    Dengue Fever
    Dengue Hemorrhagic Fever
    Dengue Shock Syndrome
Diphtheria
Ehrlichiosis/Anaplasmosis
    Ehrlichia chaffeensis
    Ehrlichia ewingii
    Anaplasma phagocytophilum
    Undetermined
Giardiasis
Gonorrhea
Haemophilus influenzae, invasive disease
Hansen disease (leprosy)
Hantavirus pulmonary syndrome
Hemolytic uremic syndrome, post-diarrheal
Hepatitis
    Hepatitis A, acute
    Hepatitis B, acute
    Hepatitis B, chronic
    Hepatitis B virus, perinatal infection
    Hepatitis C, acute
    Hepatitis C, chronic
HIV infection*
    HIV infection, adult/adolescent (age ≥13 years)
    HIV infection, child (age ≥18 months and <13 years)
    HIV infection, pediatric (age < 18 months)
Influenza-associated pediatric mortality
Legionellosis
Listeriosis
Lyme disease
Malaria
Measles
Meningococcal disease
Mumps
Novel influenza A virus infections
Pertussis
Plague
Poliomyelitis, paralytic
Poliovirus infection, nonparalytic
Psittacosis
Q Fever
    Acute
    Chronic
Rabies
    Rabies, animal
    Rabies, human
Rubella
Rubella, congenital syndrome

TABLE 7.1

Nationally notifiable infectious diseases, 2010 [CONTINUED]

Salmonellosis
Severe Acute Respiratory Syndrome-associated Coronavirus (SARS-CoV) disease
Shiga toxin-producing Escherichia coli (STEC)
Shigellosis
Smallpox
Spotted Fever Rickettsiosis
Streptococcal toxic-shock syndrome
Streptococcus pneumoniae, invasive disease
Syphilis
    Primary
    Secondary
    Latent
    Early latent
    Late latent
    Latent, unknown duration
    Neurosyphilis
    Late, non-neurological
    Stillbirth
    Congenital
Tetanus
Toxic-shock syndrome (other than Streptococcal)
Trichinellosis (Trichinosis)
Tuberculosis
Tularemia
Typhoid fever
Vancomycin—intermediate Staphylococcus aureus (VISA)
Vancomycin—resistant Staphylococcus aureus (VRSA)
Varicella (morbidity)
Varicella (deaths only)
Vibriosis
Viral Hemorrhagic Fevers
    Arenavirus
    Crimean-Congo Hemorrhagic Fever virus
    Ebola virus
    Lassa virus
    Marburg virus
Yellow fever

*AIDS has been reclassified as HIV stage III

SOURCE: "Nationally Notifiable Infectious Diseases: United States 2010," in *National Notifiable Diseases Surveillance System*, U.S. Department of Health and Human Services, Centers for Disease Control and Prevention, December 2009, http://www.cdc.gov/ncphi/disss/nndss/PHS/infdis2010.htm (accessed January 11, 2010)

usually involves the lungs, but other organs also may be involved

RESISTANT STRAINS OF BACTERIA

Antibiotics have generally been considered "miracle drugs" that control or cure many bacterial infectious diseases. However, during the last decade nearly all major bacterial infections in the world have become increasingly resistant to the most commonly prescribed antibiotic treatments, primarily because of repeated and improper uses of antibiotics. Decreasing inappropriate antibiotic use is the best way to control this resistance.

Bacteria such as pneumococcus, which causes pneumonia and children's ear infections—diseases long considered common and treatable—are evolving into strains that are proving to be untreatable with commonly used antibiotics. Pneumococcal bacteria cause many hundreds of thousands of cases of pneumonia and bacterial meningitis (inflammation of the tissue covering the brain and

- Giardiasis (19,417 cases)—a common protozoal infection of the small intestine, spread via contaminated food and water and direct person-to-person contact

- Tuberculosis (13,299 cases)—an infection caused by the bacterium *Mycobacterium tuberculosis* that

TABLE 7.2

Reported cases of notifiable diseases[a], by month, 2007

Disease	Jan	Feb	Mar	Apr	May	Jun	Jul	Aug	Sep	Oct	Nov	Dec	Total
AIDS[b]	2,179	2,323	3,577	2,947	2,616	4,112	2,358	3,125	3,464	2,679	1,782	6,341	37,503
Anthrax	—	—	—	—	—	—	—	—	1	—	—	—	1
Botulism													
foodborne	—	—	2	1	3	1	4	12	—	1	1	7	32
infant	5	8	8	7	9	11	7	6	8	4	5	7	85
other (wound & unspecified)	—	2	1	—	3	3	2	5	3	2	2	4	27
Brucellosis	9	8	13	8	15	12	6	15	11	8	8	18	131
Chancroid[c]	—	1	1	3	2	1	2	2	2	2	2	5	23
Chlamydia[c, d]	69,148	81,289	110,160	85,292	91,968	99,883	83,002	86,902	109,130	88,688	81,391	121,521	1,108,374
Cholera	—	—	—	—	—	—	1	—	3	3	—	—	7
Coccidioidomycosis	644	547	733	556	552	862	503	582	591	597	651	1,303	8,121
Cryptosporidiosis	254	204	305	237	285	441	703	2,096	3,964	1,379	668	634	11,170
Cyclosporiasis	9	6	3	6	6	24	14	10	8	5	1	1	93
Domestic arboviral diseases[f]													
California serogroup virus disease													
neuroinvasive	—	—	—	—	1	5	7	18	12	6	1	—	50
nonneuroinvasive	—	—	—	—	1	1	1	—	1	1	—	—	5
Eastern equine encephalitis virus disease													
neuroinvasive	—	—	—	—	—	—	1	2	—	—	—	—	3
nonneuroinvasive	—	—	—	—	—	—	—	—	—	1	—	—	1
Powassan virus disease, neuroinvasive	—	—	—	1	2	1	1	—	—	—	2	—	7
St. Louis encephalitis virus disease													
neuoinvasive	—	—	—	—	1	—	1	1	3	1	1	—	8
nonneuroinvasive	—	—	—	—	—	—	—	1	—	—	—	—	1
West Nile virus disease													
neuroinvasive	—	—	4	1	3	36	175	555	356	85	7	5	1,227
nonneuroinvasive	1	—	—	1	11	73	539	1,168	509	84	15	2	2,403
Ehrlichiosis													
human granulocytic	6	3	3	4	36	92	135	72	95	78	52	258	834
human monocytic	6	4	14	11	51	130	138	120	85	64	37	168	828
human (other and unspecified)	2	1	4	12	35	86	66	28	39	24	18	22	337
Giardiasis	1,016	1,138	1,428	1,143	1,067	1,406	1,438	1,944	2,617	1,920	1,626	2,674	19,417
Gonorrhea[c]	23,795	25,854	34,829	26,752	28,384	32,427	27,070	28,758	35,921	28,179	26,125	37,897	355,991
Haemophilus influenzae, invasive disease													
all ages, serotypes	218	211	254	250	180	227	179	166	168	143	164	381	2,541
age <5 years													
serotype[b]	3	1	2	1	—	2	1	2	2	4	—	4	22
nonserotype[b]	14	15	19	22	13	20	16	12	14	9	13	32	199
unknown serotype	18	15	25	12	18	15	16	15	9	9	10	18	180
Hansen disease (Leprosy)	5	8	13	10	7	12	5	5	11	10	7	8	101
Hantavirus pulmonary syndrome	2	—	1	3	2	5	6	2	3	5	2	1	32
Hemolytic uremic syndrome, postdiarrheal	9	10	8	16	9	34	29	42	31	30	22	52	292
Hepatitis, viral, acute													
A	161	204	266	225	212	281	248	244	368	206	174	390	2,979
B	268	328	445	323	343	418	322	326	433	364	337	612	4,519
C	40	68	80	55	55	70	66	51	75	62	70	153	845
Influenza-associated pediatric mortality[f]	8	14	17	12	13	2	3	2	2	—	3	1	77
Legionellosis	118	117	145	103	122	277	260	325	425	244	234	346	2,716
Listeriosis	62	29	49	47	42	70	74	84	119	86	50	96	808
Lyme disease	559	516	786	736	1,383	4,901	6,000	3,787	2,972	1,822	1,550	2,432	27,444
Malaria	79	62	83	82	85	144	119	142	155	115	99	243	1,408
Measles, total	—	2	1	4	9	5	2	2	7	2	1	8	43
Meningococcal disease													
all serogroups	92	93	134	107	91	104	73	60	74	72	60	117	1,077
serogroup A, C, Y, & W-135	23	30	48	33	25	30	15	16	26	26	13	40	325
serogroup B	14	13	12	16	12	17	16	12	11	9	13	22	167
other serogroup	—	4	6	4	—	3	2	1	3	4	5	3	35
serogroup unknown	55	46	68	54	54	54	40	31	34	33	29	52	550
Mumps	61	78	136	85	67	57	40	42	49	39	51	95	800
Novel influenza A virus infections	—	—	—	—	—	—	—	2	2	—	—	—	4
Pertussis	653	743	853	697	690	890	899	929	911	810	720	1,659	10,454
Plague	—	—	—	1	1	2	—	—	2	—	1	—	7
Psittacosis	1	2	1	—	—	—	—	1	1	2	2	2	12
Q fever	9	9	16	14	18	23	15	15	14	8	14	16	171

spinal cord). It also causes otitis media (OM; middle-ear infection), which, according to Peter S. Morris and Amanda J. Leach in a report published in *Pediatric Clinics of North America* ("Acute and Chronic Otitis Media," vol. 56, no. 6, December 2009), remains the most common indication for antibiotic prescribing in young children despite the fact that it is usually a mild condition that resolves spontaneously without any treatment.

In "Streptococcus Pneumoniae: Does Antimicrobial Resistance Matter?" (*Seminars in Respiratory and Critical Care Medicine*, vol. 30, no. 2, April 2009), Joseph P. Lynch and George G. Zhanel indicate that during the past three

TABLE 7.2

Reported cases of notifiable diseases[a], by month, 2007 [CONTINUED]

Disease	Jan	Feb	Mar	Apr	May	Jun	Jul	Aug	Sep	Oct	Nov	Dec	Total
Rabies													
animal	402	311	520	502	534	599	476	608	699	496	334	381	5,862
human	—	—	—	—	—	—	—	—	—	—	—	1	1
Rocky Mountain spotted fever	24	30	62	96	150	337	307	314	327	140	100	334	2,221
Rubella	4	—	3	1	—	1	3	—	—	—	—	—	12
Salmonellosis	2,621	2,189	2,798	2,468	3,128	4,562	4,733	5,040	6,299	5,093	3,578	5,486	47,995
Shiga toxin-producing E. coli (STEC)	200	125	212	260	256	444	655	693	739	534	326	403	4,847
Shigellosis	861	750	1,099	1,172	1,407	1,917	1,697	1,604	2,090	2,180	1,848	3,133	19,758
Streptococcal disease, invasive, group A	343	460	800	577	517	547	372	258	304	216	293	607	5,294
Streptococcal toxic-shock syndrome	7	4	19	7	14	10	9	5	4	9	6	38	132
Streptococcus pneumoniae, invasive disease, drug-resistant													
all ages	327	328	432	306	219	223	145	102	191	153	261	642	3,329
age <5 yrs	40	61	72	55	37	35	23	17	37	36	55	95	563
Streptococcus pneumoniae, invasive disease, nondrug-resistant <5	127	172	228	153	156	177	94	72	91	149	197	416	2,032
Syphilis[c]													
all stages[g]	2,417	2,786	3,847	3,182	3,300	3,874	3,100	3,299	4,189	3,346	2,941	4,639	40,920
congenital (age <1 yr)	37	22	44	39	32	40	32	35	34	29	45	41	430
primary and secondary	665	729	1,010	840	849	1,091	813	961	1,216	1,007	888	1,397	11,466
Tetanus	—	1	2	—	2	3	1	3	4	4	3	5	28
Toxic-shock syndrome	5	4	6	7	9	11	8	6	12	9	2	13	92
Trichinellosis	—	1	—	—	—	2	1	—	—	1	—	—	5
Tuberculosis[h]	620	784	984	974	1,148	1,166	1,107	1,143	1,153	1,111	1,126	1,983	13,299
Tularemia	—	—	1	4	8	33	36	17	11	4	4	19	137
Typhoid fever	28	28	30	34	29	29	32	35	79	30	24	56	434
Vancomycin-intermediate Staphylococcus aureus	—	—	3	1	1	4	—	1	11	7	4	5	37
Vancomycin-resistant Staphylococcus aureus	—	—	—	—	—	—	—	—	—	1	—	1	2
Varicella (morbidity)	3,346	3,982	5,720	4,514	4,746	3,142	965	876	2,139	2,824	2,848	5,044	40,146
Varicella (mortality)[i]	1	—	—	1	—	—	1	—	—	1	2	—	6
Vibriosis	26	10	17	25	37	49	57	80	82	88	41	37	549

[a]No cases of diphtheria; neuroinvasive or non-neuroinvasive western equine encephalitis virus disease; poliomyelitis, paralytic; poliovirus infection, nonparalytic; rubella, congenital syndrome; severe acute respiratory syndrome-associated coronavirus syndrome (SARS-CoV); smallpox; and yellow fever were reported in 2007. Data on chronic hepatitis B and hepatitis C virus infection (past or present) are not included because they are undergoing data quality review. Data on human immunodeficiency virus (HIV) infections are not included because HIV infection reporting has been implemented on different dates and using different methods than for AIDS case reporting.
[b]Total number of AIDS cases reported to the Division of HIV/AIDS Prevention, National Center for HIV/AIDS, Viral Hepatitis, Sexually Transmitted Disease (STD), and TB Prevention (NCHHSTP) through December 31, 2007.
[c]Totals reported to the Division of STD Prevention, NCHHSTP, as of May 9, 2008.
[d]Chlamydia refers to genital infections caused by Chlamydia trachomatis.
[e]Totals reported to the Division of Vector-Borne Infectious Diseases, National Center for Zoonotic, Vector-Borne, and Enteric Diseases (NCZVED) (ArboNET Surveillance), as of June 1, 2008.
[f]Totals reported to the Influenza Division, National Center for Immunization and Respiratory Diseases (NCIRD), as of December 31, 2007.
[g]Includes the following categories: primary, secondary, latent (including early latent, late latent, and latent syphilis of unknown duration), neurosyphilis, late (including late syphilis with clinical manifestations other than neurosyphilis), and congenital syphilis.
[h]Totals reported to the Division of TB Elimination, NCHHSTP, as of May 16, 2008.
[i]Death counts provided by the Division of Viral Diseases, NCIRD, as of March 31, 2008.

SOURCE: Patsy A. Hall-Baker et al. "Table 1. Reported Cases of Notifiable Diseases, by Month—United States, 2007," in "Summary of Notifiable Diseases—United States, 2007," *Morbidity and Mortality Weekly Report*, vol. 56, no. 53, July 9, 2009, http://www.cdc.gov/mmwr/preview/mmwrhtml/mm5653a1.htm (accessed January 11, 2010)

decades, antimicrobial resistance among *Streptococcus pneumoniae*, the most common cause of community-acquired pneumonia, escalated significantly, with 15% to 30% of infections being multidrug-resistant (MDR), meaning they were resistant to three or more classes of antibiotics. Lynch and Zhanel point to a 2006 survey revealing that the national rate of MDR was 15.2%, with the highest MDR rate in the Southeast and lowest in the Northeast. Lynch and Zhanel explain that prior antibiotic use is the most common risk factor associated with antibiotic drug-resistance.

To treat patients with penicillin-resistant pneumococcus infections, physicians use a combination of other antibiotics, such as vancomycin, imipenem, and rifampin for resistant pneumonia and clindamycin or cefuroxime for ear infections. Another strategy to combat the illness is the pneumococcal vaccine. One of the reasons that public health professionals advocate widespread use of the pneumococcal vaccine is the hope that it will produce "herd immunity"—when a large proportion of the population is immune, the likelihood of person-to-person spread is so small that the disease does not proliferate and even nonimmune individuals are protected from disease. Unfortunately, Lynch and Zhanel observe that some of the reduction in the occurrence of illness anticipated from the introduction of the pneumococcal vaccine has been offset by the increased prevalence of resistant infections that are not prevented by the current vaccine.

Methicillin-Resistant *Staphylococcus Aureus*

Methicillin-resistant *Staphylococcus aureus* (MRSA) are bacterial infections that resist treatment with customary antibiotics. According to the CDC, they are most common in hospitalized patients with weakened immune systems as well as in nursing home residents; however, they can also appear in people living in the community at large. MRSA infections vary from life-threatening illnesses to minor skin infections.

The CDC reports in "Overview of Healthcare-associated MRSA" (March 3, 2010, http://www.cdc.gov/ncidod/dhqp/ar_mrsa.html) and "*S. Aureus* and MRSA Surveillance Summary 2007" (October 17, 2007, http://www.cdc.gov/ncidod/dhqp/ar_mrsa_surveillanceFS.html) that suspected staph and MRSA infections are responsible for about 12 million visits to physicians each year. In 1974 MRSA infections were just 2% of the total number of staph infections; in 2004 they accounted for 63% of staph infections.

In "An Update on Community-Associated MRSA Virulence" (*Current Opinions In Pharmacology*, vol. 9, no. 5, October 2009), Scott D. Kobayashi and Frank R. DeLeo observe that *Staphylococcus aureus* is the leading cause of bacterial infections in the United States, thus becoming a major health problem worldwide. The success of this microbe as a cause of disease has been facilitated by its strong tendency to develop antibiotic resistance, with multidrug-resistant strains most common in hospitals and other health care facilities. By the 21st century MRSA has emerged as a widespread cause of community infections—as opposed to infections confined to hospitals or other institutions where they were first reported in the 1990s—and now spreads rapidly among healthy individuals. MRSA strains are epidemic in the United States.

MRSA can be prevented by following infection control guidelines. In *Management of Multidrug-Resistant Organisms in Healthcare Settings, 2006* (2006, http://www.cdc.gov/ncidod/dhqp/pdf/ar/MDROGuideline2006.pdf), Jane D. Siegel et al. of the Healthcare Infection Control Practices Advisory Committee describe the prevention and management of multidrug-resistant organisms (MDROs) such as MSRA. Table 7.3 describes the education, monitoring, prudent use of antimicrobial drugs, surveillance, and precautions to prevent the transmission of infection that can control MDROs in health care settings.

Educating Physicians and Patients about Appropriate Use of Antibiotics

According to the CDC, antibiotic resistance is among the most urgent public health problems in the world. In 1995 the CDC Division of Foodborne Bacterial and Mycotic Diseases began a national campaign to reduce antimicrobial resistance by encouraging the appropriate use of antibiotics.

Didier Guillemot et al. explain in "Reduction of Antibiotic Use in the Community Reduces the Rate of Colonization with Penicillin G-Nonsusceptible *Streptococcus Pneumoniae*" (*Clinical Infectious Diseases*, vol. 41, no. 7, October 1, 2005) that reducing antibiotic use lowers rates of drug-resistant bacteria. The researchers tested two methods intended to reduce the rate of penicillin-resistant pneumococci present in kindergarten students. The first prescription-reduction method involved not prescribing antibiotics for respiratory tract infections that were thought to be viral, because antibiotics work against bacteria, not viruses. The second approach, a dose/duration method, entailed using only recommended doses of antibiotics for no longer than 5 days. Guillemot et al. also targeted physicians, pharmacists, parents, and children in the groups receiving both types of treatment with an information campaign about antibiotic resistance and appropriate antibiotic use. A control group of children and their doctors received no specific information about antibiotic use.

At the conclusion of the study, antibiotic use had declined by more than 15% in both treatment groups, compared with less than 4% in the control group. Even though colonization (the formation of groups of the same type of microorganism that develop) by regular pneumococci was higher in the treatment groups than in the control group, colonization by penicillin-resistant pneumococci was lower in the treatment groups than in the control group. The prescription-reduction group saw the greatest decline in penicillin-resistant colonization—from 53% to 35%—and the dose/duration group dropped from 55% to 44%. The control group remained virtually unchanged. This indicates that reduced antibiotic use permits drug-susceptible bacteria to reestablish themselves as dominant colonizers of the respiratory tract. Guillemot et al. conclude that reducing the number of prescriptions and the dose and duration of needed antibiotics can generate significant and rapid reductions of penicillin-resistant pneumococcal colonization in areas that have high rates of drug-resistant bacteria.

These findings highlight the need for professional and public awareness and understanding of the need to assume active roles in preventing antibiotic resistance. The consequences of the failure of antibiotics to treat formerly treatable illnesses could be dire: longer-lasting illnesses, more physician office visits or longer hospital stays, the need for more expensive and toxic medications, and even death.

In "Can a Nationwide Media Campaign Affect Antibiotic Use?" (*American Journal of Managed Care*, vol. 15, no. 8, August 2009), Beatriz Hemo et al. evaluated the effectiveness of a media campaign to reduce antibiotic overuse among children in Israel by reducing the parents' demands for antibiotics. During the winter of 2006, Israel's second-largest health maintenance organization (HMO),

TABLE 7.3

Recommendations for prevention and control of multidrug-resistant organisms (MDROs) in health care settings

Administrative measures/adherence monitoring	MDRO education	Judicious antimicrobial use	Surveillance	Infection control precautions to prevent transmission	Environmental measures	Decolonization
Make MDRO prevention/control an organizational priority. Provide administrative support and both fiscal and human resources to prevent and control MDRO transmission. (IB) Identify experts who can provide consultation and expertise for analyzing epidemiologic data, recognizing MDRO problems, or devising effective control strategies, as needed. (II) Implement systems to communicate information about reportable MDROs to administrative personnel and state/local health departments. (II) Implement a multi-disciplinary process to monitor and improve HCP adherence to recommended practices for standard and contact precautions. (IB) Implement systems to designate patients known to be colonized or infected with a targeted MDRO and to notify receiving healthcare facilities or personnel prior to transfer of such patients within or between facilities. (IB) Support participation in local, regional and/or national coalitions to combat emerging or growing MDRO problems. (IB) Provide updated feedback at least annually to healthcare providers and administrators on facility and patient-care unit MDRO infections. Include information on changes in prevalence and incidence, problem assessment and performance improvement plans. (IB)	Provide education and training on risks and prevention of MDRO transmission during orientation and periodic educational updates for HCP; include information on organizational experience with MDROs and prevention strategies. (IB)	In hospitals and LTCFs, ensure that a multi-disciplinary process is in place to review local susceptibility patterns (antibiograms), and antimicrobial agents included in the formulary, to foster appropriate antimicrobial use. (IB) Implement systems (e.g., CPOE, susceptibility report comment, pharmacy or unit director notification) to prompt clinicians to use the appropriate agent and regimen for the given clinical situation. (IB) Provide clinicians with antimicrobial susceptibility reports and analysis of current trends, updated at least annually, to guide antimicrobial prescribing practices. (IB) In settings with limited electronic communication system infrastructures to implement physician prompts, etc., at a minimum implement a process to review antibiotic use. Prepare and distribute reports to providers. (II)	Use standardized laboratory methods and follow published guidelines for determining antimicrobial susceptibilities of targeted and emerging MDROs. Establish systems to ensure that clinical micro labs (in-house and outsourced) promptly notify infection control or a medical director/designee when a novel resistance pattern for that facility is detected. (IB) In hospitals and LTCFs: · . develop and implement laboratory protocols for storing isolates of selected MDROs for molecular typing when needed to confirm transmission or delineate epidemiology of MDRO in facility. (IB) · . establish laboratory-based systems to detect and communicate evidence of MDROs in clinical isolates (IB) · . prepare facility-specific antimicrobial susceptibility reports as recommended by CLSI; monitor reports for evidence of changing resistance that may indicate emergence or transmission of MDROs (IA/IC) · . develop and monitor special-care unit-specific antimicrobial susceptibility reports (e.g., ventilator-dependent units, ICUs, oncology units). (IB) · . monitor trends in incidence of target MDROs in the facility over time to determine if MDRO rates are decreasing or if additional interventions are needed. (IA)	Follow standard precautions in all healthcare settings. (IB) Use of contact precautions (CP): — In *acute care settings*. Implement CP for all patients known to be colonized/infected with target MDROs.(IB) —In *LTCFs: Consider the individual patient's clinical situation and facility resources in deciding whether to implement CP (II)* —In *ambulatory and home care settings, follow standard precautions (II)* —In *hemodialysis units*: Follow dialysis specific guidelines (IC) No recommendation can be made regarding when to discontinue CP. (*unresolved issue*) Masks are not recommended for routine use to prevent transmission of MDROs from patients to HCWs. Use masks according to standard precautions when performing splash-generating procedures, caring for patients with open tracheostomies with potential for projectile secretions, and when there is evidence for transmission from heavily colonized sources (e.g., burn wounds). Patient placement in hospitals and LTCFs: When single-patient rooms are available, assign priority for these rooms to patients with known or suspected MDRO colonization or infection. Give highest priority to those patients who have conditions that may facilitate transmission, e.g., uncontained secretions or excretions. When single-patient rooms are not available, cohort patients with the same MDRO in the same room or patient-care area. (IB)	Follow recommended cleaning, disinfection and sterilization guidelines for maintaining patient care areas and equipment. Dedicate non-critical medical items to use on individual patients known to be infected or colonized with an MDRO. Prioritize room cleaning of patients on contact precautions. Focus on cleaning and disinfecting frequently touched surfaces (e.g., bedrails, bedside commodes, bathroom fixtures in patient room, doorknobs) and equipment in immediate vicinity of patient.	Not recommended routinely

TABLE 7.3

Recommendations for prevention and control of multidrug-resistant organisms (MDROs) in health care settings [CONTINUED]

Administrative measures/ adherence monitoring	MDRO education	Judicious antimicrobial use	Surveillance	Infection control precautions to prevent transmission	Environmental measures	Decolonization
				When cohorting patients with the same MDRO is not possible, place MDRO patients in rooms with patients who are at low risk for acquisition of MDROs and associated adverse outcomes from infection and are likely to have short lengths of stay. *(II)*		

Notes: MDRO=multidrug-resistant organism. HCP=health care provider. LTCF=long term care facility. CPOE=computerized provider order entry. CLSI=Clinical and Laboratory Standards Institute. ICU=intensive care unit. HCW=health care worker.

SOURCE: Jane D. Siegel et al., "Table 3. Tier 1. General Recommendations for Routine Prevention and Control of MDROs in Healthcare Settings," in *Management of Multidrug-Resistant Organisms in Healthcare Settings, 2006*, Centers for Disease Control and Prevention, Healthcare Infection Control Practices Advisory Committee, 2006, http://www.cdc.gov/ncidod/dhqp/pdf/ar/MDROGuideline2006.pdf (accessed January 11, 2010)

which provides health care services for 1.7 million people, launched a nationwide media campaign intended to heighten awareness of the misuse of antibiotics among the general public. The campaign focused on the inappropriate use of antibiotics in the treatment of influenza and upper respiratory infections caused by viruses. Hemo et al. found "a significant decrease in antibiotic purchases for the treatment of the conditions studied subsequent to the campaign and greater knowledge regarding appropriate antibiotic use among parents exposed to the campaign." Their findings suggest that the media campaign had a favorable impact on parents' attitudes and the actual use of antibiotics.

PREVENTION THROUGH IMMUNIZATION

Many infectious diseases can be prevented by immunizations. According to the CDC's National Immunization Program, in "List of Vaccine-Preventable Diseases" (May 8, 2009, http://www.cdc.gov/vaccines/vpd-vac/vpd-list.htm), there are 27 diseases that can be prevented by vaccination. Immunization against only a portion of those

diseases, however, is recommended for the general public. Even though the other portion is preventable by vaccination, widespread administration of the vaccines is not recommended because the risk of contracting these diseases—anthrax, meningococcal infection, rotavirus, and smallpox, for example—is not great enough to warrant it. (For the 2009 schedule of childhood and adolescent immunizations, see Figure 2.1 in Chapter 2; Figure 7.1 lists the 2009 adult immunization recommendations, and Figure 7.2 lists vaccines that may be administered to adults based on their medical histories, lifestyles, occupational exposures, or other indications.) The vaccine-preventable diseases that the majority of adults should receive are:

- Diphtheria—this bacterial infection causes potentially fatal respiratory infections that are treated with antibiotics. People diagnosed with diphtheria are isolated until cultures are negative, to prevent the spread of the disease.

- Haemophilus influenza type b—this bacterial infection causes respiratory infections and other diseases, such as meningitis.

FIGURE 7.1

Recommended adult immunization schedule, by vaccine and age group, 2009

▨ For all persons in this category who meet the age requirements and who lack evidence of immunity (e.g., lack documentation of vaccination or have no evidence of prior infection)	▨ Recommended if some other risk factor is present (e.g., on the basis of medical, occupational, lifestyle, or other indications)	☐ No recommendation

Vaccine ▼ Age group ▶	19–26 years	27–49 years	50–59 years	60–64 years	≥65 years
Tetanus, diphtheria, pertussis (Td/Tdap) vaccination*	Substitute 1-time dose of Tdap for Td booster; then boost with Td every 10 yrs				Td booster every 10 yrs
Human papillomavirus (HPV) vaccination*	3 doses (females)				
Varicella vaccination*	2 doses				
Zoster vaccination				1 dose	
Measles, mumps, rubella (MMR) vaccination*	1 or 2 doses		1 dose		
Influenza vaccination*	1 dose annually				
Pneumococcal (polysaccharide) vaccination	1 or 2 doses				1 dose
Hepatitis A vaccination*	2 doses				
Hepatitis B vaccination*	3 doses				
Meningococcal vaccination*	1 or more doses				

*Covered by the Vaccine Injury Compensation Program

SOURCE: Adapted from "Figure 1. Recommended Adult Immunization Schedule, by Vaccine and Age Group—United States, 2009," in "Recommended Adult Immunization Schedule—United States, 209," *MMWR*, vol. 57, no. 53, January 9, 2009, http://www.cdc.gov/mmwr/PDF/wk/mm5753-Immunization.pdf (accessed January 11, 2010).

FIGURE 7.2

Vaccines recommended for some adults based on medical and other indications, 2009

☐ For all persons in this category who meet the age requirements and who lack evidence of immunity (e.g., lack documentation of vaccination or have no evidence of prior infection) ☐ Recommended if some other risk factor is present (e.g., on the basis of medical, occupational, lifestyle, or other indications) ☐ No recommendation

Vaccine ▼　Indication ▶	Pregnancy	Immuno-compromising conditions (excluding human immuno-deficiency virus [HIV])	HIV infection CD4+ T lymphocyte count <200 cells/µL	HIV infection CD4+ T lymphocyte count ≥200 cells/µL	Diabetes, heart disease, chronic lung disease, chronic alcoholism	Asplenia (including elective splenectomy and terminal complement component deficiencies)	Chronic liver disease	Kidney failure, end-stage renal disease, receipt of hemodialysis	Health-care personnel
Tetanus, diphtheria, pertussis (Td/Tdap)*	Td	Substitute 1-time dose of Tdap for Td booster; then boost with Td						every 10 yrs	
Human papillomavirus (HPV)*		3 doses for females through age 26 yrs							
Varicella*	Contraindicated				2 doses				
Zoster	Contraindicated				1 dose				
Measles, mumps, rubella (MMR)*	Contraindicated				1 or 2 doses				
Influenza*		1 dose TIV annually							1 dose TIV or LAIV annually
Pneumococcal (polysaccharide)		1 or 2 doses							
Hepatitis A*		2 doses							
Hepatitis B*		3 doses							
Meningococcal*		1 or more doses							

*Covered by the Vaccine Injury Compensation Program

SOURCE: "Figure 2. Vaccines That Might Be Indicated for Adults Based on Medical and Other Indications—United States, 2009," in "Recommended Adult Immunization Schedule—United States, 2009," *MMWR*, vol. 57, no. 53, January 9, 2009, http://www.cdc.gov/mmwr/PDF/wk/mm5753-Immunization.pdf (accessed January 11, 2010).

- Hepatitis A—this virus is spread through fecal (stool) or oral routes, although it may also be transmitted via blood or sexual contact. Outbreaks usually occur from contaminated food and water; military workers, children in day care centers, and their care providers are considered at high risk.

- Hepatitis B—it is transmitted by blood, sexual contact, or from mother to unborn child; intravenous drug users, gay men, and health care workers are at high risk.

- Human papillomavirus (HPV)—HPV is transmitted by sexual contact, and ideally the vaccine is administered before potential exposure to HPV.

- Influenza—this viral infection produces sudden fever, muscle aches, and respiratory infection symptoms.

- Measles—this highly contagious viral disease produces red circular spots on the skin.

- Meningitis—meningococcal vaccine was added to the 2005–06 schedule for select populations such as college students living in dormitories to prevent bacterial meningitis caused by infection with Neisseria meningitides. Meningitis means inflammation of the meninges (the covering of the brain and the spinal cord) and it is characterized by fever, vomiting, intense headache, and stiff neck.

- Mumps—this highly contagious viral disease produces swelling of the parotid glands (salivary glands that occur below and in front of the ear).

- Pertussis (whooping cough)—this bacterial infection causes illness marked by spasms of coughing.

- Pneumococcal—this bacteria causes pneumonia, an inflammation of the lungs.

- Poliomyelitis (polio)—a viral disease that causes fever, atrophy (wasting) of skeletal muscles, and paralysis.

- Rubella (German measles)—this viral infection is usually mild in children but can seriously harm an unborn child when contracted by a woman early in her pregnancy.

- Tetanus—the bacteria from this disease produce a toxin that causes victims to have painful muscle spasms.

- Varicella (chickenpox)—this is a highly contagious viral disease marked by skin eruptions of fluid-filled lesions that itch.

INFLUENZA

Influenza (the flu) is a contagious respiratory disease caused by a virus. When a person infected with the flu sneezes, coughs, or even talks, the virus is expelled in droplets into the air and may be inhaled by anyone nearby. It can also be transmitted by direct hand contact. The flu primarily affects the lungs, but the whole body experiences symptoms. The infected person usually becomes acutely ill, with fever, chills, weakness, loss of appetite, and aching muscles in the head, back, arms, and legs. The person with an influenza infection may also have a sore throat, a dry cough, nausea, and burning eyes. The accompanying fever increases quickly—sometimes reaching 104 degrees Fahrenheit—but usually subsides after two or three days. Influenza leaves the patient exhausted.

For healthy individuals, the flu is typically a moderately severe illness, with most adults and children back to work or school within a week. However, for the very young, the very old, and people who are not in good general health, the flu can be extremely severe and even fatal. Complications such as secondary bacterial infections may develop, taking advantage of the body's weakened condition and lowered resistance. The most common bacterial complication is pneumonia, but sinuses, bronchi (lung tubes), or inner ears can also become secondarily infected with bacteria. Less common but very serious complications include viral pneumonia, encephalitis (inflammation of the brain), acute renal (kidney) failure, and nervous system disorders. These complications can be fatal.

Who Gets the Flu?

Anyone can get the flu, especially if there is an epidemic in the community. (An epidemic is a period when the number of cases of a disease exceeds the number expected based on past experience.) During an epidemic year, 20% to 30% of the population may contract influenza. Not surprisingly, people who are not healthy are considered at high risk for most strains of influenza and their complications. The high-risk population includes those who have chronic lung conditions, such as asthma, emphysema,

chronic bronchitis, tuberculosis, or cystic fibrosis (an inherited disease characterized by chronic respiratory and digestive problems); those with heart disease, chronic kidney disease, diabetes, or severe anemia; people residing in nursing homes; those over the age of 65; and some health care workers.

Vaccines

Influenza can be prevented by inoculation with a current influenza vaccine, which is formulated annually so that it contains the influenza viruses expected to cause the flu the next year. The viruses are killed or inactivated to prevent those who are vaccinated from getting influenza from the vaccine. After being immunized, the person develops antibodies to the influenza viruses. The antibodies are most effective after one or two months. High-risk people should be vaccinated early in the fall because peak flu activity usually occurs around the beginning of the new calendar year. The flu season usually runs from October to May and peaks in December and January.

Each year's flu vaccine protects against only the viruses that were included in its formulation. If another strain of flu appears, people can still catch the new strain even though they were vaccinated for the primary expected strains.

Most people have little or no noticeable reaction to the vaccine; about a quarter may have a swollen, red, tender area where the vaccination was injected. Children may suffer a slight fever for 24 hours or have chills or a headache. Those who already suffer from a respiratory disease may experience worsened symptoms. Usually, these reactions are temporary. Because the egg in which the virus is grown cannot be completely extracted, people with egg protein allergies should consult their physicians before receiving the vaccine and, if vaccinated, should be closely observed for any indications of an allergic reaction.

Older Adults Benefit from Flu Vaccinations

Influenza is a major cause of illness and death among people aged 65 and older. According to Janet E. McElhaney, in "Influenza Vaccination in the Elderly: Seeking New Correlates of Protection and Improved Vaccines" (*Aging Health*, vol. 4, no. 6, December 1, 2008), every year influenza and its complications are responsible for an estimated 60% of the nearly 300,000 excess hospitalizations for respiratory and circulatory problems and 85% to 90% or more of the 31,000 to 51,000 unexpected deaths in this population. McElhaney asserts, "Given their high risk for these serious, influenza-associated complications, the elderly are included among the high-priority groups for annual influenza vaccination in many countries." She also observes that influenza vaccination is a cost-saving intervention in older adults, at least in part because it prevents costly hospitalizations.

Recent research confirms that adults aged 65 and older who obtain influenza vaccinations significantly reduce their risk of death from any cause and hospitalization from complications of the flu. In "Effectiveness of Influenza Vaccine in the Community-Dwelling Elderly" (*New England Journal of Medicine*, vol. 357, no. 14, October 4, 2007), Kristin L. Nichol et al. examined the medical records of 713,872 older adults in 5 states over 10 flu seasons—from 1990 to 2000. They find that subjects who had received flu vaccinations had a 27% lower risk for hospitalization and a 48% lower risk for death than those who had not.

Pandemic Influenza

In "Pandemic Flu: Key Facts" (January 17, 2006, http://www.cdc.gov/flu/pandemic/pdf/pandemicflufacts.pdf), the CDC defines pandemic flu as "a global outbreak of disease that occurs when a new influenza A virus appears or 'emerges' in the human population, causes serious illness, and then spreads easily from person to person worldwide." Pandemics are different from seasonal outbreaks or even epidemics of influenza. Seasonal outbreaks are caused by influenza viruses that already move from person to person, whereas pandemics are caused by new viruses, subtypes of viruses that have never passed between people, or subtypes that have not circulated among people for a very long time.

In the past, influenza pandemics have produced high levels of illness, death, social disruption, and economic loss. The 20th century saw three pandemics. The CDC reports that the 1918–19 "Spanish flu" claimed half a million lives in the United States and as many as 50 million people throughout the world. Nearly half of the deaths were young, healthy adults. In 1957–58 the "Asian flu" was responsible for 70,000 deaths in the United States. The 1968–69 "Hong Kong flu" proved fatal for 34,000 people in the United States. All three pandemics involved avian influenza, or bird flu. The 1957–58 and 1968–69 pandemics were caused by viruses containing a combination of genes from a human influenza virus and an avian influenza virus; the 1918–19 pandemic virus also appears to have been an avian flu.

AVIAN INFLUENZA. Avian influenza is an infectious disease of birds caused by type A strains of the influenza virus. The disease, which was first identified in Italy more than 100 years ago, occurs worldwide. Because these viruses usually do not infect humans, there is little or no immune protection against them. If an avian influenza virus infected people and gained the ability to spread easily from person to person, an influenza pandemic could begin. The first cases in humans probably resulted from contact with infected birds or surfaces contaminated with excretions from infected birds. The disease usually only affects birds and pigs; the first documented infection of humans occurred in Hong Kong in 1997. An outbreak of avian flu has affected bird populations in countries throughout Asia and Europe. It has affected humans as well—according to the WHO (April 3, 2008, http://www.who.int/csr/disease/

avian_influenza/country/cases_table_2008_04_03/en/index.html), as of April 2008 human cases of influenza A (H5N1) infection had been reported in 14 countries (Azerbaijan, Cambodia, China, Djibouti, Egypt, Indonesia, Iraq, Lao People's Democratic Republic, Myanmar, Nigeria, Pakistan, Thailand, Turkey, and Vietnam).

Even though the spread of H5N1 virus from person to person has been rare, by late 2007 researchers were concerned that the virus had mutated to infect humans more easily. Maggie Fox reports in "H5N1 Bird Flu Virus Mutations Facilitate Human Infection" (Reuters Health Information, October 5, 2007) that there remains considerable cause for concern and vigilance, because the recent avian flu outbreaks in Asia and Europe have killed more than half of those infected. Even more frightening, most cases have occurred in previously healthy children and young adults as opposed to the old and infirm, who generally succumb to influenza. Although attention had turned in 2009 and 2010 to another influenza virus, H1N1, the WHO continued vigilantly to monitor cases of H5N1 throughout the world. A December 18, 2009, WHO report ("Avian Influenza—Situation in Cambodia," http://www.who.int/csr/don/2009_12_18/en/index.html) confirmed a new case of human infection with H5N1 in Cambodia, bringing that country's total number of confirmed cases to nine, seven of which have been fatal.

In efforts to prepare for an avian flu pandemic, in April 2007 the U.S. Food and Drug Administration (FDA) approved the first human H5N1 vaccine, which could help protect people at the highest risk of exposure during the early critical months of a pandemic. Even though the vaccine is not available commercially, Michael O. Leavitt (1951–), the former secretary of the U.S. Department of Health and Human Services (HHS), noted in *Pandemic Planning Update VI* (January 8, 2009, http://www.flu.gov/professional/panflureport6.html) that at the end of 2008 the U.S. government had reached its "goal of stockpiling enough pandemic influenza antivirals to cover 44 million people, which will help slow the spread of an emerging pandemic."

Four different influenza antiviral medications (amantadine, rimantadine, oseltamivir, and zanamivir) are approved by the FDA for the treatment and/or prevention of influenza. All four usually work against influenza A viruses. However, the drugs are not always effective because influenza virus strains can become resistant to one or more of these medications.

The HHS supports pandemic influenza activities in the areas of surveillance, vaccine development and production, strategic stockpiling of antiviral medications, research, and risk communications. The HHS aims to have sufficient antiviral courses of drug treatment on hand in anticipation of a possible pandemic. There are also plans in place for pandemic preparedness for health care facilities, schools, local governments, businesses, and law enforcement agencies. Individuals and families can prepare for a pandemic flu by stockpiling nonperishable food and regular prescription medication.

SWINE FLU. In April 2009, H1N1, sometimes called swine flu because it has two genes from flu viruses that normally circulate in pigs as well as avian and human genes, was detected in people in the United States. On June 11, 2009, the WHO declared that the 2009 H1N1 influenza was a pandemic. In "Questions & Answers: 2009 H1N1 Flu ('Swine Flu') and You" (February 10, 2010, http://www.cdc.gov/h1n1flu/qa.htm), the CDC describes the illness caused by H1N1 as ranging from mild to severe, with typical influenza symptoms—fever, cough, sore throat, runny or stuffy nose, body aches, headache, chills and fatigue. Severe illness, hospitalizations, and deaths from H1N1 were reported. Figure 7.3 shows laboratory-confirmed hospitalizations and deaths attributable to all types of influenza, including H1N1, from August 30, 2009, through January 2, 2010.

Because initial supplies of H1N1 vaccine were limited as manufacturers shifted from seasonal flu vaccine production to H1N1 vaccine production, the CDC Advisory Committee on Immunization Practices (ACIP; "Recommendations for Vaccine against 2009 H1N1 Influenza Virus," December 22, 2009, http://www.cdc.gov/h1n1flu/vaccination/public/vaccination_qa_pub.htm) recommended that people at highest risk for complications from this virus, or those caring for high-risk individuals, receive the vaccine first. These target populations included pregnant women, people who live with or care for children younger than 6 months old, health care and emergency medical services workers, anyone 6 months through 24 years of age, and people ages 25 through 64 at higher risk for H1N1 influenza because of certain chronic health conditions or compromised immune systems. The ACIP advised that once these target groups had been vaccinated, programs and providers should begin vaccinating everyone from age 25 through 64. Because research indicated that, unlike seasonal flu, the risk for H1N1 infection among people 65 years and older was less than the risk for younger age groups, older adults were not initially targeted to receive early doses of the vaccine. As vaccine supply increased, the ACIP advised vaccination of people over the age of 65. By December 2009 many states were offering vaccination to people of all

FIGURE 7.3

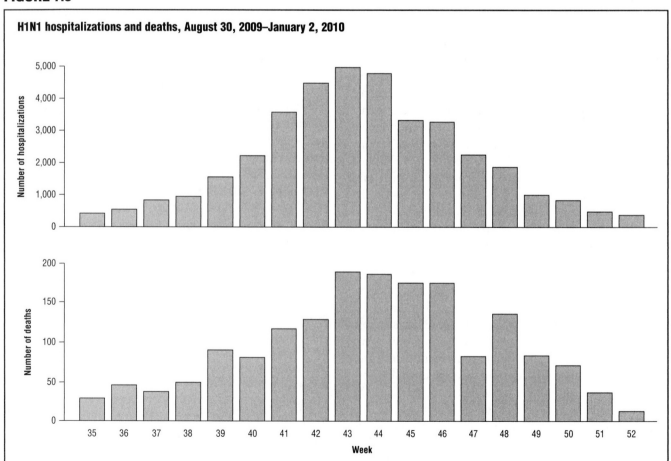

H1N1 hospitalizations and deaths, August 30, 2009–January 2, 2010

Note: H1N1 (Hemagglutinin Type 1 and Neuraminidase Type 1) is also known as the swine flu.

SOURCE: "Weekly Laboratory-Confirmed Influenza-Associated Hospitalizations and Deaths, National Summary, August 30, 2009–January 2, 2010," in "2009–2010 Influenza Season Week 52 Ending January 2, 2010," in *FluView*, Centers for Disease Control and Prevention, January 8, 2010, http://www.cdc.gov/flu/weekly/pdf/External_F0952.pdf (accessed January 11, 2010)

FIGURE 7.4

Flu activity by state, week ending October 17, 2009

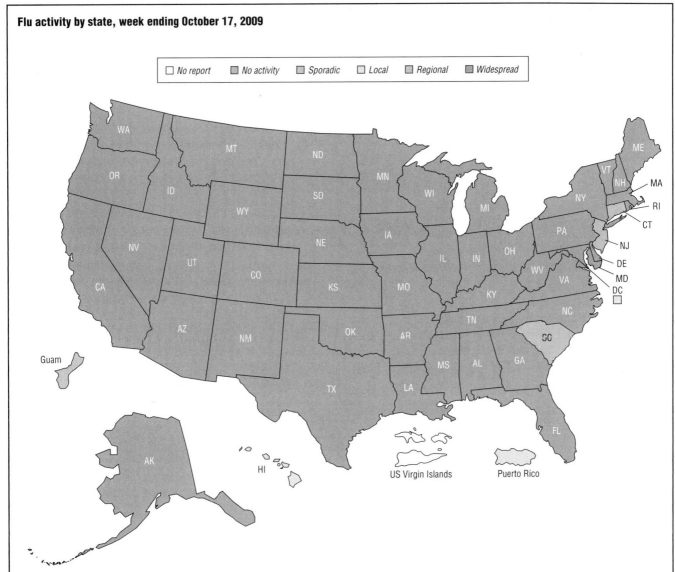

Legend: ☐ No report | No activity | Sporadic | ☐ Local | Regional | Widespread

SOURCE: "2009–2010 Influenza Season Week 41 ending October 17, 2009," in *FluView: A Weekly Influenza Surveillance Report Prepared by the Influenza Division*, Centers for Disease Control and Prevention, October 16, 2009, http://www.cdc.gov/flu/weekly/weeklyarchives2009–2010/weekly41.htm (accessed March 28, 2010)

ages, and, while older adults still appeared less likely to become ill with H1N1, severe infections and deaths had occurred in every age group, including older people.

The CDC reports that during the week of October 11–17, 2009, 46 states reported geographically widespread influenza activity. Guam and three states reported regional influenza activity, and one state, the District of Columbia, and Puerto Rico reported local influenza activity. (See Figure 7.4.) By the close of 2009, 60 million Americans had received the H1N1 vaccine, and 111 million additional doses were being made available to the states for distribution ("CDC: 60 Million in U.S. Had H1N1 Vaccine," UPI, December 22, 2009, http://www.upi.com/Health_News/2009/12/22/CDC-60-million-in-US-had-H1N1-vaccine/UPI-87811261526103/). At year's end just one state, Alabama,

still had widespread influenza activity, while Nebraska reported no influenza activity at all. (See Figure 7.5.)

Along with vaccination, the CDC encouraged other, general preventive measures including:

• Covering the nose and mouth with a tissue when coughing or sneezing and throwing the tissue in the trash after using it

• Washing hands often with soap and water and, when soap and water are unavailable, using an alcohol-based hand rub

• Avoiding touching the eyes, nose, and mouth to prevent the spread of virus

• Staying home from work or school when sick, in order to limit contact with others and keep from infecting them

FIGURE 7.5

Flu activity by state, week ending January 2, 2010

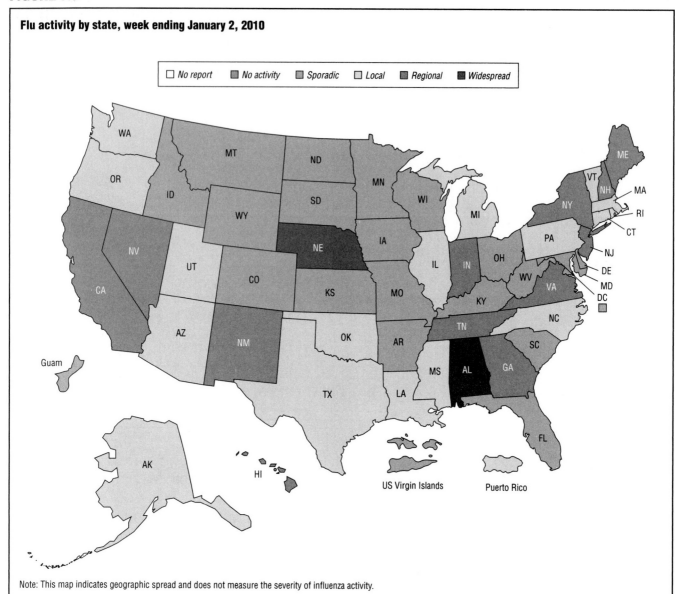

Note: This map indicates geographic spread and does not measure the severity of influenza activity.

SOURCE: "Weekly Influenza Activity Estimates Reported by State and Territorial Epidemiologists, Week Ending January 2, 2010—Week 52," in "FluView: A Weekly Influenza Surveillance Report Prepared by the Influenza Division," Centers for Disease Control and Prevention, January 8, 2010, http://www .cdc.gov/h1n1flu/updates/us/ (accessed January 11, 2010)

The CDC also advised the use of prescription antiviral drugs—oseltamivir and zanamivir—especially for persons at high risk of developing serious flu-related complications. In a December 22, 2009, press briefing ("CDC 2009 H1N1 Flu Media Briefing," http://www.cdc.gov/media/transcripts/2009/t091222.htm), the CDC's director of National Center for Immunization and Respiratory Diseases, Anne Schuchat, reported that hospitalizations for H1N1 influenza were largely among persons with asthma or other chronic lung disease.

According to the CDC, during the 2009–10 flu season, the vast majority of influenza cases were attributable to H1N1, and H1N1 flu caused more illness in people age 25 years and younger than in older people. As reported by Reuters ("Some Immunity Building Up against Pandemic Flu: WHO," January 8, 2010, http://www.reuters.com/article/idUSTRE5BL2ZT20100108), the WHO notes that by January 8, 2010, the H1N1 flu was responsible for 12,799 deaths, more than half of which occurred in Mexico, the United States, and Canada, where H1N1 disease activity appeared to have peaked in October 2009. The WHO also observed that southern hemisphere countries that experienced H1N1 in 2009 went on to display considerable population immunity, which means the virus spreads much more slowly and less easily.

TUBERCULOSIS

Tuberculosis (TB), a communicable disease caused by the bacterium *Mycobacterium tuberculosis*, is spread from person to person through the inhalation of airborne particles containing *M. tuberculosis*. The particles, called droplet nuclei, are produced when a person with infectious TB of the lungs or larynx forcefully exhales, such as when coughing, sneezing, speaking, or singing. These infectious particles can remain suspended in the air and may be inhaled by someone sharing the same air.

The CDC fact sheet "What Is TB?" (June 1, 2009, http://www.cdc.gov/tb/publications/faqs/qa_introduction .htm#Intro1) notes that most TB occurs in the lungs (pulmonary TB). The risk of transmission is increased where ventilation is poor and when susceptible people share air for prolonged periods with a person who has untreated pulmonary TB. However, the disease may occur at any site of the body, such as the larynx, the lymph nodes, the brain, the kidneys, or the bones. This type of TB infection, which occurs outside the lungs, is referred to as extrapulmonary. Except for laryngeal TB, people with extrapulmonary TB are usually not considered infectious to others.

In "The Difference between Latent TB Infection and Active TB Disease" (June 1, 2009, http://www.cdc.gov/ tb/publications/factsheets/general/LTBIandActiveTB .htm), the CDC explains that TB does not develop in everyone infected with the bacteria. In the United States about 90% of infected people never show symptoms of TB, but they are considered to have latent TB infections. The only indication of a latent TB infection is a positive reaction to the tuberculin skin test or special TB blood test. Between 5% and 10% of those infected develop active disease later in life, and about half of those who develop active TB do so within the first two years of infection. Table 7.4 shows the differences between latent TB infection and TB disease. People with compromised immune systems are at greater risk of developing TB than those with healthy immune systems. For example, Elizabeth L. Corbett et al. note in "The Growing Burden of Tuberculosis: Global Trends and Interactions with the HIV Epidemic" (*Archives of Internal Medicine*, vol. 163, no. 9, May 12, 2003) that more than 10% of those infected with both TB and HIV develop full-blown TB symptoms within a year.

Ancient Enemy and Continuing Threat

According to the CDC, in the fact sheet "Data and Statistics" (September 18, 2009, http://www.cdc.gov/tb/ statistics/default.htm), TB is among the world's deadliest diseases. Overall, one-third of the world's population is infected with the TB bacillus. Each year 2 million people worldwide die from TB, and each year more than 9 million people become sick with TB. This has increased dramatically since the HIV/AIDS epidemic swept through many countries. TB is a leading cause of death among people infected with HIV.

After several decades of decline, TB made a comeback in the United States in the late 1980s and early 1990s. (See Figure 7.6.) In 1992 the CDC reported 26,673 cases of TB, up from 22,201 in 1985. Since 1992 the number of cases has declined steadily, and by 2008 it had decreased by approximately 50% to 12,904—a prevalence rate of 4.2 per 100,000 people.

In "Reported Tuberculosis in the United States, 2008" (September 2009, http://www.cdc.gov/tb/statistics/reports/

TABLE 7.4

Distinguishing Latent TB infection from TB disease

A person with Latent TB infection	A person with TB Disease
• Has no symptoms	• Has symptoms that may include: - a bad cough that lasts 3 weeks or longer - pain in the chest - coughing up blood or sputum - weakness or fatigue - weight loss - no appetite - chills - fever - sweating at night
• Does not feel sick	• Usually feels sick
• Cannot spread TB bacteria to others	• May spread TB bacteria to others
• Usually has a skin test or blood test result indicating TB infection	• Usually has a skin test or blood test result indicating TB infection
• Has a normal chest x-ray and a negative sputum smear	• May have an abnormal chest x-ray, or positive sputum smear or culture
• Needs treatment for latent TB infection to prevent active TB disease	• Needs treatment to treat active TB disease

TB = Tuberculosis

SOURCE: "The Difference between Latent TB Infection and TB Disease," in *Basic TB Facts*, Centers for Disease Control and Prevention, Division of Tuberculosis Elimination, June 1, 2009, http://www.cdc.gov/tb/topic/ basics/default.htm (accessed January 11, 2010)

FIGURE 7.6

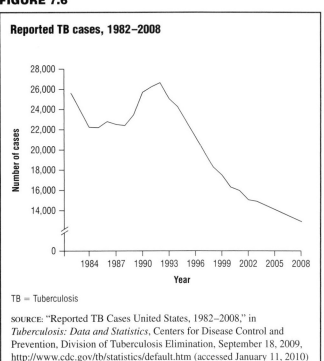

Reported TB cases, 1982–2008

TB = Tuberculosis

SOURCE: "Reported TB Cases United States, 1982–2008," in *Tuberculosis: Data and Statistics*, Centers for Disease Control and Prevention, Division of Tuberculosis Elimination, September 18, 2009, http://www.cdc.gov/tb/statistics/default.htm (accessed January 11, 2010)

2008/pdf/2008report.pdf), the CDC reports that the proportion of TB cases in foreign-born persons has increased steadily since 1993 and in 2008 accounted for 59% of all TB cases in the United States. (See Figure 7.7.) Persons born outside the United States have accounted for the majority of TB cases in this country every year since 2001. (See Figure 7.8.)

Treatment has become increasingly difficult because new strains of multidrug-resistant (MDR) TB have developed. If the disease is not properly treated or if treatment is not completed, some TB can become resistant to drugs, making it much harder to cure. According to the CDC, in 2008 the proportion of patients with MDR TB decreased from 2.5% in 1993 to 1.0% in 2008. However, the propor-

FIGURE 7.7

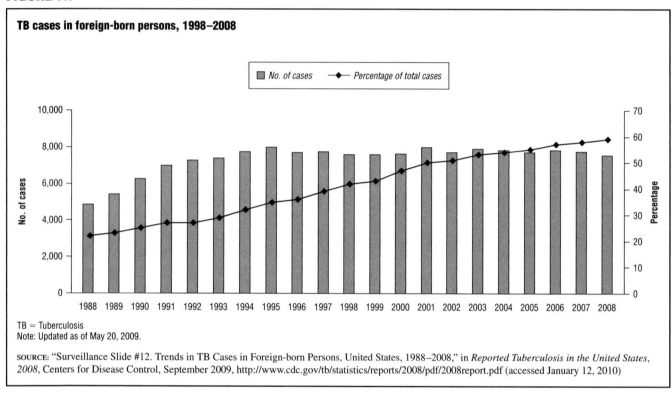

TB cases in foreign-born persons, 1998–2008

TB = Tuberculosis
Note: Updated as of May 20, 2009.

SOURCE: "Surveillance Slide #12. Trends in TB Cases in Foreign-born Persons, United States, 1988–2008," in *Reported Tuberculosis in the United States, 2008*, Centers for Disease Control, September 2009, http://www.cdc.gov/tb/statistics/reports/2008/pdf/2008report.pdf (accessed January 12, 2010)

FIGURE 7.8

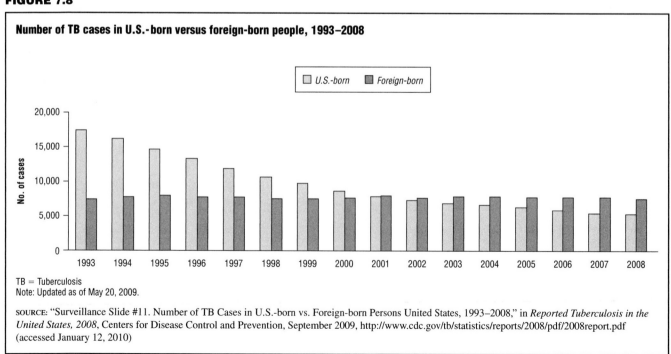

Number of TB cases in U.S.-born versus foreign-born people, 1993–2008

TB = Tuberculosis
Note: Updated as of May 20, 2009.

SOURCE: "Surveillance Slide #11. Number of TB Cases in U.S.-born vs. Foreign-born Persons United States, 1993–2008," in *Reported Tuberculosis in the United States, 2008*, Centers for Disease Control and Prevention, September 2009, http://www.cdc.gov/tb/statistics/reports/2008/pdf/2008report.pdf (accessed January 12, 2010)

TABLE 7.5

Multidrug-resistant tuberculosis (TB) in persons with no previous TB, by origin of birth, 1993–2008

Year	Resistance to isoniazid[a]						Resistance to isoniazid and rifampin[a]					
	Total cases[b, c]		U.S.-born		Foreign-born[d, e]		Total cases[b, c]		U.S.-born		Foreign-born[d, e]	
	No.	(%)	No.	(%)	No.	(%)	No.	(%)	No.	(%)	No.	(%)
1993	1399	(8.4)	804	(6.8)	579	(12.4)	407	(2.5)	301	(2.6)	103	(2.2)
1994	1360	(8.3)	711	(6.5)	635	(12.0)	353	(2.2)	238	(2.2)	110	(2.1)
1995	1174	(7.3)	555	(5.4)	618	(11.0)	254	(1.6)	169	(1.6)	85	(1.5)
1996	1137	(7.4)	495	(5.2)	639	(11.3)	207	(1.3)	105	(1.1)	101	(1.8)
1997	1079	(7.5)	435	(5.0)	640	(11.2)	155	(1.1)	76	(0.9)	79	(1.4)
1998	1013	(7.5)	367	(4.8)	644	(11.3)	132	(1.0)	55	(0.7)	76	(1.3)
1999	899	(7.1)	283	(4.0)	614	(11.0)	127	(1.0)	39	(0.6)	88	(1.6)
2000	890	(7.5)	269	(4.4)	618	(10.9)	120	(1.0)	40	(0.7)	80	(1.4)
2001	802	(7.0)	243	(4.4)	558	(9.5)	115	(1.0)	34	(0.6)	81	(1.4)
2002	825	(7.7)	205	(4.1)	619	(10.9)	132	(1.2)	35	(0.7)	97	(1.7)
2003	822	(7.7)	215	(4.5)	604	(10.4)	94	(0.9)	24	(0.5)	70	(1.2)
2004	801	(7.6)	214	(4.6)	587	(10.2)	100	(1.0)	26	(0.6)	74	(1.3)
2005	764	(7.6)	188	(4.3)	570	(10.1)	98	(1.0)	20	(0.5)	77	(1.4)
2006	771	(7.8)	172	(4.2)	597	(10.4)	101	(1.0)	18	(0.4)	83	(1.4)
2007	719	(7.5)	166	(4.3)	552	(9.6)	104	(1.1)	19	(0.5)	85	(1.5)
2008	726	(8.2)	173	(4.9)	550	(10.3)	86	(1.0)	20	(0.6)	66	(1.2)

Note: Resistance to at least isoniazid and rifampin.
[a]Isolates may be resistant to other drugs.
[b]All cases were culture positive, and initial drug susceptibility testing done.
[c]Includes persons of unknown country of birth.
[d]Includes persons born outside the United States, American Samoa, the Federated States of Micronesia, Guam, the Republic of the Marshall Islands, Midway Island, the Commonwealth of the Northern Mariana Islands, Puerto Rico, the Republic of Palau, the U.S. Virgin Islands, and U.S. minor and outlying Pacific islands.
[e]Includes Not Specified for Country of Origin. Excludes missing.
Note: Data for all years updated through May 20, 2009. Percentages are of total cases for given year with no previous history of TB, culture positive, and initial drug susceptibility testing done (total cases not shown). More than 95% of all persons in each group had drug-susceptibility test results reported for an initial isolate.

SOURCE: "Table 10. Tuberculosis Cases and Percentages, by Resistance to INH or Multidrug Resistance in Persons with No Previous History of TB, by Origin of Birth: United States, 1993–2008," in *Reported Tuberculosis in the United States, 2008*, Centers for Disease Control and Prevention, September 2009, http://www.cdc.gov/tb/statistics/reports/2008/pdf/2008report.pdf (accessed January 12, 2010).

tion of MDR TB in foreign-born people increased from 25.3% (103 of 407 MDR TB patients) in 1993 to 76.7% (66 of 86 MDR TB patients) in 2008. Table 7.5 shows the rates of MDR TB, termed "resistance to Isoniazid and Rifampin," among U.S.-born and foreign-born people. Table 7.6 shows that the rates of MDR TB are even higher among people with a previous history of TB.

March 24 of each year has been designated World TB Day by the CDC to recognize and increase awareness of the global threat to health posed by the disease. This annual event, first sponsored by the WHO, honors the date in 1882 when Dr. Robert Koch (1843–1910) announced his discovery of *Mycobacterium tuberculosis*.

HIV/AIDS

AIDS is the late stage of an infection caused by HIV, a retrovirus that attacks and destroys certain white blood cells, which weakens the body's immune system and makes it susceptible to infections and diseases that ordinarily would not be life threatening. AIDS is considered a blood-borne STD because HIV is spread through contact with blood, semen, or vaginal fluids from an infected person.

Around the World

AIDS and HIV were virtually unknown before 1981, when testing and reporting of the disease became mandatory, but awareness grew as the annual number of diagnosed cases and deaths steadily increased. In *AIDS Epidemic Update 2009* (November 30, 2009, http://www.who.int/hiv/pub/epidemiology/epidemic/en/index.html), the Joint United Nations Programme on HIV/AIDS and the WHO note that in 2008, 33.42 million people worldwide were estimated to be living with HIV/AIDS and about 2 million deaths were attributable to AIDS. Over two-thirds of all people infected with HIV lived in sub-Saharan Africa. An estimated 22.4 million people in this region were living with HIV and 1.9 million were newly infected.

In the United States

The CDC reports in *HIV/AIDS Surveillance Report: Cases of HIV Infection and AIDS in the United States and Dependent Areas, 2007* (2009, http://www.cdc.gov/hiv/topics/surveillance/resources/reports/2007report/pdf/2007SurveillanceReport.pdf) that at the end of 2007 there were an estimated 455,636 people living with AIDS. In 2007 an estimated 37,041 diagnoses of AIDS in the United States were made. Of these diagnosed cases, 26,355 were in males and 9,579 cases in females. An estimated 28 AIDS cases were diagnosed in children under age 13.

Although the *HIV/AIDS Surveillance Report* revealed a 15% increase in the number of HIV diagnoses from

TABLE 7.6

Multidrug-resistant tuberculosis (TB) in persons with previous history of TB, by origin of birth, 1993–2008

Year	Resistance to isoniazid[a]						Resistance to isoniazid and rifampin[a]					
	Total cases[b, c]		U.S.-born		Foreign-born[d, e]		Total cases[b, c]		U.S.-born		Foreign-born[d, e]	
	No.	(%)	No.	(%)	No.	(%)	No.	(%)	No.	(%)	No.	(%)
1993	164	(16.6)	85	(12.7)	76	(25.0)	76	(7.7)	30	(4.5)	46	(15.3)
1994	176	(17.0)	81	(11.7)	94	(27.9)	74	(7.2)	35	(5.1)	38	(11.3)
1995	168	(17.5)	77	(13.0)	91	(25.1)	70	(7.3)	28	(4.7)	42	(11.6)
1996	142	(16.5)	67	(12.0)	74	(24.4)	43	(5.0)	20	(3.6)	22	(7.3)
1997	109	(14.7)	35	(7.7)	74	(25.9)	44	(5.9)	12	(2.6)	32	(11.2)
1998	98	(13.0)	38	(7.8)	60	(22.8)	23	(3.1)	6	(1.2)	17	(6.5)
1999	82	(12.3)	25	(6.5)	55	(19.4)	28	(4.2)	6	(1.6)	22	(7.8)
2000	84	(13.2)	22	(6.1)	62	(22.8)	26	(4.1)	2	(0.6)	24	(8.8)
2001	86	(13.7)	28	(8.6)	58	(19.3)	32	(5.1)	7	(2.2)	25	(8.3)
2002	80	(14.1)	23	(7.6)	57	(21.6)	26	(4.6)	3	(1.0)	23	(8.7)
2003	65	(12.5)	16	(6.4)	49	(18.1)	21	(4.0)	2	(0.8)	19	(7.0)
2004	64	(11.9)	15	(5.5)	49	(18.6)	27	(5.0)	4	(1.5)	23	(8.7)
2005	70	(13.8)	18	(7.6)	52	(19.3)	22	(4.4)	1	(0.4)	21	(7.8)
2006	67	(13.6)9		(4.4)	57	(19.7)	21	(4.3)	1	(0.5)	20	(6.9)
2007	71	(14.3)	14	(6.8)	57	(19.7)	19	(3.8)	3	(1.4)	16	(5.5)
2008	53	(13.0)	12	(7.6)	41	(16.3)	17	(4.2)	2	(1.3)	15	(6.0)

Note: Resistance to at least isoniazid and rifampin

[a] Isolates may be resistant to other drugs.
[b] All cases were culture positive, and initial drug susceptibility testing done.
[c] Includes persons of unknown country of birth.
[d] Includes persons born outside the United States, American Samoa, the Federated States of Micronesia, Guam, the Republic of the Marshall Islands, Midway Island, the Commonwealth of the Northern Mariana Islands, Puerto Rico, the Republic of Palau, the U.S. Virgin Islands, and U.S. minor and outlying Pacific islands.
[e] Includes Not Specified for Country of Origin. Excludes missing.
Note: Data for all years updated through May 20, 2009. Percentages are of total cases for given year with previous history of TB, culture positive, and initial drug susceptibility testing done (total cases not shown). More than 95% of all persons in each group had drug-susceptibility test results reported for an initial isolate.

SOURCE: "Table 11. Tuberculosis Cases and Percentages, by Resistance to INH or Multidrug Resistance in Persons with Previous History of TB, by Origin of Birth: United States, 1993–2008," in *Reported Tuberculosis in the United States, 2008*, Centers for Disease Control and Prevention, September 2009, http://www.cdc.gov/tb/statistics/reports/2008/pdf/2008report.pdf (accessed January 12, 2010)

2004 to 2007 in the 34 states with name-based reporting, this increase is attributable to a 15% increase in annual HIV/AIDS diagnoses from 2006 to 2007. There was a 26% increase in HIV/AIDS diagnoses among men who have sex with men, a 9% increase among heterosexual males, and an increase among persons age 50 and older. It is not entirely clear, however, whether these data represent an actual increase in the number of HIV diagnoses or whether they are attributable to changes in state reporting requirements and regulations; an increase in the number of people being tested; or a combination of these factors. Compounding the difficulty in establishing the number of persons affected by the epidemic is the fact that an estimated 25% of cases are undiagnosed, according to the CDC in "Panel Presentations on Issues Impacting the Strategic Plan" (December 28, 2007, http://www.cdc.gov/hiv/resources/reports/psp/CHAC_meeting/panel_presentation.htm).

The CDC's analysis of the groups most affected by HIV/AIDS confirms that the majority of infections (53%) continues to be diagnosed in men who have sex with men. The analysis pinpoints the age groups as well as racial and ethnic distribution of new HIV infections. For example, African-American and Hispanic/Latino men ages 13 to 29 who have sex with men were most affected. In contrast, among white men who have sex with men, most new infections occurred in those age 30 to 39. Nearly one quarter of new infections in women were diagnosed in Hispanic and Latina women, and rates of infection in this group were four times the rates reported for white women.

The CDC observes that in 2007 males accounted for nearly 74% of all HIV/AIDS cases among adults and adolescents. Rates of AIDS cases in 2007 were 21.6 per 100,000 among males and 7.5 per 100,000 among females. (See Table 7.7.) From the beginning of the AIDS epidemic through 2007, a total of 1,030,832 people in the United States and dependent areas had been reported as having AIDS. Since its recognition in 1981, the disease has killed 583,298 people in the United States.

How Is AIDS Spread?

HIV/AIDS is not transmitted through casual contact with an infected person. The CDC has identified several behavioral risk factors that greatly increase the likelihood of a person's chances of being infected. Table 7.8 shows the estimated numbers of those diagnosed with AIDS by year of diagnosis and selected characteristics of patients, including the ways in which they contracted the disease.

More than 25 years of research and observation have definitively concluded that the HIV infection can only be transmitted by the following methods:

TABLE 7.7

Estimated numbers of cases and rates (per 100,000 population) of AIDS, by race/ethnicity, age category, and sex, 2007

| | Adults or adolescents | | | | | | Children (<13 yrs) | | Total, all[a] | |
| Race/ethnicity | Males | | Females | | Total[a] | | | | | |
	No.	Rate	No.	Rate	No.	Rate	No.	Rate	No.	Rate
American Indian/Alaska Native	112	12.5	46	5.0	158	8.6	0	0.0	158	6.9
Asian[b]	381	7.3	93	1.6	475	4.3	0	0.0	475	3.6
Black/African American	11,243	81.3	6,243	39.8	17,486	59.2	21	0.3	17,507	47.3
Hispanic/Latino[c]	5,466	31.0	1,452	8.9	6,918	20.4	2	0.0	6,921	15.2
Native Hawaiian/other Pacific Islander	64	37.5	12	7.1	76	22.3	0	0.0	76	18.3
White	8,802	10.6	1,600	1.8	10,402	6.1	5	0.0	10,407	5.2
Total[d]	**26,355**	**21.6**	**9,579**	**7.5**	**35,934**	**14.4**	**28**	**0.1**	**35,962[e]**	**11.9**

Note: These numbers do not represent reported case counts. Rather, these numbers are point estimates, which result from adjustments of reported case counts. The reported case counts have been adjusted for reporting delays, but not for incomplete reporting.

Data exclude cases in persons whose state or area of residence is unknown, as well as cases from U.S. dependent areas, for which U.S. census information about race and age categories is lacking.

[a]Because row totals were calculated independently of the values for the subpopulations, the values in each row may not sum to the row total.

[b]Includes Asian/Pacific Islander legacy cases.

[c]Hispanics/Latinos can be of any race.

[d]Includes person of unknown race or multiple races. Because column totals were calculated independently of the values for the subpopulations, the values in each column may not sum to the column total.

[e]Includes 418 persons of unknown race or multiple races.

SOURCE: "Table 6b. Estimated Numbers of Cases and Rates (per 100,000 Population) of AIDS, by Race/Ethnicity, 2007—50 States and the District of Columbia," in *HIV/AIDS Surveillance Report: Cases of HIV Infection and AIDS in the United States and Dependent Areas, 2007,* vol. 19, Centers for Disease Control and Prevention, 2009, http://www.cdc.gov/hiv/topics/surveillance/resources/reports/2007report/pdf/2007SurveillanceReport.pdf (accessed January 12, 2010)

- By oral, anal, or vaginal sex with an infected person; worldwide, heterosexual sex is the most common mode of transmission

- By sharing drug needles or syringes with an infected person

- From an infected mother to her baby at the time of birth and possibly through breast milk

- By receiving a transplanted organ or bodily fluids, such as blood transfusions or blood products, from an infected person

Because avoiding these methods of transmission virtually eliminates the possibility of becoming infected with HIV, unlike some other infectious diseases, AIDS is considered almost entirely preventable.

High concentrations of HIV have been found in blood, semen, and cerebrospinal fluid. Concentrations one thousand times less have been found in saliva, tears, vaginal secretions, breast milk, and feces. There have been no reports, however, of HIV transmission from saliva, tears, or human bites. Research, such as that done by Julián Campo et al. ("Oral Transmission of HIV, Reality or Fiction? An Update," *Oral Diseases*, vol. 12, no. 3, May 2006), confirms that the risk of transmission from these other body fluids is very low.

Opportunistic Infections

Once HIV has destroyed the immune system, the body can no longer protect itself against bacterial, fungal, parasitic, or viral agents that take advantage of the compro-

mised condition, causing opportunistic infections (OIs). OIs are illnesses caused by organisms that would not normally harm a healthy person. Because the patient is considered to have AIDS if at least one OI appears, OIs are considered "AIDS-defining events." OIs are not the only AIDS-defining events; the diagnosis of malignancies such as Kaposi's sarcoma (a rare skin carcinoma that is capable of spreading to internal organs), Burkitt's lymphoma, invasive cervical cancer, and primary brain lymphoma are also considered AIDS-defining events.

One of the most common opportunistic infections is *Pneumocystis carinii* pneumonia, a lung infection caused by a fungus. Other infections to which patients with AIDS are susceptible are toxoplasmosis (a contagious disease caused by a one-cell parasite), oral candidiasis (thrush), esophageal candidiasis (an infection of the esophagus), extrapulmonary cryptococcosis (a systemic fungus that enters the body through the lungs and may invade any organ of the body), pulmonary TB, extrapulmonary TB, *Mycobacterium avium* complex (a serious bacterial infection that can occur in one part of the body, such as the liver, bone marrow, and spleen, or can spread throughout the body), and cytomegalovirus disease (a member of the herpes virus group).

Treatment of AIDS

The first drug thought to delay symptoms was azidothymidine (now called zidovudine [ZDV]), but its effects have been found to be temporary at best. Several other drugs work on the same principle as ZDV, but until the advent of protease inhibitors (PIs), a class of drugs that became available in the mid-1990s, it seemed that there

TABLE 7.8

Estimated numbers of AIDS cases, by year of diagnosis and selected characteristics of persons, 2004–07

	Year of diagnosis			
	2004	**2005**	**2006**	**2007**
Data for 34 states				
Age at diagnosis (year)				
<13	212	189	169	159
13–14	41	40	45	40
15–19	1,081	1,216	1,409	1,703
20–24	3,714	3,875	4,184	4,907
25–29	4,524	4,547	4,884	5,771
30–34	5,353	5,024	4,686	5,089
35–39	6,359	5,907	5,678	6,088
40–44	6,011	5,889	6,003	6,554
45–49	4,286	4,338	4,377	5,172
50–54	2,645	2,698	2,862	3,489
55–59	1,473	1,531	1,512	1,938
60–64	771	729	741	942
≥65	696	657	643	803
Race/ethnicity				
American Indian/Alaska Native	177	180	163	228
Asian[a]	308	329	332	455
Black/African American	19,309	18,479	18,975	21,549
Hispanic/Latino[b]	6,183	6,383	6,590	7,484
Native Hawaiian/other Pacific Islander	39	43	49	46
White	10,836	10,818	10,815	12,556
Transmission category				
Male adult or adolescent				
Male-to-male sexual contact	17,898	18,333	18,894	22,472
Injection drug use	3,198	2,990	2,931	3,133
Male-to-male sexual contact and injection drug use	1,413	1,308	1,195	1,260
High-risk heterosexual contact[c]	4,167	3,923	4,029	4,551
Other[d]	140	120	132	102
Subtotal	26,814	26,673	27,182	31,518
Transmission category				
Female adult or adolescent				
Injection drug use	2,065	1,834	1,729	1,806
High-risk heterosexual contact[c]	7,967	7,852	8,033	9,076
Other[d]	103	90	80	96
Subtotal	10,135	9,775	9,842	10,977
Child (<13 years at diagnosis)				
Perinatal	177	162	134	139
Other[e]	37	30	36	20
Subtotal	214	192	170	159
Subtotal for 34 states	37,164	36,640	37,193	42,655
Data for U.S. dependent areas	1,234	1,391	1,338	1,429
Total[f]	**38,398**	**38,032**	**38,531**	**44,084**

Note: These numbers do not represent reported case counts. Rather, these numbers are point estimates, which result from adjustments of reported case counts. The reported case counts have been adjusted for reporting delays and missing risk-factor information, but not for incomplete reporting. Data include persons with a diagnosis of HIV infection (not AIDS), a diagnosis of HIV infection and a later diagnosis of AIDS, or concurrent diagnoses of HIV infection and AIDS.
[a]Includes Asian/Pacific Islander legacy cases.
[b]Hispanics/Latinos can be of any race.
[c]Heterosexual contact with a person known to have, or to be at high risk for, HIV infection.
[d]Includes hemophilia, blood transfusion, perinatal exposure, and risk factor not reported or not identified.
[e]Includes hemophilia, blood transfusion, and risk factor not reported or not identified.
[f]Includes persons of unknown race or multiple races and persons of unknown sex. Because column totals were calculated independently of the values for the subpopulations, the values in each column may not sum to the column total.

SOURCE: "Table 1. Estimated Numbers of HIV/AIDS Cases, by Year of Diagnosis and Selected Characteristics, 2004–2007—34 States and 5 U.S. Dependent Areas with Confidential Name-Based HIV Infection Reporting," in *HIV/AIDS Surveillance Report: Cases of HIV Infection and AIDS in the United States and Dependent Areas, 2007*, Centers for Disease Control and Prevention, 2009, http://www.cdc.gov/hiv/topics/surveillance/resources/reports/2007report/pdf/2007SurveillanceReport.pdf (accessed January 12, 2010)

was no way of stopping HIV. PIs appear to keep HIV from reproducing, unlike ZDV and similar drugs, which help keep HIV out of the cell's chromosomes. Even if the PIs are not entirely effective long term in reducing patients' viral "loads," they have improved patients' prospects simply by creating more roadblocks for HIV. However, HIV mutates so rapidly that it eventually becomes resistant to most drugs when they are used alone.

Treatment recommendations change rapidly in response to the development of new drugs and clinical trials indicating the effectiveness of different combinations of antiretroviral drugs. Researchers are acting quickly to develop new mixtures of the recently approved and older drugs. Because HIV mutates to resist any drug it faces, including all PIs, researchers have found that varying the combination of drugs prescribed can "fool" the virus before it has time to mutate.

Still, there are reasons for optimism in the battle against HIV/AIDS. National Institute of Allergy and Infectious Diseases director Anthony S. Fauci and his colleagues, in "Emerging Infectious Diseases: A 10-Year Perspective from the National Institute of Allergy and Infectious Diseases" published in the CDC's *Emerging Infectious Diseases* in April 2005, report that because of the use of combinations of drugs that target different proteins involved in HIV pathogenesis (a treatment strategy known as highly active antiretroviral therapy), the rates of death and illness in the United States and other industrialized countries have been dramatically reduced. The death rate due to HIV/AIDS in Europe and North America has fallen by 80%. As of 2010 more than 20 antiretroviral medications were approved by the FDA that target HIV, and researchers were pursuing novel strategies for prevention and vaccine development. Even if a cure for the disease is not imminent, new and better drugs used in various combinations have made HIV infection a chronic but manageable disease, much like diabetes.

COMPLICATIONS AND SIDE EFFECTS OF TREATMENT. Patients undergoing therapy with new drugs or drug combinations must be highly disciplined. For instance, indinavir must be taken on an empty stomach, every eight hours, not less than two hours before or after a meal, and with large amounts of water to prevent the development of kidney stones. Patients must also be careful to never skip doses of indinavir, otherwise HIV will quickly grow immune to its effect. (Indinavir has been found to generate cross-resistance, meaning it made patients resistant to other PIs.) Saquinavir mesylate must be taken in large doses. Ritonavir must be carefully prescribed and administered because it interacts negatively with some antifungals and antibiotics used by AIDS patients. Because there are many minor and serious risks associated with use of these drugs, patients must be closely monitored.

The drug regimens are complicated, and many produce severe side effects in a substantial number of patients. The difficulty of dealing with a complicated regimen of daily medication and maintaining the personal resolve to continue the regimen are ongoing issues for many HIV/AIDS patients. When effective AIDS drugs were introduced, patients sometimes had to wake up in the middle of the night to take pills, and some treatment regimens consisted of as many as 50 or 60 pills administered several times a day. Even with intense pressure to simplify treatment regimens, pharmaceutical companies remained skeptical about an effective once-a-day pill despite the consensus opinion that it would help more people start, and stick with, treatment. As recently as 2005, many combined HIV/AIDS medication regimens were administered two to three times per day. Once-a-day regimens were sought after but were not available until 2006.

In 2006 Joel E. Gallant et al. indicated in "Tenofovir DF, Emtricitabine, and Efavirenz vs. Zidovudine, Lamivudine, and Efavirenz for HIV" (*New England Journal of Medicine*, vol. 354, no. 3, January 19, 2006) that a once-daily combination of three antiretroviral drugs is more effective as initial treatment for HIV infection than the previous and widely used three-drug combination. The researchers found that after one year of treatment, a regimen of antiretroviral pills, called tenofovir DF and emtricitabine, plus efavirenz, improved patients' ability to suppress the virus by 14%. Even more promising, the new regimen produced fewer side effects and researchers were optimistic that the simpler, more convenient regimen would encourage more people to seek treatment and increase adherence to prescribed treatment.

In "Epidemiology of Treatment Failure: A Focus on Recent Trends" (*Current Opinion in HIV and AIDS*, vol. 4, no. 6, November 2009), Mark W. Hull et al. observe that the development of more potent antiretroviral drugs that are better tolerated (with fewer side effects) and simpler treatment regimens have resulted in fewer instances of treatment failure. Hull et al. assert, "Improved tolerability has aided adherence, which remains a key determinant of treatment success."

LYME DISEASE

Spread by the bites of infected deer ticks, Lyme disease is the most commonly reported vector-borne disease in the United States. (Vector-borne means the indirect transmission of an infectious agent that occurs when any animal that transmits human disease touches or bites an individual.) Lyme disease is caused by the *Borrelia burgdorferi* organism and produces early symptoms such as skin rashes, headache, fever, and general illness; if untreated, the disease can cause arthritis and heart damage.

The CDC began to track Lyme disease in 1982, and the disease was added to the list of nationally notifiable diseases in 1990. In 2008 the CDC received reports of 28,921 confirmed cases of Lyme disease and 6,277 probable cases, with most cases occurring in northeastern and north-central states. (See Figure 7.9 and Figure 7.10.) Although there is some variability from year to year, there has been a considerable increase in the number of reported cases from 1994 to 2008.

In December 1998 the FDA announced approval for the world's first vaccine against Lyme disease. Doctors warned, however, that even though the vaccine would

FIGURE 7.9

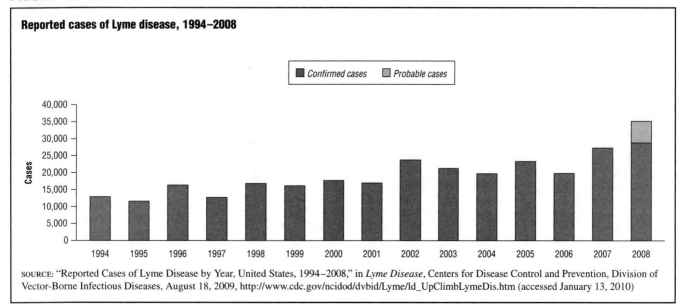

Reported cases of Lyme disease, 1994–2008

SOURCE: "Reported Cases of Lyme Disease by Year, United States, 1994–2008," in *Lyme Disease*, Centers for Disease Control and Prevention, Division of Vector-Borne Infectious Diseases, August 18, 2009, http://www.cdc.gov/ncidod/dvbid/Lyme/ld_UpClimbLymeDis.htm (accessed January 13, 2010)

help prevent Lyme disease, it would not eliminate the threat entirely. To achieve the best immunity, a person must receive a series of three shots of the vaccine over the course of a full year. The CDC reports that as of 2002, the vaccine was no longer available. The manufacturer reportedly discontinued vaccine production because of insufficient demand. Because the protection afforded by the vaccine diminishes over time, even persons who received it before 2002 are probably no longer protected against the disease

The FDA and CDC warn that people must take precautions against ticks. Wearing long-sleeved shirts and long pants, tucking pant legs into socks, and spraying the skin and/or clothing with tick repellents can keep ticks away from the skin. If a tick is found on the body, it should be removed promptly, and the affected individual should be alert for early symptoms of the disease. Immediate medical care, which consists of antibiotic treatment, is imperative to prevent long-term health damage from Lyme disease.

WEST NILE VIRUS

The West Nile virus (WNV) is common in Africa, West Asia, and the Middle East, and it can infect birds, mosquitoes, horses, humans, and other mammals. It is spread by bites from infected mosquitoes, and even though most people who become infected have few or no symptoms, some develop serious and even fatal illnesses. The virus was first reported in the United States in 1999, and the CDC has tracked its westward spread across the United States. In "West Nile Virus: Statistics, Surveillance, and Control" (December 8, 2009, http://www.cdc.gov/ncidod/dvbid/westnile/surv&controlCaseCount09_detailed.htm),

the CDC indicates that in 2009 WNV caused 663 cases of human illness and 30 deaths in the United States.

According to the CDC, the presence of WNV in either humans or infected mosquitoes is permanently established in the United States. Even though human illness from the virus is relatively rare, the disease is more likely to be fatal in older adults and young children. Figure 7.11 shows the distribution of human WNV cases by state as well as by infection of birds, animals, or mosquitoes.

The CDC advises taking precautions against mosquito bites, such as using insect repellent; wearing long pants and long-sleeved shirts treated with insect repellent; remaining indoors during dawn, dusk, and early evening, the hours when mosquitoes are the most likely to bite; and removing standing water to prevent mosquitoes from laying eggs and breeding near homes and other populated areas.

SEVERE ACUTE RESPIRATORY SYNDROME

In "Frequently Asked Questions about SARS" (May 3, 2005, http://www.cdc.gov/ncidod/sars/faq.htm), the CDC explains that severe acute respiratory syndrome (SARS) is a viral respiratory illness caused by a coronavirus that was first reported in southern China in November 2002. The illness spread to more than 24 countries in North America, South America, Europe, and Asia before the global outbreak was contained in July 2003. SARS seems to be transmitted primarily by person-to-person contact, through respiratory droplets, which travel via coughs or sneezes to the mucous membranes of other people or to surfaces that others touch. Symptoms of the disease may include high fever, body aches, malaise (overall discomfort), diarrhea,

FIGURE 7.10

Geographic distribution of Lyme disease cases, 2008

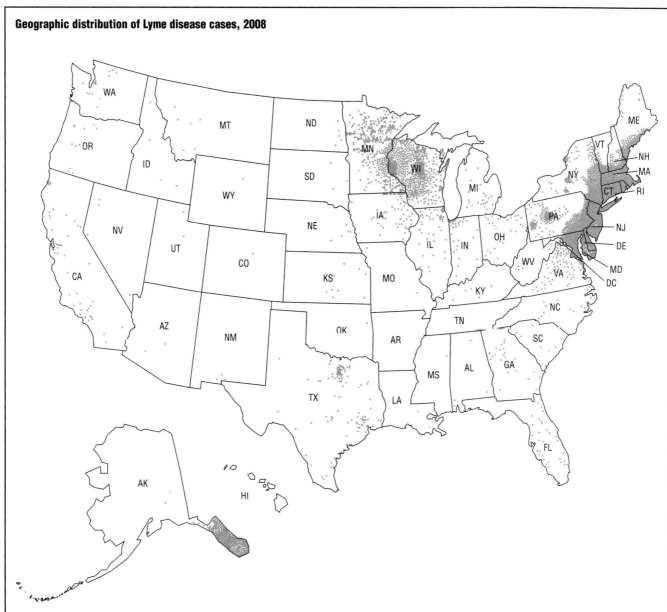

Note: 1 dot placed randomly within county of residence for each confirmed case.

SOURCE: "Reported Cases of Lyme Disease—United States, 2008," in Lyme Disease, Centers for Disease Control and Prevention, Division of Vector-Borne Infectious Diseases, September 15, 2009, http://www.cdc.gov/ncidod/dvbid/Lyme/ld_Incidence.htm (accessed January 13, 2010)

and mild respiratory symptoms; after two to seven days the infected person may develop a dry cough. The disease then progresses to pneumonia in most people.

According to the CDC, 8,098 people worldwide became sick with SARS during the outbreak, and 774 died. In the United States eight people—all of whom had traveled to parts of the world where the virus was present—contracted the disease.

In 2005 the National Institute of Allergy and Infectious Diseases (NIAID) applied its resources to establishing diagnostics, developing vaccines, and identifying antiviral compounds to combat SARS-associated coronavirus

(SARS-CoV). Among the many projects that have received NIAID support are the development of a SARS chip, a deoxyribonucleic acid (DNA) microarray to rapidly identify SARS sequence variants, and a SARS diagnostic test based on polymerase chain reaction (PCR) technology. (PCR is a technique for amplifying DNA sequences by as many as one billion times, and it is important in biotechnology, medicine, and genetic research.)

The CDC reports in "Current SARS Situation" (May 3, 2005, http://www.cdc.gov/ncidod/sars/situation.htm) that there has been no known SARS transmission anywhere in the world since April 2004; as of early 2010 this situation remained unchanged. The outbreak of human cases of

FIGURE 7.11

Geographic distribution of West Nile virus activity, 2009

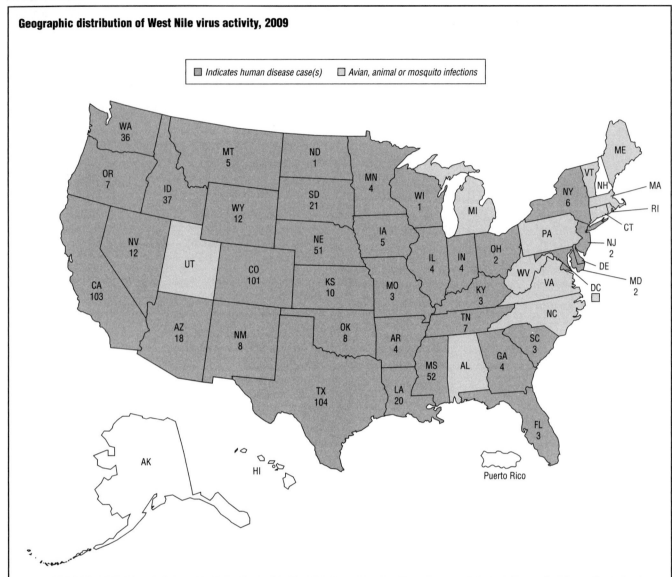

☐ Indicates human disease case(s)   ☐ Avian, animal or mosquito infections

SOURCE: "2009 West Nile Virus Activity in the United States," in *West Nile Virus: Statistics, Surveillance, and Control*, Centers for Disease Control and Prevention, Division of Vector-Borne Infectious Diseases, December 8, 2009, http://www.cdc.gov/ncidod/dvbid/westnile/Mapsactivity/surv&control09Maps_PrinterFriendly.htm (accessed January 13, 2010)

SARS-CoV infection occurred in China, and the cases were considered to be laboratory-acquired infections. The WHO (http://www.who.int/csr/sars/country/en/index.html) noted that by the time SARS had run its course, just 27 cases were reported in the United States, and there were no U.S. SARS-related deaths.

RESPONDING TO BIOLOGIC TERRORISM: INTENTIONAL EPIDEMICS

Healthy nations are secure and stable nations.

—Anthony S. Fauci, director of the National Institute of Allergy and Infectious Diseases, *The Edge of Discovery: A Portrait of the National Institute of Allergy and Infectious Diseases* (NIAID, June 2009, http://www3.niaid.nih.gov/about/whoWeAre/pdf/NIAIDEDGE.pdf)

In September and October 2001, in an unprecedented event, 22 letters containing *Bacillus anthracis* spores sent through the U.S. Postal Service caused anthrax outbreaks in 7 states: Connecticut, 1 case; Pennsylvania, 1 case; Florida, 2 cases; Virginia, 2 cases; Maryland, 3 cases; New Jersey, 5 cases; and New York City, 8 cases (includes a case of a New Jersey resident exposed in New York City). Five of the letters resulted in fatal cases of anthrax.

In "The Power of Biomedical Research" (*Washington Times*, July 9, 2003), NIAID director Anthony S. Fauci states that these anthrax attacks "starkly exposed the vulnerability of the United States—and, indeed, the rest of the world—to bioterrorism." Accordingly, the NIAID devotes one-third of its research portfolio to accelerated programs to prevent, diagnose, and treat possible intentional epidemics. Efforts focus on Category A agents (anthrax, botulinum toxin, smallpox, plague, tularemia, and hemorrhagic fever viruses such as Ebola) considered to be the worst bioterror threats and on Category B and C priority agents that also pose significant threats to human health.

NIAID biodefense initiatives include 11 regional centers of excellence for biodefense and emerging infectious diseases research. These facilities provide the secure space needed to carry out the nation's expanded biodefense research program. Researchers have sequenced the genomes of all biological agents considered to pose the most severe threats, and the NIAID has awarded contracts to screen new chemical compounds as possible treatments for bioterror attacks. In a June 8, 2009, press release ("NIAID Renews Funding for National Emerging Infectious Diseases Research Network," June 8, 2009, http://www3.niaid.nih.gov/news/newsreleases/2009/RCEs_ARRA.htm), the NIAID announced that it had renewed funding for the 11 centers, which totals approximately $455 million over 5 years.

The NIAID has also been active in vaccine development as a biodefense countermeasure. The institute, as well as the U.S. Department of Defense, supports the development of a next-generation anthrax vaccine, which has been undergoing clinical trials since 2007. In "Vaccines for Preventing Anthrax" (*Cochrane Reviews*, no. 4, 2009), Sarah Donegan, Richard Bellamy, and Carrol L. Gamble review the benefits and harms of the different anthrax vaccines available in 2009—a live-attenuated vaccine, an alum-precipitated cell-free filtrate vaccine, and a recombinant protein vaccine. Donegan, Bellamy, and Gamble find limited evidence that a live-attenuated vaccine is effective in preventing anthrax and some evidence that inactivated vaccines stimulate good immune responses. Ongoing clinical trials are evaluating the safety and efficacy of recombinant protein vaccines.

CHAPTER 8
MENTAL HEALTH AND ILLNESS

Mental health may be measured in terms of an individual's ability to think and communicate clearly, to learn and grow emotionally, to deal productively and realistically with change and stress, and to form and maintain fulfilling relationships with others. Mental health is a principal component of wellness—self-esteem, resilience, and the ability to cope with adversity influence how people feel about themselves and whether they choose lifestyles and behaviors that promote or jeopardize their health.

Mental illness refers to all identifiable mental health disorders and mental health problems. In the landmark study *Mental Health: A Report of the Surgeon General, 1999* (1999, http://www.surgeongeneral.gov/library/mentalhealth/home.html), the U.S. Department of Health and Human Services (HHS) defines mental disorders as "health conditions that are characterized by alterations in thinking, mood, or behavior (or some combination thereof) associated with distress and/or impaired functioning." The HHS distinguishes mental disorders from mental problems, describing the signs and symptoms of mental health problems as less intense and of shorter duration than those of mental health disorders. However, it acknowledges that both mental health disorders and problems may be distressing and disabling.

The symptoms of mental disorders differentiate one type of problem from another; however, the symptoms of mental illness vary far more widely in both type and intensity than do the symptoms of most physical illnesses. In general, people are usually considered mentally healthy if they are able to maintain their mental and emotional balance in times of crisis and stress and cope effectively with the problems of daily life. When coping ability is lost, then there is some degree of mental dysfunction. The goals of diagnosis and treatment of mental disorders are to recognize and understand the conditions, to reduce their underlying causes, and to work toward regaining mental and emotional equilibrium.

HOW MANY PEOPLE ARE MENTALLY ILL?

It is complicated to determine how many people suffer from mental illness due to changing definitions of mental illness and difficulties classifying, diagnosing, and reporting mental disorders. There are social stigmas attached to mental illness, such as being labeled "crazy," being treated as a danger to others, and being denied a job or health insurance coverage, that keep some sufferers from seeking help, and many of those in treatment do not reveal it on surveys. Some patients do not realize that their symptoms are caused by mental disorders. Because knowledge about the way the brain works is relatively narrow, mental health professionals must continually reassess how mental illnesses are defined and diagnosed. In addition, what might be considered, for example, delusional thinking in one culture may well be widely accepted in another; the symptoms of mental illness are notoriously fluid, and diagnosis may be skewed by cultural differences or other bias on the part of both patient and practitioner.

In *The Numbers Count: Mental Disorders in America* (August 10, 2009, http://www.nimh.nih.gov/health/publications/the-numbers-count-mental-disorders-in-america/index.shtml), the National Institute of Mental Health (NIMH; one of the National Institutes of Health) estimates that 26.2% of Americans age 18 and older are affected by mental disorders and that 6% suffer from serious mental illness. Community surveys estimate that as many as 30% of the adult population in the United States suffer from mental disorders. The National Center for Chronic Disease Prevention and Health Promotion (one of the Centers of Disease Control and Prevention) reports that from 2003 to 2008 about 10% of American adults say they experience frequent mental distress, as defined by "14 or more mentally unhealthy days." (See Figure 8.1.) The Harvard School of Medicine in its National Comorbidity Survey (July 2007, http://www.hcp.med.harvard.edu/ncs/) uses a national sample of 10,000 respondents to assess the prevalence of mental disorders in the United States. The survey

FIGURE 8.1

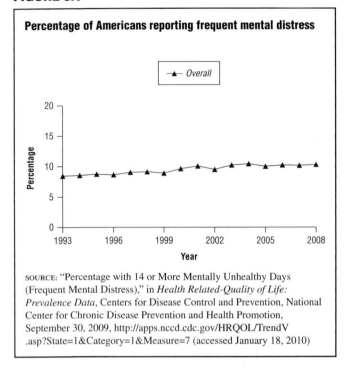

Percentage of Americans reporting frequent mental distress

SOURCE: "Percentage with 14 or More Mentally Unhealthy Days (Frequent Mental Distress)," in *Health Related-Quality of Life: Prevalence Data*, Centers for Disease Control and Prevention, National Center for Chronic Disease Prevention and Health Promotion, September 30, 2009, http://apps.nccd.cdc.gov/HRQOL/TrendV .asp?State=1&Category=1&Measure=7 (accessed January 18, 2010)

FIGURE 8.2

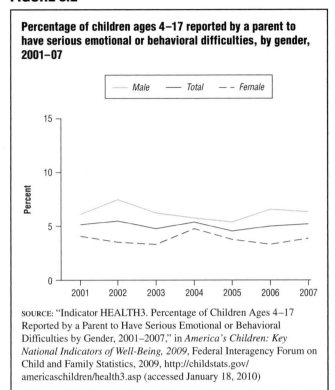

Percentage of children ages 4–17 reported by a parent to have serious emotional or behavioral difficulties, by gender, 2001–07

SOURCE: "Indicator HEALTH3. Percentage of Children Ages 4–17 Reported by a Parent to Have Serious Emotional or Behavioral Difficulties by Gender, 2001–2007," in *America's Children: Key National Indicators of Well-Being, 2009*, Federal Interagency Forum on Child and Family Statistics, 2009, http://childstats.gov/ americaschildren/health3.asp (accessed January 18, 2010)

indicates that in any given year 32.4% of all Americans meet the criteria for having a mental illness and that the lifetime prevalence of any diagnosable mental disorder is 57.4%.

How Many Children Suffer from Mental Illness?

Data describing the prevalence of mental disorders in children vary. The National Health and Nutrition Examination Survey (NHANES) conducted by NIMH and the National Center for Health Statistics of the Centers for Disease Control and Prevention (CDC) surveyed 3,042 children ages 8 through 15 between 2001 and 2004 to determine the prevalence of mental health problems in this population. The NHANES found that 13% of children had at least one mental disorder in the year prior to the survey and close to 2% of respondents had more than one disorder. In an analysis of the NHANES data in "Prevalence and Treatment of Mental Disorders among US Children in the 2001–2004 NHANES" (*Pediatrics*, vol. 125, no. 1, January 2010), Kathleen Merikangas et al. find that boys were more than twice as likely as girls to have attention deficit/hyperactivity disorder, whereas girls were twice as likely to suffer from mood disorders (primarily depression). There were no differences between boys and girls in the rates of anxiety disorders or conduct disorders. Merikangas et al. observe that while these prevalence rates are lower than many of those previously reported, just half of children with mental health disorders sought treatment from a mental health professional.

The National Health Interview Study (NHIS), a continuing, nationwide survey conducted by the National

Center for Health Statistics (NCHS), reported lower rates—from 2001 to 2007 the percentage of children with serious emotional or behavioral difficulties was stable at about 5%. During this same period the percentage of children with serious emotional or behavioral difficulties differed by gender and age. Parents reported that more boys than girls had difficulties. (See Figure 8.2.)

Many mental disorders that begin during childhood and adolescence recur or continue into adulthood. Children and teens with mood and anxiety disorders suffer from unfounded fears, prolonged sadness or tearfulness, withdrawal, low self-esteem, and feelings of worthlessness and hopelessness. These children and adolescents often suffer from more than one mental health problem (e.g., symptoms of depression and anxiety together). From 2004 to 2007 the percentage of adolescents ages 12 through 17 that had a major depressive episode (MDE; defined as a period of at least 2 weeks of depressed mood or loss of interest or pleasure in daily activities plus at least 4 additional symptoms of depression such as problems with sleep, eating, energy, concentration, and feelings of self-worth) decreased from 9% to 8%. (See Figure 8.3.) The prevalence of MDE was more than twice as high among girls and higher in older teens than younger ones.

Some Americans Experience Serious Mental Distress

The NHIS poses questions about psychological distress. These questions ask how often a respondent experienced

FIGURE 8.3

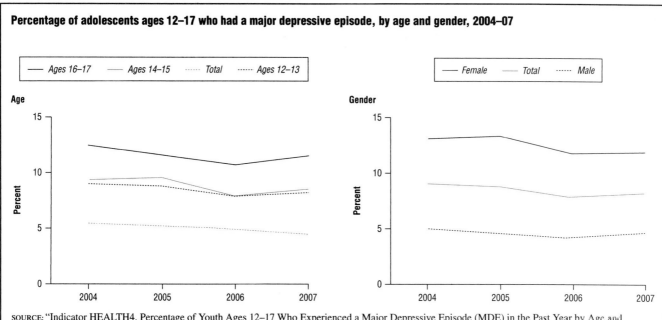

Percentage of adolescents ages 12–17 who had a major depressive episode, by age and gender, 2004–07

SOURCE: "Indicator HEALTH4. Percentage of Youth Ages 12–17 Who Experienced a Major Depressive Episode (MDE) in the Past Year by Age and Gender, 2004–2007," in *America's Children: Key National Indicators of Well-Being, 2009*, Federal Interagency Forum on Child and Family Statistics, 2009, http://childstats.gov/americaschildren/health4.asp (accessed January 18, 2010)

FIGURE 8.4

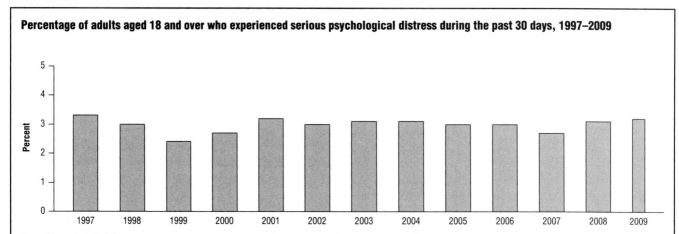

Percentage of adults aged 18 and over who experienced serious psychological distress during the past 30 days, 1997–2009

Notes: Six psychological distress questions are included in the National Health Interview Survey's (NHIS) Sample Adult Core component. These questions ask how often a respondent experienced certain symptoms of psychological distress during the past 30 days. The response codes (0–4) of the six items for each person are summed to yield a scale with a 0–24 range. A value of 13 or more for this scale is used here to define serious psychological distress (15). Beginning with the 2003 data, NHIS transitioned to weights derived from the 2000 census. In this early release, estimates for 2000–2002 were recalculated using weights derived from the 2000 census.

SOURCE: "Figure 13.1. Percentage of Adults Aged 18 Years and over Who Experienced Serious Psychological Distress during the Past 30 Days: United States, 1997–June 2009," in *Early Release of Selected Estimates Based on Data from the January–June 2009 National Health Interview Survey*, Centers for Disease Control and Prevention, National Center for Health Statistics, December 2009, http://www.cdc.gov/nchs/data/nhis/earlyrelease/200912_13.pdf (accessed January 18, 2010)

certain symptoms of psychological distress during the 30 days preceding the survey. In the first half of 2009, slightly more than 3% of adults aged 18 and older said they had experienced serious psychological distress during the past 30 days. Figure 8.4 shows that the percentage of adults reporting serious psychological distress declined from 3.3% in 1997 to 2.4% in 1999, but it increased to 3.2% in 2001 and, with the exception of a drop in 2007 to 2.7%, has not varied significantly since.

The NHIS reveals that people aged 65 and older (2.1%) were less likely to have experienced serious psychological distress during the 30 days preceding the survey than people aged 45 to 64 (3.5%). (See Figure 8.5.) Among people aged 18 to 44, women were more likely than men to report serious psychological distress during the 30 days preceding the survey.

The percentage of adults in the first half of 2009 that experienced serious psychological distress during the 30

FIGURE 8.5

Percentage of adults aged 18 and over who experienced serious psychological distress during the past 30 days, by age group and sex, January–June 2009

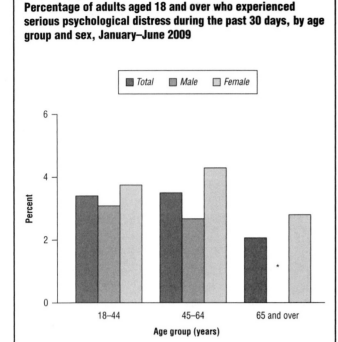

*Estimate does not meet standards of reliability or precision.

Notes: Six psychological distress questions are included in the National Health Interview Survey's (NHIS) Sample Adult Core component. These questions ask how often a respondent experienced certain symptoms of psychological distress during the past 30 days. The response codes (0–4) of the six items for each person are summed to yield a scale with a 0–24 range. A value of 13 or more for this scale is used here to define serious psychological distress (15).

SOURCE: "Figure 13.2. Percentage of Adults Aged 18 Years and over Who Experienced Serious Psychological Distress during the Past 30 Days, by Age Group and Sex: United States, January–June 2009," in *Early Release of Selected Estimates Based on Data from the January–June 2009 National Health Interview Survey*, Centers for Disease Control and Prevention, National Center for Health Statistics, December 2009, http://www.cdc.gov/nchs/data/nhis/earlyrelease/200912_13.pdf (accessed January 18, 2010)

FIGURE 8.6

Age-sex-adjusted percentage of adults aged 18 and over who experienced serious psychological distress during the past 30 days, by race/ethnicity, January–June 2009

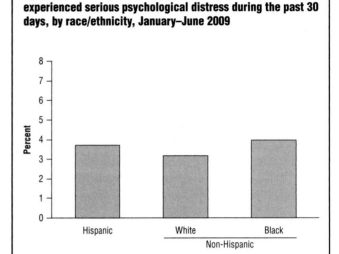

Notes: Six psychological distress questions are included in the National Health Interview Survey's (NHIS) Sample Adult Core component. These questions ask how often a respondent experienced certain symptoms of psychological distress during the past 30 days. The response codes (0–4) of the six items for each person are summed to yield a scale with a 0–24 range. A value of 13 or more for this scale is used here to define serious psychological distress (15). Estimates are age-sex adjusted using the projected 2000 U.S. population as the standard population and using three age groups: 18–44 years, 45–64 years, and 65 years and over.

SOURCE: "Figure 13.3. Age-Sex-Adjusted Percentage of Adults Aged 18 Years and over Who Experienced Serious Psychological Distress during the Past 30 Days, by Race/Ethnicity: United States, January–June 2009," in *Early Release of Selected Estimates Based on Data from the January–June 2009 National Health Interview Survey*, Centers for Disease Control and Prevention, National Center for Health Statistics, December 2009, http://www.cdc.gov/nchs/data/nhis/earlyrelease/200912_13.pdf (accessed January 18, 2010)

days preceding the survey varied by ethnicity—Hispanic and African-American people were more likely to report such distress than were white people. (See Figure 8.6.) The age-sex-adjusted prevalence of serious psychological distress was 3.7% for Hispanic people, 3.2% for non-Hispanic white people, and 3.9% for African-American people.

Not All People Need or Seek Treatment

The NIMH observes that not all mental disorders require treatment, because many people with mental disorders have relatively brief, self-limiting illnesses that are not disabling enough to warrant treatment. However, Philip S. Wang et al. indicate in "Twelve-Month Use of Mental Health Services in the United States: Results from the National Comorbidity Survey Replication" (*Archives of General Psychiatry*, vol. 62, no. 6, June 2005) that less than half of people in need of mental health treatment receive it. Those who seek treatment generally delay pursuing help for a decade or more, and during this time they are likely to develop additional problems. Nonethe-

less, the researchers reveal that the percent of the population treated for mental illness over a 12-month period had increased from 13% a decade ago to 17% in 2003. Wang et al. theorize that the increase in people seeking treatment might be attributable to direct-to-consumer advertisements for antidepressants and other drugs, and to the diminishing stigma associated with obtaining mental health treatment. Regardless, the researchers find that the treatment received is frequently inadequate. Wang et al. attribute delays in seeking treatment to inattention to early warning signs, to insufficient health insurance, and to the lingering stigma that surrounds mental illness.

In "Perceived Barriers to Mental Health Service Utilization in the United States, Ontario, and the Netherlands," (*Psychiatric Services*, vol. 58, March 2007), Jitender Sareen et al. observe that considerable research confirms the finding that "most people with mental disorders do not receive even minimally adequate treatment." Although attitudinal barriers—such as fear of stigmatization and wishing to solve one's own mental health problems without assistance—are frequently cited as barriers to seeking treatment, Sareen et al. assert that in the United States the financial cost of mental health treatment may affect its use, especially among people with low incomes.

In "Depression Care in the United States: Too Little for Too Few" (*Archives of Psychiatry*, vol. 67, no. 1, January 2010), Hector M. González et al. find that a low number of Americans with major depressive disorders receive adequate depression care and that the likelihood of receiving adequate care for mental health disorders such as depression varies among different racial and ethnic groups. Mexican-Americans and African-Americans were the least likely to receive adequate therapy for depression.

TYPES OF DISORDERS

Psychiatrists have identified a wide range of mental disorders, from phobias (intense, irrational, and persistent fears) to depression to schizophrenia. Psychiatric diagnoses are made based on criteria described in the fourth edition of the *Diagnostic and Statistical Manual of Mental Disorders* (*DSM-IV*) by the American Psychiatric Association (APA). Some disorders are relatively mild and affect an individual's life in only a minor way. Others can be overwhelming, completely debilitating, and life-threatening.

Anxiety disorders, which include phobias, and depression are the two most common mental disorders. The NIMH publication *The Numbers Count* notes that an estimated 40 million Americans have an anxiety disorder. Nearly 21 million American adults—close to 10% of the population—suffer from some form of depression. The types of anxiety disorders suffered by Americans aged 18 and older include panic disorder (experienced by an estimated 6 million people), obsessive-compulsive disorder (2.2 million), post-traumatic stress disorder (7.7 million), generalized anxiety disorder (6.8 million), and phobias—social phobia (15 million), agoraphobia (1.8 million), and specific phobia (19.2 million). Many people suffer from more than one mental disorder at a time (comorbidity); for example, millions of Americans suffer from substance (drug or alcohol) abuse combined with one or more other mental disorders.

Children suffer from many of the same mental disorders that afflict adults, but they may also be affected by developmental disorders. Children with disorganized thinking and difficulty communicating verbally, and those who have trouble understanding and navigating the world around them, may be diagnosed with autism or another pervasive developmental disorder. These disorders may be among the most disabling because they are associated with serious learning difficulties and impaired intelligence. Examples of pervasive developmental disorders include autism, Asperger's disorder, and Rett's disorder.

AUTISM SPECTRUM DISORDERS (PERVASIVE DEVELOPMENTAL DISORDERS)

Autism is a spectrum of disorders affecting a person's ability to communicate and interact with others.

Autism spectrum disorders (ASDs), also known as pervasive developmental disorders, are conditions that result from a neurological disorder that typically appears during the first three years of childhood and continues throughout life. These disorders were first described in 1943 by Leo Kanner (1894–1981), who reported on 11 children who displayed an unusual lack of interest in other people but were extremely interested in unusual aspects of the inanimate environment. Autistic children appear unattached to parents or caregivers, assume rigid or limp body postures when held, suffer impaired language, and exhibit behavior such as head banging, violent tantrums, and screaming. They are often self-destructive and uncooperative and experience delayed mental and social skills. Autism is associated with a variety of neurological symptoms such as seizures and persistence of reflexes—involuntary muscle reactions and responses, such as the sucking reflex when the area around the mouth is stimulated, that are normal in infancy but usually disappear during normal child development. Autism is the most common of the pervasive developmental disorders, and the NIMH reports in *The Numbers Count* that its prevalence in 3- to 10-year-olds is about 3.4 cases per 1,000 children and its prevalence is 4 times more frequent in boys than in girls.

In "Prevalence of Autism Spectrum Disorders—Autism and Developmental Disabilities Monitoring Network, United States, 2006" (*Morbidity and Mortality Weekly Report*, vol. 58, December 18, 2009), Catherine Rice et al. find that in the United States nearly 1 in 100 8-year-old children has some autism spectrum disorder. Although autism affects people of all races and ethnicities, it occurs between four and five times more frequently in boys than in girls. In the year 2000 the CDC began the Autism and Developmental Disabilities Monitoring (ADDM) Network to collect and analyze prevalence data in the United States. Comparing 2002 and 2006 ASD prevalence at 10 sites, the ADDM Network found the prevalence of ASDs increased 57% across all the sites, with the increases ranging from 27% to 95%. (See Figure 8.7.) According to the CDC in *ADDM: Autism and Developmental Disabilities Monitoring Network* (2009, http://www.cdc.gov/ncbddd/autism/states/ADDMCommunityReport2009.pdf), although these data confirm that the prevalence of children identified with ASDs has been rising, it is not yet known whether a true increase in risk exists or if the increase is largely attributable to improved identification and reporting of cases.

Even though ASDs were once thought to have psychological origins or occur as the result of bad parenting, both of these hypotheses have been discarded in favor of biological and genetic explanations of causality. The cause of autism remains unknown, but the disorder has been associated with maternal rubella infection, phenylketonuria

FIGURE 8.7

Changes in prevalence of autism spectrum disorder in 8-year-olds, 2002–06

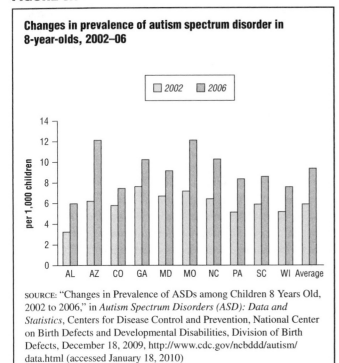

SOURCE: "Changes in Prevalence of ASDs among Children 8 Years Old, 2002 to 2006," in *Autism Spectrum Disorders (ASD): Data and Statistics*, Centers for Disease Control and Prevention, National Center on Birth Defects and Developmental Disabilities, Division of Birth Defects, December 18, 2009, http://www.cdc.gov/ncbddd/autism/data.html (accessed January 18, 2010)

(an inherited disorder of metabolism), tuberous sclerosis (an inherited disease of the nervous system and skin), lack of oxygen at birth, and encephalitis (inflammation of the brain). There is considerable evidence of the heritability of autism. Christine M. Freitag of Saarland University Hospital, Homburg, Germany, notes in "The Genetics of Autistic Disorders and Its Clinical Relevance: A Review of the Literature" (*Molecular Psychiatry*, vol. 12, no. 1, 2007) that it affects approximately 0.2% of children in the general population, but that the risk of bearing a second child with autism rises to between 12% and 20%.

Several genes and mutations associated with autism have been identified. In "Association of Autism with Polymorphisms in the Paired-Like Homeodomain Transcription Factor 1 (*PITX1*) on Chromosome 5q31: A Candidate Gene Analysis" (*BMC Medical Genetics*, vol. 8, no. 1, December 6, 2007), Anne Philippi et al. suggest that at least three genes may be implicated in the development of autism. One is a regulator of the pituitary-hypothalamic axis (the pituitary is a small gland in the brain that produces hormones, and the hypothalamus is a part of the brain that controls body temperature, hunger, sleep, and thirst). Another is involved in the development of nerves, and a third is involved in X-chromosome inactivation in females, which may explain the disproportionate (four-to-one) number of males affected by autism.

In "Genomic and Epigenetic Evidence for Oxytocin Receptor Deficiency in Autism" (*BMC Medicine*, vol. 7, no. 22, October 2009), Simon G. Gregory et al. report the identification of an inherited disruption of gene expression

in a part of the brain system that mediates the disturbed social behavior observed in autism. Gregory et al. found the same disruption in the oxytocin receptor gene in both a person with autism and his mother; the mother had obsessive-compulsive disorder, which, like autism, often involves repetitive behaviors. This genetic variant may prove to be a biomarker for autism that would enable the diagnosis to be made with a blood test. This finding also supports other research suggesting that treatment with oxytocin, a hormone produced by the pituitary gland that is involved in reproduction and social behavior, may help people with autism.

Autism varies from mild to quite severe, and the prognosis depends on the extent of the individual's disabilities and whether he or she receives the early, intensive interventions associated with improved outcomes. A diagnosis of "atypical autism" or "pervasive developmental disorder not otherwise specified" (PDD-NOS) is generally used to refer to mild cases of autism or children with impaired social interaction and verbal and nonverbal communication who are not asocial enough to be considered autistic. Treatment of autism is individualized and may include applied behavior analysis, medications, dietary management and supplements, music therapy, occupational therapy, physical therapy, speech and language therapy, and vision therapy.

Asperger's disorder is a milder form of autism, and sufferers are sometimes called "high functioning children with autism." The disorder is named for the Austrian physician Hans Asperger (1906–1980), who first described it in 1944. The *DSM-IV* states that Asperger's disorder appears to be more common in boys. Affected children tend to be socially isolated and behave oddly. They have impaired social interactions, are unable to express pleasure in others' happiness, and lack social and emotional reciprocity. They are below average in nonverbal communication, and their speech is marked by peculiar abnormalities of inflection and a repetitive pattern. Unlike autism, however, cognitive and communicative development is normal or near normal during the first years of life, and verbal skills are usually relatively strong. Sufferers also have impaired gross motor skills, tend to be clumsy, and may engage in repetitive finger flapping, twisting, or awkward whole-body movements. They usually have very narrow areas of interest that are highly specific, idiosyncratic, and so consuming that they do not pursue age-appropriate activities. Examples of such interests include train schedules, spiders, or telegraph pole insulators.

Rett's disorder (also known as Rett's syndrome) is sometimes mistaken for autism when diagnosed in very young children (and is linked to autism, Asperger's syndrome, attention deficit hyperactivity disorder, and schizophrenia), but it is much less prevalent and has a distinctive onset and course. The condition occurs primarily in girls who, after early normal development, experience slower-than-expected head growth in the first months of life and a loss of purposeful hand motions between ages five and thirty months. Affected children are usually profoundly mentally retarded and exhibit stereotypical repetitive behaviors such as hand wringing or hand washing. Interest in socialization diminishes during the first few years of the disorder but may resume later in life, despite severe impairment in expressive and receptive language development. Affected individuals experience problems in the coordination of gait or trunk movements, and walking may become difficult.

DEPRESSION

According to the NIMH in *The Numbers Count*, major depressive disorders afflict about 14.8 million American adults—about 6.7% of the U.S. population. Women are affected more often than men. Depression can strike at any age; however, the median (average) age when it begins is 32.

Defining Depression

Depression is a "whole body" illness, involving physical, mental, and emotional problems. A depressive disorder is not a temporary sad mood, and it is not a sign of personal weakness or a condition that can be willed away. People with depressive illness cannot just "pull themselves together" and hope they will become well. Without treatment, the symptoms can persist for months or even years. Table 8.1 is a list of symptoms that characterize depression. Not everyone who is depressed experiences all the symptoms. Some people have few symptoms, and some have many. Like other mental illnesses, the severity and duration of the symptoms of depression vary.

TABLE 8.1

Symptoms of depression

Persistent sad, anxious or "empty" feelings

Feelings of hopelessness and/or pessimism

Feelings of guilt, worthlessness and/or helplessness

Irritability, restlessness

Loss of interest in activities or hobbies once pleasurable, including sex

Fatigue and decreased energy

Difficulty concentrating, remembering details and making decisions

Insomnia, early-morning wakefulness, or excessive sleeping

Overeating, or appetite loss

Thoughts of suicide, suicide attempts

Persistent aches or pains, headaches, cramps or digestive problems that do not ease even with treatment

SOURCE: "What Are the Signs and Symptoms of Depression?" in *Depression*, National Institute of Mental Health, January 30, 2009, http://www.nimh.nih.gov/health/publications/depression/what-are-the-signs-and-symptoms-of-depression.shtml (accessed January 18, 2010)

There are several types of depressive disorders. The most common form is dysthymic disorder (dysthymia), a less severe but chronic form of depression that by definition lasts at least two years in adults or at least one year in children. Dysthymic disorders commonly appear for the first time in children, teens, and young adults, and even though they may not disable people as severely as other forms of depression, these disorders can ruin lives by robbing them of joy, energy, and productivity. According to the NIMH in *The Numbers Count*, 1.5% of American adults suffer from dysthymia, and many also suffer from major depression during the course of their life.

Major depression is a more severe and disabling form. In fact, it is a leading cause of disability among Americans aged 15 to 44.

Causes of Depression

Combinations of genetic, psychological, and environmental factors are involved in the development of depressive disorders. Some types of depression run in families, and research studies of twins demonstrate that genetic factors determine susceptibility to depression. Major depression seems to recur in generation after generation of some families, but it also occurs in people with no family history of depression.

Studies of the brain support the premise that depression may have a biological and chemical basis. Even though brain imaging studies clearly indicate that there are differences in the brain between those who suffer from depression and those who do not, it is not yet known if these differences cause the depression or result from it. Researchers speculate that the problem may be caused by the complex neurotransmission (chemical messaging) system of the brain and that people suffering depression have either too much or too little of certain neurochemicals in the brain. Researchers believe depressed patients with normal levels of neurotransmitters may suffer from an inability to regulate them. Most antidepressant drugs currently used to treat the disorder attempt to correct these chemical imbalances.

A person's psychological makeup is another factor in depressive disorders. People who are easily overwhelmed by stress or who suffer from low self-esteem or a pessimistic view of life, of themselves, and of the world tend to be prone to depression. Events outside the person's control can also trigger a depressive episode. A major change in the patterns of daily living—such as a serious loss, a chronic illness, a difficult relationship, or financial problems—can trigger the onset of depression.

Treatment of Depression

Antidepressant medications that alter brain chemistry have been used to treat depressive disorders effectively.

TABLE 8.2

Side effects of antidepressants

The most common side effects associated with SSRIs and SNRIs include:

Headache—usually temporary and will subside.
Nausea—temporary and usually short-lived.
Insomnia and nervousness (trouble falling asleep or waking often during the night)—may occur during the first few weeks but often subside over time or if the dose is reduced.
Agitation (feeling jittery).
Sexual problem—both men and women can experience sexual problems including reduced sex drive, erectile dysfunction, delayed ejaculation, or inability to have an orgasm.

Tricyclic antidepressants also can cause side effects including:

Dry mouth—it is helpful to drink plenty of water, chew gum, and clean teeth daily.
Constipation—it is helpful to eat more bran cereals, prunes, fruits, and vegetables.
Bladder problems—emptying the bladder may be difficult, and the urine stream may not be as strong as usual. Older men with enlarged prostate conditions may be more affeced. The doctor should be notified if it is painful to urinate.
Sexual problems—sexual functioning may change, and side effects are similar to those from SSRIs.
Blurred vision—often passes soon and usually will not require a new corrective lenses prescription.
Drowsiness during the day—usually passes soon, but driving or operating heavy machinery should be avoided while drowsiness occurs. The more sedating antidepresants are generally taken at bedtime to help sleep and minimize daytime drowsiness.

Note: SSRI is selective serotonin reuptake inhibitor. SNRI is serotonin and norepinephrine reuptake inhibitor.

SOURCE: "Side Effects," in *Depression*, National Institute of Mental Health, 2008, http://www.nimh.nih.gov/health/publications/depression/nimhdepression.pdf (accessed January 18, 2010)

Antidepressant medications—including selective serotonin reuptake inhibitors (SSRIs) such as fluoxetine hydrochloride, tricyclic antidepressants such as amitriptyline, and monoamine oxidase inhibitors—work by influencing the function of neurotransmitters such as dopamine or norepinephrine. The SSRIs have fewer reported side effects (such as sedation, headache, weight gain or loss, and nausea) than tricyclic antidepressants.

Antidepressants do not offer immediate relief from symptoms; most take full effect in about four weeks, and some take up to eight weeks to achieve optimal therapeutic effect. Patients must be closely monitored by health professionals for side effects, dosage, and effectiveness. Table 8.2 lists the most common side effects of antidepressants. In cases of chronic depression, medication may be needed continuously and on a long-term basis to prevent the recurrence of the disease.

In 2004 the U.S. Food and Drug Administration (FDA) issued a warning that depression may worsen or suicidal thoughts may occur in people, particularly children and adolescents, who take any of the popular antidepressants. This is most likely to occur at the beginning of treatment or when the doses are increased or decreased. The FDA ordered manufacturers to revise the labeling of antidepressants to increase awareness of these side effects. The NIMH reports in *Depression* (2007, http://www.nimh.nih.gov/health/publications/depression/nimhdepression.pdf) that research conducted between 1988 and 2006 suggests that the benefits of antidepressant medications likely outweigh their risks to children and adolescents with major depression and anxiety disorders.

Psychotherapy has also been demonstrated as effective therapy for mild to moderate depression. Talking about problems with mental health professionals can help patients better understand their feelings. Two types of short-term therapy lasting 10 to 20 weeks appear to improve symptoms of depression. Interpersonal psychotherapy concentrates on helping patients improve personal relationships with family and friends. Cognitive behavioral therapy (CBT) attempts to help patients replace negative thoughts and feelings with more positive, optimistic approaches and actions.

Some people respond well to psychotherapy, and others respond well to antidepressants. Many do best with a combination of treatment—drugs for relatively quick relief of symptoms and therapy to learn how to cope with life's problems more effectively. John S. March et al. find in "The Treatment for Adolescents with Depression Study (TADS): Long-Term Effectiveness and Safety Outcomes" (*Archives of General Psychiatry*, vol. 64, no. 10, October 2007) that depressed adolescents recovered more quickly when they received drug treatment (fluoxetine) alone or in combination with CBT than those who received CBT alone.

The results of a meta-analysis—a review of the results of 6 studies spanning 30 years of antidepressant drug treatment—published in the January 6, 2010, issue of the *Journal of the American Medical Association* (Fournier, Jay C. et al., "Antidepressant Drug Effects and Depression Severity," vol. 303, no. 1) suggest that people with severe depression benefit most from antidepressant medications, while there is little or no benefit for persons with the less-severe symptoms of mild depression. Fournier et al. assert that the benefit of antidepressant medication is comparable to placebo for people with mild or moderate symptoms.

Electrical stimulation of the brain, known as electroconvulsive therapy (ECT), may also be used to treat people with severe depression that has not responded to medication. Electric shocks administered to one side of the patient's head while he or she is under general anesthesia cause brain seizures that somehow relieve depression. The mechanism by which ECT works is as yet unknown. The treatment requires multiple sessions to achieve results; patients usually receive one, sometimes two, treatments per week over the course of 9 to 12 weeks. Because ECT has the potential for serious side effects (e.g., reactions to anesthesia and memory loss) and because of the history of abuses of the treatment, ECT is a controversial treatment of last resort for people with the most refractory (treatment-resistant) depression.

Children Suffer from Depression Too

The most frequently diagnosed mood disorders in children and adolescents are major depressive disorder, dysthymic disorder, and bipolar disorder. Children who are depressed are not unlike their adult counterparts. They may be teary and sad, lose interest in friends and activities, and become listless, self-critical, and hypersensitive to criticism from others. They feel unloved, helpless, and hopeless about the future, and they may think about suicide. Depressed children and adolescents may also be irritable, aggressive, and indecisive. They may have problems concentrating and sleeping and often become careless about their appearance and hygiene. In *Mental Health*, the HHS distinguishes childhood depression from adult depression, noting that children display fewer psychotic symptoms, such as hallucinations and delusions, and more anxiety symptoms, such as clinging to parents or unwillingness to go to school. Depressed children also experience more somatic symptoms, such as general aches and pains, stomachaches, and headaches, than adults with depression.

Dysthymic disorder usually begins in childhood or early adolescence and is a chronic but milder depressive disorder with fewer symptoms. The child or adolescent is depressed on a daily basis for at least one year. Because the average duration of the disorder is about four years, some children become so accustomed to feeling depressed that they may not identify themselves as depressed or complain about symptoms. Nearly three-quarters of children and adolescents with dysthymic disorder experience at least one major depressive episode in the course of their life.

Reactive depression is the most common mental health problem in children and adolescents. It is not considered a mental disorder, and many health professionals consider occasional bouts of reactive depression as entirely consistent with normal adolescent development. It is characterized by transient depressed feelings in response to some negative experience, such as a rejection from a boyfriend or girlfriend or a failing grade. Sadness or listlessness spontaneously resolves in a few hours or may last as long as two weeks. Generally, distraction, in the form of a change of activity or setting, helps improve the mood of affected individuals.

BIPOLAR DISORDER

Bipolar disorder, also known as manic depression, is characterized by alternating periods of persistently elevated, expansive, or irritable mood—called mania—and periods of depression. During a manic episode, a person may feel inflated self-esteem, decreased need for sleep, unusually talkative or pressure to keep talking, and easily distracted. He or she may also have flights of ideas, racing thoughts, increased goal-directed activity

such as shopping, and excessive involvement in high-risk activities. According to the NIMH in *The Numbers Count*, bipolar disorder affects about 5.7 million adult Americans, and the median age of onset is 25.

In the early stages of the illness, patients may experience few symptoms or even symptom-free periods between relatively mild episodes of mania and depression. As the illness progresses, however, manic and depressive episodes become more serious and more frequent. Patients are less likely to experience intermissions, manic euphoria is increasingly replaced by irritability, and depressions deepen. Some individuals suffer psychotic episodes during periods of mania or depression. Bipolar disorder is one of the most lethal illnesses. According to Frederick K. Goodwin and Kay Redfield Jamison in *Manic-Depressive Illness* (2007), "Patients with depressive and manic-depressive illnesses are far more likely to commit suicide than individuals in any other psychiatric or medical risk group. The mortality rate for untreated manic-depressive patients is higher than it is for most types of heart disease and many types of cancer."

The onset of bipolar illness is usually a depressive episode during adolescence. Manic episodes may not appear for months or even years. During manic episodes adolescents are tireless, overly confident, and tend to have rapid-fire or pressured speech. They may perform tasks and schoolwork quickly and energetically but in a wildly disorganized manner. Manic adolescents may seriously overestimate their capabilities, and the combination of bravado and loosened inhibitions may prompt them to participate in high-risk behaviors, such as vandalism, drug abuse, or unsafe sex.

Nitin Gogtay et al. indicate in "Dynamic Mapping of Cortical Development before and after the Onset of Pediatric Bipolar Illness" (*Journal of Child Psychology and Psychiatry*, vol. 48, no, 9, September 2007) that imaging studies of the brains of children and adolescents with bipolar disorder and those diagnosed with schizophrenia show that they have different patterns of development compared with that seen in their healthy age peers. The similarities between the brain scans of children who develop bipolar disease and those who suffer from schizophrenia lead Gogtay et al. to speculate that "both disorders might stem from the same underlying illness process."

There appear to be rising rates of diagnosis of bipolar disorder in children and teens. In "National Trends in the Outpatient Diagnosis and Treatment of Bipolar Disorder in Youth" (*Archives of Psychiatry*, vol. 64, no. 9, September 2007), Carmen Moreno et al. report that from 1994 to 1995 the number of physician visits resulting in a diagnosis of bipolar disorder for people aged 19 and younger was 25 out of every 100,000 people. Between 2002 and 2003 this number had soared to 1,003 office visits resulting in bipolar diagnoses per 100,000 people.

In "Trends in Antipsychotic Drug Use by Very Young, Privately Insured Children" (*Journal of the American Academy of Child & Adolescent Psychiatry*, vol. 49, no. 1, January 2010), Mark Olfsen et al. confirm that from 2001 to 2007 the number of very young children—ages two to five—diagnosed with bipolar disorder and other mental disorders and prescribed powerful antipsychotic drugs increased. During the same period there was a slight decrease in the proportion of very young children who received psychotherapy. Olfsen et al. observed, "Most very young children treated with antipsychotic medications did not receive a mental health assessment, a psychotherapy visit, or treatment from a psychiatrist during the year of antipsychotic use" and that 1 in 70 privately insured children in 2007 received a prescription drug intended to treat a mental disorder.

Treatments for Bipolar Disorder

Lithium has been widely used to treat bipolar disorder since the 1960s, and it is still the medication of choice for controlling the illness. In the 1970s psychiatrists also began using anticonvulsant drugs, including valproate, carbamazepine, and clonazepam, to treat patients who could not tolerate lithium or for whom the drug did not work. Other anticonvulsants, such as oxcarbazepine, lamotrigine, and gabapentin, also have been evaluated to treat the mania associated with bipolar disorder. Chlorpromazine and haloperidol, both antipsychotics, are also helpful in some cases. Antimanic and other antipsychotic agents, such as olanzapine, risperidone, and zipraisidone, are often combined with antidepressants to relieve depressive symptoms and promote better sleep patterns, an important factor in maintaining patients' mood stability. These medication strategies have proven highly effective in treating bipolar disorder; however, many patients still experience a residual pattern of ups and downs.

Medications may become less effective over time and have to be changed. Another major concern among practitioners and patients are medication side effects, especially of lithium. Because therapeutic blood levels of the drug are close to fatal levels, patients taking lithium must consume adequate amounts of water and salt to prevent dehydration, which would cause lithium blood levels to rise to toxic levels. People who take lithium must have their blood level of the drug checked frequently, and they must also be aware of the signs of lithium poisoning. Long-term usage of the drug has been shown to cause kidney damage; however, adequate consumption of water and careful dosage monitoring are believed to reduce the risk of kidney disease.

SCHIZOPHRENIA

A person who hears voices, becomes violent, and sometimes ends up as a homeless person, muttering and shouting incomprehensibly, frequently suffers from schizophrenia.

This disease generally presents in adolescence, causing hallucinations, paranoia, delusions, and social isolation. The effects begin slowly and, initially, are often considered the normal behavioral changes of adolescence. Gradually, voices take over in the schizophrenic's mind, obliterating reality and directing the person to all kinds of erratic behaviors. Suicide attempts and violent attacks are not uncommon to schizophrenics. In an attempt to escape the torment inflicted by their brains, many schizophrenics turn to drugs. The NIMH observes in "Schizophrenia" (March 12, 2010, http://www.nimh.nih.gov/health/publications/schizophrenia/complete-publication.shtml) that people who have schizophrenia abuse alcohol and/or drugs more often than the general population.

In *The Numbers Count*, the NIMH reports that 2.4 million Americans suffer from schizophrenia and similar disorders. Even though the precise causes of schizophrenia are unknown, for years researchers have hypothesized that genetic susceptibility is a risk factor for schizophrenia and bipolar disorder. The disease affects an estimated 1% of the U.S. population, but according to Undine E. Lang et al., in "Molecular Mechanisms of Schizophrenia" (*Cellular Physiology and Biochemistry*, vol. 20, no. 6, 2007), "family, twin and adoption studies have demonstrated a high heritability of the disease."

Imaging studies of the brain reveal abnormal brain development in children who have schizophrenia, and imaging studies of adults with the disease find enlargement of the ventricles of the brain. Some studies suggest that the brain of a person with schizophrenia manufactures too much dopamine, a chemical vital to normal nerve activity. Conventional drug treatment focuses on blocking dopamine receptors in the brain, but not all people with schizophrenia respond to treatment. This type of treatment can produce serious side effects. Newer antipsychotic medications used to treat the disorder, such as risperidone, have fewer side effects than previously used medications. Patients who take these medications must be monitored closely for serious side effects such as the loss of the white blood cells that fight infection.

ANXIETY DISORDERS

Everyone experiences some degree of anxiety almost every day. In the 21st century, a certain amount of anxiety is unavoidable and, in some cases, may even be beneficial. For example, mild anxiety before an exam or a job interview may actually improve performance. Anxiety before a surgical operation, giving a speech, or driving in bad weather is normal.

Nevertheless, when anxiety becomes extreme or when an attack of anxiety strikes suddenly, without an apparent external cause, it can be both debilitating and destructive. Its symptoms may include nervousness, fear, a "knot" in the stomach, rapid heartbeat, or increased blood pressure.

If the anxiety is severe and long lasting, more serious problems may develop. People suffering from anxiety over an extended period may have headaches, ulcers, irritable bowel syndrome, insomnia, and depression. Because anxiety tends to create various other emotional and physical symptoms, a "snowball" effect can occur in which these problems produce even more anxiety.

Chronic anxiety can interfere with an individual's ability to lead a normal life. Mental health professionals consider a person who has prolonged anxiety as having an anxiety disorder. The NIMH estimates in *The Numbers Count* that approximately 40 million Americans suffer from anxiety disorders.

Panic Disorder

Extremely high levels of anxiety may produce panic attacks that are both unanticipated and seemingly without cause. In one type of panic attack, called unexpected, the sufferer is unable to predict when an attack will occur. Other types of panic attacks are linked to a particular location, circumstance, or event and are called situationally bound or situationally predisposed panic attacks. These panic episodes can last as long as 30 minutes and are marked by an overwhelming sense of impending doom while the person's heart races and breathing quickens to the point of gasping for air. Sweating, weakness, dizziness, terror, and feelings of unreality are also typical. Individuals undergoing a panic attack fear they are going to lose control, "lose their mind," or even die. In *The Numbers Count* the NIMH estimates that about 6 million Americans suffer from panic disorders, which usually begin in early adulthood.

Repeated panic attacks may be called a panic disorder. According to the APA, in "Answers to Your Questions about Panic Disorder" (2010, http://www.apa.org/topics/anxiety/panic-disorder.aspx), panic disorder occurs twice as often among women than men and it can run in families. Research reveals that people who experience panic attacks tend to suppress their emotions. Investigators hypothesize that this tendency leads to an emotional buildup for which a panic attack is a form of release. Interestingly, most people who suffer from panic attacks do not experience anxiety between attacks.

The usual treatment for panic disorder is CBT combined with antianxiety drugs to treat the fear of the attacks. Sometimes antidepressant medications are used, even though people suffering from anxiety disorders are usually not clinically depressed. Relaxation therapy has also proved beneficial.

Phobias

Phobias are defined as unreasonable fears associated with a particular situation or object. The most common of the many varieties of phobias are specific phobias. Fear of bees, snakes, rodents, heights, odors, blood, injections, and storms are examples of common specific phobias. Specific phobias, especially animal phobias, are common in children, but they can occur at any age. The NIMH indicates in *The Numbers Count* that 19.2 million American adults suffer from specific phobias. Most people with a phobia understand that their fears are unreasonable, but this awareness does not make them feel any less anxious.

Some specific phobias, such as a fear of heights, usually do not interfere with daily life or cause as much distress as more severe forms, such as agoraphobia (see below). People suffering from severe phobias may rearrange their life drastically to avoid the situations they fear will trigger panic attacks.

SOCIAL PHOBIAS. Social phobias (also called social anxiety disorders) can be more serious than specific phobias. The person with a social phobia is intensely afraid of being judged by others. At social gatherings the person with social phobia expects to be singled out, scrutinized, judged, and found lacking. People with social phobias are usually very anxious about feeling humiliated or embarrassed. They are often so crippled by their own fears that they may have a hard time thinking clearly, remembering facts, or carrying on normal conversations. The individual with social phobia may tremble, sweat, or blush and often fears fainting or losing bladder or bowel control in social settings. In response to these overwhelming fears, the person with social phobia tries to avoid public situations and gatherings of people. The NIMH estimates in *The Numbers Count* that about 15 million adults suffer from social phobia. Social phobias tend to start at around age 13 and, if not treated, can continue throughout life.

Because social phobics fear being the center of attention or the subject of criticism, public speaking, asking questions, eating in front of others, or even attending social events create anxiety. Social phobias should not be confused with shyness, which is considered a normal variation in personality. Social phobias can be disabling, preventing sufferers from attending school, working, and having friends.

AGORAPHOBIA. Many people who experience panic attacks go on to develop agoraphobia—the fear of crowds and open spaces. The term comes from the Greek word *agora*, which means "marketplace." This type of phobia is a severely disabling disorder that often traps its victims, rendering them virtual prisoners in their own homes, unable to work, shop, or attend social activities.

Agoraphobia normally develops slowly, following an initial unexpected panic attack. For example, on an ordinary day, while shopping, driving to work, or doing errands, the individual is suddenly struck by a wave of terror characterized by symptoms such as trembling, a pounding heart, profuse sweating, and difficulty in breathing normally. The person desperately seeks safety, reassurance from friends and family, or a physician. The panic subsides and all is well—until another panic attack occurs.

The person with agoraphobia begins to avoid all places and situations where an attack occurred and then begins to avoid places where an attack could possibly occur or where it might be difficult to escape and get help. Gradually, the victim becomes more and more limited in the choice of places that are "safe." Eventually, the person with agoraphobia cannot venture outside the immediate neighborhood or leave the house. The fear ultimately expands to touch every aspect of life.

In *The Numbers Count* the NIMH estimates that about 1.8 million adults suffer from agoraphobia, and it usually begins during the late teens or twenties.

PHOBIA TREATMENT PROGRAMS. Phobia treatment programs use a wide variety of CBT techniques to help patients face and overcome their fears. In addition, drugs may be used to ease the symptoms of anxiety, fear, and depression and to help the person return to a normal life more quickly. Antidepressants have been shown to help people who suffer from panic attacks and agoraphobia. In addition, antianxiety drugs are useful in treating the generalized anxiety that frequently accompanies phobias.

Deborah C. Beidel et al. indicate in "SET-C Versus Fluoxetine in the Treatment of Childhood Social Phobia" (*Journal of the American Academy of Child and Adolescent Psychiatry*, vol. 46, no. 12, December 2007) that behavioral therapy was more effective than drug treatment in helping children overcome social phobias. Even though many children were helped by treatment with fluoxetine, the behavioral therapy appeared to offer more global benefits by also helping the children to improve their social skills and overall functioning.

In "Attention Training in Individuals with Generalized Social Phobia: A Randomized Controlled Trial" (*Journal of Consulting and Clinical Psychology*, vol. 77, no. 5, October 2009), Nader Amir et al. considered whether people suffering from social phobia could be conditioned to divert their attention from perceived threat and thus reduce symptoms of social anxiety. In the study's Attention Modification Program (AMP), participants were shown pictures of faces with either threatening or neutral emotional expressions placed at different locations on a computer screen. Participants in this group were given a prompt on the screen that directed them to neutral faces, thereby directing attention away from the threatening ones. In the control group, the prompt appeared with equal frequency in the position of the threatening and neutral faces. The results of the study, which measured clinician-observed and self-reported symptoms, show the AMP

group had reduced symptoms of anxiety and suggest that such training may be helpful for treating social phobia.

Obsessive-Compulsive Disorder

Obsessive-compulsive disorder (OCD) is an anxiety disorder marked by unwanted, often unpleasant recurring thoughts (obsessions) and repetitive, often mechanical behaviors (compulsions). The repetitive behaviors, such as continually checking to be certain windows and doors are locked or repeated hand washing, are intended to dispel the obsessive thoughts that trigger them—that an intruder will enter the house through an unlocked door or window, or that disease will be prevented by hand washing. The vicious cycle of obsessions and compulsions only serves to heighten anxiety; OCD can debilitate those who have the disorder.

The NIMH estimates in *The Numbers Count* that about 2.2 million adults over age 18 suffer from OCD. Its symptoms generally appear during childhood or adolescence. Imaging studies using positron emission tomography (PET) reveal that people with OCD have different patterns of brain activity than those without the disorder. Furthermore, the PET scans show that the part of the brain most affected by OCD (the striatum) changes and responds to both medication and behavioral therapy.

Many of the medications used to treat other anxiety disorders appear effective for patients with OCD, as has a behavioral type of therapy called "exposure and response prevention," during which patients with OCD learn new ways to manage their obsessive thoughts without resorting to compulsive behaviors.

Anxiety among Children and Adolescents

Children and adolescents suffer from many of the same anxiety disorders as do adults. Taken together, the different types of anxiety disorders constitute the mental disorders most prevalent among children and adolescents. In their "Prevalence and Treatment of Mental Disorders among US Children in the 2001–2004 NHANES," Merikangas et al. find that 0.7% of children suffer from generalized anxiety or panic disorders.

Separation anxiety disorder is a type of anxiety disorder found specifically in children. It is normal for infants, toddlers, and very young children to experience anxiety when separated from their parents or caregivers. For example, nearly every child experiences at least a momentary pang of separation anxiety on the first day of preschool or kindergarten. When this condition occurs in older children or adolescents and it is severe enough to impair social, academic, or job functioning for at least one month, it is considered separation anxiety disorder. The risk factors associated with separation anxiety disorder include stress, such as the illness or death of a family member, geographic relocation, and physical or sexual assault.

Children with separation anxiety may be clingy, and often they harbor fears that accidents or natural disasters will forever separate them from their parents. Because they fear being apart from their parents, they may resist attending school or going anywhere without a parent. Separation anxiety can produce physical symptoms such as dizziness, nausea, or palpitations. It is often associated with symptoms of depression. Young children with separation anxiety may have difficulty falling asleep alone in their room and may have recurrent nightmares.

According to the HHS, research suggests that some children develop OCD following an infection with a specific type of streptococcus. This condition is known as pediatric autoimmune neuropsychiatric disorders associated with streptococcal (PANDAS) infections. It is believed that antibodies intended to combat the strep infection mistakenly attack a region of the brain and trigger an inflammatory reaction, which in turn leads to development of OCD. In "The PANDAS Subgroup of Tic Disorders and Childhood-Onset Obsessive-Compulsive Disorder" (*Journal of Psychosomatic Research*, vol. 67, no. 6, December 2009), Davide Martino et al. suggest that in addition to childhood-onset obsessive-compulsive disorder, the PANDAS spectrum also may include attention deficit/hyperactivity disorder. SSRIs are effective in reducing or even eliminating the symptoms of OCD in many affected children and adolescents. However, side effects such as dry mouth, sleepiness, dizziness, fatigue, tremors, and constipation are common and may themselves impair functioning.

ATTENTION DEFICIT HYPERACTIVITY DISORDER

Attention deficit disorder (ADD) and attention deficit hyperactivity disorder (ADHD) are relatively new names for psychiatric disorders that usually begin or become apparent in children going to preschool and elementary school. Children with ADHD cannot sit still, have difficulty controlling their impulsive actions, and are unable to focus on projects long enough to complete them; those diagnosed with ADD have the same symptoms but do not display hyperactivity. Even though teachers originally dubbed ADHD a "learning problem," the disorder affects more than just schoolwork. Children with ADHD have trouble socializing, are often unable to make friends, and suffer from low self-esteem. If left untreated, ADHD can leave children unable to cope academically or socially, possibly leading to depression.

According to the NIMH in *The Numbers Count*, 4.1% of adults suffer from ADHD. The condition frequently coexists with other mental health problems such as substance abuse, anxiety disorders, depression, or antisocial behavior. In "America's Children: Key National Indicators of Well-Being, 2009" (http://www.childstats.gov/

americaschildren/special1.asp), the Federal Interagency Forum on Child and Family Statistics indicates that ADD and ADHD are reported in 30% of children with special health care needs. The NHANES, as described by Merikangas et al., finds that higher rates of ADHD were reported in children of lower socioeconomic status. Children diagnosed with ADHD are usually affected into their teen years, but for most, symptoms subside in adulthood and adults become more adept at controlling their behavior. Regardless, vigilance is warranted because research reveals an increased incidence in juvenile delinquency and subsequent encounters with the criminal justice system among adults who were diagnosed with ADHD in their youth.

The reported incidence of ADHD has increased over the past 25 years, possibly because of better diagnosis, changing expectations, or insufficient supportive social structures. In the absence of clear criteria for ADHD or guidelines by which to diagnose it, researchers fear that the disorder may be under- or overdiagnosed. The cause of ADHD is as yet unknown. According to the NIMH ("What Causes ADHD?" January 23, 2009, http://www.nimh.nih.gov/health/publications/attention-deficit-hyperactivity-disorder/what-causes-adhd.shtml), "many studies suggest that genes play a large role." The NIMH also notes that ADHD is likely caused by a combination of things and suggests that environmental factors, brain injuries, nutrition, and social environment may play a role. A biological explanation of ADHD arose because its symptoms respond to treatment with stimulants such as methylphenidate, which increase the availability of dopamine—the neurotransmitter that is vital for purposeful movement, motivation, and alertness. As a result, researchers theorize that ADHD may be caused by unavailability of dopamine in the central nervous system.

While genes have been offered as a cause of ADHD, the evidence of a genetic component has been inconclusive. There is an increased incidence of ADHD in children with a first-degree relative with ADHD, conduct disorders, antisocial personality, substance abuse, and others, but this observation does not resolve the question of whether nature (genetics) or nurture (family and environmental influences) contributes more strongly to the origins of ADHD. Twin studies find that when ADHD is present in one twin, it is significantly more likely to be present in an identical twin than in a fraternal twin. These findings support inheritance as an important risk in a proportion of children with ADHD.

Even though imaging studies reveal differences in the brains of children with ADHD, and scientists have found a link between the inability to pay attention and the diminished utilization of glucose in parts of the brain, some researchers question whether these changes cause the disorder. They argue that the observed changes may result from the disorder, or simply coexist with it. As a result, some mental health professionals and educators concede that some children are legitimately diagnosed with ADHD, and others are mislabeled. They speculate that the latter group may be simply high-spirited, undisciplined, or misbehaving.

Treatment for ADHD

Much controversy about ADHD has focused on its treatment. NIMH research indicates that there are two effective treatment methods for elementary-school children with ADHD: a closely monitored medication regimen and a combination of medication and behavioral interventions. Behavioral interventions include psychotherapy, CBT, social skills training, support groups, and parent-educator skills training.

Even though some researchers still question the wisdom of treatment with potentially addicting, powerful stimulants, prescription stimulants (such as methylphenidate, dextromethamphetamine, and amphetamine) have proved to be safe and effective for short-term treatment of ADHD. Peter Jensen et al. confirm in "3-Year Follow-up of the NIMH MTA Study" (*Journal of the American Academy of Child and Adolescent Psychiatry*, vol. 46, no. 8, August 2007) the efficacy of medication and behavioral treatment alone or in combination, and the children in the study showed sustained improvement after three years. In another study, "A One Year Trial of Methylphenidate in the Treatment of ADHD" (*Journal of Attention Disorders*, January 13, 2010), Paul H. Wender et al. find that adults with ADHD who responded well to short-term treatment with methylphenidate also benefited from long-term treatment. Wender et al. report that long-term drug treatment resulted in "marked improvements in ADHD symptoms and psychosocial functioning."

DISRUPTIVE DISORDERS

Children and adolescents with disruptive disorders, which include oppositional defiant disorder and conduct disorder, display antisocial behaviors. Like separation anxiety, the diagnosis of a disruptive disorder largely depends on assessing whether behavior is age appropriate. For example, just as clinging may be considered normal for a toddler but abnormal behavior in an older child, toddlers and very young children often behave aggressively (e.g., grabbing toys and even biting one another). When, however, a child older than age five displays such aggressive behavior, it may indicate an emerging oppositional defiant or conduct disorder.

It is important to distinguish isolated acts of aggression or the normal childhood and adolescent phases of testing limits from the pattern of ongoing, persistent defiance, hostility, and disobedience that is the hallmark of

oppositional defiant disorder (ODD). Children with ODD are argumentative, lose their temper, refuse to adhere to rules, blame others for their own mistakes, and are spiteful and vindictive. Their behaviors often alienate them from family and peers and cause problems at school.

Family strife, volatile marital relationships, frequently changing caregivers, and inconsistent child-rearing practices may increase the risk for the disorder. Some practitioners consider ODD a gateway condition to conduct disorder. According to the HHS in *Mental Health*, estimates of the prevalence of ODD range from 1% to 6%, depending on the population and the way the disorder is evaluated. Prepubescent boys are diagnosed more often with ODD than girls of the same age, but after puberty the rates in both genders are equal.

Children or adolescents with conduct disorder are aggressive. They may fight, sexually assault, or behave cruelly to people or animals. Because lying, stealing, vandalism, truancy, and substance abuse are common behaviors, adults, social service agencies, and the criminal justice system often view affected young people as "bad" rather than as mentally ill. The American Academy of Child and Adolescent Psychiatry describes in "Conduct Disorders" (July 2004, http://www.aacap.org/cs/root/facts_for_families/conduct_disorder) an array of generally antisocial behaviors that when exhibited by children or adolescents suggest a diagnosis of conduct disorder. These actions and behaviors include:

- Bullies, threatens, or intimidates others
- Often initiates physical fights
- Uses a weapon such as a bat, brick, knife, or gun that could cause serious physical harm
- Is physically cruel to people or animals
- Steals from a victim while confronting them
- Engages in coercive or forced sexual activity
- Deliberately sets fires with the intention to cause damage
- Deliberately destroys others' property
- Breaks into a building, house, or car
- Lies to obtain goods or favors, or to avoid obligations
- Steals items without confronting a victim
- Often stays out at night despite parental objections
- Runs away from home
- Often truant from school

Conduct disorder severely compromises the lives of affected children and adolescents. Their schoolwork suffers, as do their relationships with adults and peers. The HHS finds that youths with conduct disorders have higher rates of injury and sexually transmitted diseases and are likely to be expelled from school and have problems with the law. Rates of depression, suicidal thoughts, suicide attempts, and suicide are all higher in children and teens diagnosed with conduct disorder. Children in whom the disorder presents before age 10 are predominantly male. Early onset places them at a greater risk for adult antisocial personality disorder. More than one-quarter of severely antisocial children become antisocial adults.

As of 2010, there were no medications that had proven effective in treating conduct disorder. Even though psychosocial interventions can reduce their antisocial behavior, living with a child or teen with a conduct disorder stresses the entire family. Support programs train parents how to positively reinforce appropriate behaviors and how to strengthen the emotional bonds between parent and child. Identifying and intervening with high-risk children to enhance their social interaction and prevent academic failure can mitigate some of the potentially harmful long-term consequences of conduct disorder. In "Five- to Six-year Outcome and Its Prediction for Children with ODD/CD Treated with Parent Training" (*Journal of Child Psychology and Psychiatry*, December 8, 2009), May B. Drugli et al. find that the combination of parent training, which educates parents about strategies for managing their child's behavior, and child treatment is effective for young children with conduct disorders.

Research demonstrates that preventive measures may help reduce conduct problems in children who exhibit the most aggressive or disruptive behaviors. In "Can a Costly Intervention Be Cost-Effective?: An Analysis of Violence Prevention" (*Archives of General Psychiatry*, vol. 63, no. 11, November 2006), E. Michael Foster et al. find that the costs of providing targeted interventions were small compared with the personal and societal costs of family strife and crime that can result from untreated conduct disorders.

EATING DISORDERS

American society is preoccupied with body image. Advertisers of many products suggest that to be thin and beautiful is to be happy. Many prominent weight-loss programs reinforce this suggestion. A well-balanced, low-fat food plan, combined with exercise, can help most overweight people achieve a healthier weight and lifestyle. Dieting to achieve a healthy weight is quite different from dieting obsessively to become "model" thin, which can have consequences ranging from mildly harmful to life threatening. In *Eating Disorders* (2007, http://www.nimh.nih.gov/health/publications/eating-disorders/nimheating disorders.pdf), the NIMH observes that eating disorders frequently coexist with other mental disorders, including depression, substance abuse, and anxiety disorders.

Preteens, teens, and college-age women are at special risk for eating disorders. In fact, most of those who develop an eating disorder are young women. However, the NIMH indicates that between 5% and 15% of people with anorexia or bulimia and about 35% of those with binge-eating disorder are male. Researchers do not know exactly how many teenage boys and men are afflicted. Until recently, there has been a lack of awareness that eating disorders can be a problem for males, perhaps because men are more likely to mask the symptoms of eating disorders with excuses and rationales such as preventing heart disease or diabetes or trying to build a more muscular physique.

Research reveals that many people believe certain foods are addictive and that some people can become addicted to such behaviors as fasting, binging, purging, and laxative use associated with disordered eating. People with bulimia may talk of being "hooked" on certain foods and needing to feed their "habits." This addictive behavior can carry over into other areas of a person's life, resulting, for example, in substance abuse. Many people with eating disorders suffer from comorbidities (having more than one disease or disorder at the same time), such as severe depression, which increases their risk for suicide. G. Terrence Wilson et al., in "Beliefs about Eating and Eating Disorders" (*Eating Behaviors*, vol. 10, no. 3, August 2009) note that because some researchers and clinicians view eating disorders as addictions, some treatment prescribed for eating disorders is comparable to substance (alcohol and drug) abuse and addiction treatment.

Anorexia Nervosa

Anorexia nervosa involves severe weight loss—a minimum of 15% below normal body weight. People with anorexia literally starve themselves, although they may be very hungry. For reasons that researchers do not yet fully understand, people with anorexia are irrationally fearful about gaining weight. They are often obsessed with food and weight and develop strange eating habits, refusing to eat with other people, and exercising strenuously to burn calories and prevent weight gain. Individuals with anorexia continue to believe they are overweight even when they are dangerously thin.

The medical complications of anorexia are similar to starvation. When the body attempts to protect its most vital organs—the heart and the brain—it goes into "slow gear." Monthly menstrual periods stop, and breathing, pulse, blood pressure, and thyroid function slow down. The nails and hair become brittle, and the skin dries. Water imbalance causes constipation, and the lack of body fat causes an inability to withstand cold temperatures. Depression, weakness, and a constant obsession with food are also symptoms of the disease. In addition, personality changes may occur. The person suffering from anorexia may have outbursts of anger and hostility or may withdraw socially. In the most serious cases, death can result.

Bulimia Nervosa

People who have bulimia nervosa eat compulsively and then purge (get rid of the food) through self-induced vomiting; use of laxatives, diuretics, strict diets, fasts, or exercise; or a combination of several of these compensatory behaviors. The NIMH reports in *The Numbers Count* that an estimated 1.1% to 4.2% of females suffer from bulimia.

Many people with bulimia are at a normal body weight or higher because of their frequent binge-purge behavior, which can occur from once or twice a week to several times a day. Those people with bulimia who maintain normal weight may manage to keep their eating disorder secret for years. As with anorexia, bulimia usually begins during adolescence, but many people with bulimia do not seek help until they are in their 30s or 40s.

Both binge eating and purging are dangerous practices. James I. Hudson et al. suggest in "The Prevalence and Correlates of Eating Disorders in the National Comorbidity Survey Replication" (*Biological Psychiatry*, vol. 61, no. 3, February 1, 2007) that binge-eating disorder (binging that is not followed by purging, often resulting in obesity) is more prevalent than bulimia, with 3.5% of women and 2% of men suffering from it at some point during their life. In rare cases, bingeing can cause stomach ruptures. Purging can result in heart failure because the body loses vital minerals. The acid in vomit wears down tooth enamel and can cause scarring on the hands when fingers are pushed down the throat to induce vomiting. The esophagus may become inflamed, and glands in the neck may become swollen.

Causes of Eating Disorders

Evidence suggests a genetic component to susceptibility to eating disorders. For example, Cynthia M. Bulik et al. indicate in "Prevalence, Heritability, and Prospective Risk Factors for Anorexia Nervosa" (*Archives of General Psychiatry*, vol. 63, no. 3, March 2006) that in the general population the chance of developing anorexia is about 1 out of 200, but when a family member has the disorder, the risk increases to 1 out of 30. In "Understanding the Relation between Anorexia Nervosa and Bulimia Nervosa in a Swedish National Twin Sample" (*Biological Psychiatry*, vol. 67, no. 1, January 2010), Bulik et al. examined the heritability of anorexia nervosa and bulimia nervosa and identified an overlap of genetic and environmental factors that influence the development of both eating disorders.

People with bulimia and anorexia seem to have different personalities. Those with bulimia are likely to be impulsive (acting without considering the consequences) and are more likely to abuse alcohol and drugs. People with anorexia tend to be perfectionists, good students, and competitive athletes. They usually keep their feelings to themselves and rarely disobey their parents. People with bulimia and anorexia share certain traits: They lack self-esteem, have feelings of helplessness, and fear gaining weight. In both disorders the eating problems appear to develop as a way of handling stress and anxiety.

The person with bulimia consumes huge amounts of food in a search for comfort and stress relief. The bingeing, however, brings only guilt and depression. On the other hand, people with anorexia restrict food to gain a sense of control and mastery over some aspect of their life. Controlling their body weight seems to offer two advantages: The victims can take control of their body and can gain approval from others.

Treatment of Eating Disorders

Generally, a physician treats the medical complications of the disorder, whereas a nutritionist advises the affected individual about specific diet and eating plans. To help the person with an eating disorder face his or her underlying problems and emotional issues, psychotherapy is usually necessary. People with eating disorders, whether they are normal weight, overweight, or obese, should seek help from a mental health professional such as a psychiatrist, psychologist, or clinical social worker for their eating behavior. Sometimes the challenge is to convince people with eating disorders to seek and obtain treatment; other times it is difficult to gain their adherence to treatment. Many anorexics deny their illness, and getting and keeping anorexic patients in treatment can be difficult. Treating bulimia is similarly difficult. Many bulimics are easily frustrated and want to leave treatment if their symptoms are not quickly relieved.

Several approaches are used to treat eating disorders. CBT teaches people how to monitor their eating and change unhealthy eating habits. It also teaches them how to change the way they respond in stressful situations. CBT is based on the premise that thinking influences emotions and behavior—that feelings and actions originate with thoughts. CBT posits that it is possible to change the way people feel and act, even if their circumstances do not change. It teaches the advantages of feeling calm when faced with undesirable situations. CBT clients learn that they will confront undesirable events and circumstances whether they become troubled about them or not. When they are troubled about events or circumstances, they have two problems: the troubling event or circumstance, and the troubling feelings about the event or circumstance. Clients learn that when they do not become troubled about trying events and circumstances, they can reduce the number of problems they face by half.

Interpersonal psychotherapy (IPT) helps people look at their relationships with friends and family and make changes to resolve problems. IPT is short-term therapy that has demonstrated effectiveness for the treatment of depression. According to the International Society for Interpersonal Psychotherapy, IPT does not assume that mental illness arises exclusively from problematical interpersonal relationships. It does emphasize, however, that mental health and emotional problems occur within an interpersonal context. For this reason, the therapy aims to intervene specifically in social functioning to relieve symptoms.

Like other forms of psychotherapy, IPT may be used in conjunction with medications. Because eating disorders frequently recur, it is recommended that successful short-term treatment be combined with ongoing maintenance therapy, such as monthly sessions following completion of the short-term phase.

Group therapy has been found helpful for bulimics, who are relieved to find that they are not alone or unique in their binge-eating behaviors. A combination of behavioral therapy and family systems therapy is often the most effective with anorexics. Family systems therapy considers the family as the unit of treatment and focuses on relationships and communication patterns within the family rather than on the personality traits or symptoms displayed by individual family members. Family systems therapy also considers the family as an entity that is more than the sum of its individual members and uses systems theory to determine family members' roles within the system as a whole. Problems are addressed by modifying the system rather than by trying to change an individual family member. People with eating disorders who also suffer from depression may benefit from antidepressant and antianxiety medications to help relieve coexisting mental health problems.

Daniel le Grange et al. find in "A Randomized Controlled Comparison of Family-Based Treatment and Supportive Psychotherapy for Adolescent Bulimia Nervosa" (*Archives of General Psychiatry*, vol. 64, no. 9, September 2007) that family-based treatment for bulimia was more effective for teens suffering from the disorder than individual therapy. Eighty teens with bulimia were randomly assigned to receive family or individual therapy, and their progress was monitored during treatment and for six months afterward. More subjects in the study recovered fully from the disorder using family-based therapy than individual counseling, and the effects of treatment appeared to take hold more quickly.

Recovery from eating disorders is uneven. The Eating Disorders Coalition for Research, Policy, and Action characterizes recovery as a process that frequently entails multiple rehospitalizations, limited ability to work or attend school, and limited capacity for interpersonal relationships.

In "Eating Behavior among Women with Anorexia Nervosa" (*American Journal of Clinical Nutrition*, vol. 82, no. 2, August 2005), Robin Sysko et al. reconfirm the finding that even though hospital treatment of people with anorexia is often successful, 30% to 70% of patients suffer relapses when they are discharged back into the community. The researchers wanted to find out whether current treatment for anorexia successfully addresses severe caloric restriction and other characteristic features of anorexia nervosa. To do this, they scrutinized eating behavior among people with anorexia nervosa before and immediately after treatment that restored their weight and compared these behaviors with those of control subjects. Sysko et al. noted that control subjects consumed significantly more than anorexic patients despite the fact that subjects treated for anorexia displayed significant decreases in psychological and eating-disordered symptoms after they had regained weight. Sysko et al. feel their findings underscore the need for continuing support for people with anorexia once they leave an intensive treatment program.

PRESCRIBING PSYCHOACTIVE MEDICATION TO CHILDREN

In *Treatment of Children with Mental Illness* (2009, http://www.nimh.nih.gov/health/publications/treatment-of-children-with-mental-illness-fact-sheet/nimh-treatment-children-mental-illness-faq.pdf), a publication aimed at parents of children with a range of mental disorders, the NIMH acknowledges public concern that psychotropic medication is being prescribed to very young children and that the safety and efficacy of most psychotropic medications, especially for children under age six, have not yet been established. Several widely used drugs have not received FDA approval for use in young children simply because there are not enough data to support their use.

The data are lacking because historically there were ethical concerns about involving children in clinical trials to determine not only the most effective treatments but also the proper dosage, the potential side effects, and the long-term effects of drug use on learning and development. Policies about research involving children affect the FDA approval process and recommendations for use. For example, methylphenidate is approved for use in children ages six and older, but its use was not evaluated in children younger than age six. In contrast, dextromethamphetamine received approval for use in children as young as three years because by the time approval was sought, study guidelines permitted participation of younger children. Highlighting the discrepancies in the approved starting ages of patients for certain drugs, Table 8.3 lists the brand and generic names of prescription medications used to treat ADHD in children and adolescents and indicates FDA approval of their use in children age six and older and age three and older. In contrast, none of the drugs prescribed to treat anxiety are FDA approved for use in persons under age 18. (See Table 8.4.)

Because the FDA approval process often requires years of research to demonstrate safety and efficacy, and practitioners are eager to provide symptom relief for

TABLE 8.3

Prescription drugs used to treat ADHD

Trade name	Generic name	FDA-approved age
ADHD medications		
(All of these ADHD medications are stimulants, except Strattera.)		
Adderall	amphetamine	3 and older
Adderall XR	amphetamine (extended release)	6 and older
Concerta	methylphenidate (long acting)	6 and older
Daytrana	methylphenidate patch	6 and older
Desoxyn	methamphetamine	6 and older
Dexedrine	dextroamphetamine	3 and older
Dextrostat	dextroamphetamine	3 and older
Focalin	dexmethylphenidate	6 and older
Focalin XR	dexmethylphenidate (extended release)	6 and older
Metadate ER	methylphenidate (extended release)	6 and older
Metadate CD	methylphenidate (extended release)	6 and older
Methylin	methylphenidate (oral solution and chewable tablets)	6 and older
Ritalin	methylphenidate	6 and older
Ritalin SR	methylphenidate (extended release)	6 and older
Ritalin LA	methylphenidate (long-acting)	6 and older
Strattera	atomoxetine	6 and older
Vyvanse	lisdexamfetamine dimesylate	

ADHD = Attention Deficit Hyperactivity Disorder
FDA = Food & Drug Administration

SOURCE: "ADHD Medications," in *Mental Health Medications: Alphabetical List of Medications*, National Institute of Mental Health, August 12, 2009, http://www.nimh.nih.gov/health/publications/mental-health-medications/alphabetical-list-of-medications.shtml (accessed January 20, 2010)

TABLE 8.4

Prescription drugs used to treat anxiety disorders

Trade name	Generic name	FDA-approved age
Antianxiety medications		
(All of these antianxiety medications are benzodiazepines, except BuSpar.)		
Ativan	lorazepam	18 and older
BuSpar	buspirone	18 and older
Klonopin	clonazepam	18 and older
Librium	chlordiazepoxide	18 and older
Oxazepam (generic only)	oxazepam	18 and older
Tranxene	clorazepate	18 and older
Valium	diazepam	18 and older
Xanax	alprazolam	18 and older

FDA = Food & Drug Administration

SOURCE: "Anti-Anxiety Medications," in *Mental Health Medications: Alphabetical List of Medications*, National Institute of Mental Health, August 12, 2009, http://www.nimh.nih.gov/health/publications/mental-health-medications/alphabetical-list-of-medications.shtml (accessed January 20, 2010)

severely troubled children, many recommend off-label use of medications. Off-label treatment may involve use of a medication that has not yet received official FDA approval for use in children or the use of a drug the FDA has approved for children to treat a specific condition for which its use has not been approved. As such, they are prescribed off-label when used in pediatric and adolescent medicine. The NIMH observes that some off-label use is supported by data from well-controlled studies but cautions that other off-label prescribing, particularly to very young children whose responses to these drugs have not been scrutinized, should be performed prudently.

In "Which Groups Have Special Needs When Taking Psychiatric Medications?" (March 18, 2010, http://www.nimh.nih.gov/health/publications/mental-health-medications/which-groups-have-special-needs-when-taking-psychiatric-medications.shtml), the NIMH notes that there is strong support for the safety and efficacy of several medications for several conditions, specifically psychostimulants for ADHD. However, the NIMH also indicates that there is a lack of information about the safety and efficacy of other medications and warns that children may have different reactions to drugs than do adults. The NIMH also cautions that antidepressants and ADHD medications carry FDA warnings about potentially dangerous side effects for young people. "In addition to medications," continues the NIMH, "other treatments for young people with mental disorders should be considered. Psychotherapy, family therapy, educational courses, and behavior management techniques can help everyone involved cope with the disorder."

SUICIDE

Suicide may be the ultimate expression or consequence of depression or another serious mental disorder. Not all people who suffer from depression contemplate suicide, nor do all those who attempt suicide suffer from depressive or other mental illnesses. Regardless, except for certain desperate medical situations, suicide in the United States is generally considered an unacceptable act. It is often referred to as a "long-term solution to a short-term problem."

Since 1970 the death rate for suicide has decreased from 13.1 suicides per 100,000 resident population to 10.9 deaths per 100,000 in 2006. (See Table 8.5.) According to the NIMH, in "Suicide in the U.S.: Statistics and Prevention" (July 27, 2009, http://www.nimh.nih.gov/health/publications/suicide-in-the-us-statistics-and-prevention.shtml), in 2006 suicide ranked as the 11th-leading cause of death in the United States. It was the 7th-leading cause of death for males and the 16th-leading cause of death for females.

TABLE 8.5

Death rates for suicide, by sex, race, Hispanic origin, and age, selected years 1950–2006

[Data are based on death certificates]

Sex, race, Hispanic origin, and race	1950[a,b]	1960[a,b]	1970[b]	1980[b]	1990[b]	2000[c]	2001[c]	2002[c]	2003[c]	2004[c]	2005[c]	2006[c]
					Deaths per 100,000 resident population							
All persons												
All ages, age-adjusted[d]	13.2	12.5	13.1	12.2	12.5	10.4	10.7	10.9	10.8	10.9	10.9	10.9
All ages, crude	11.4	10.6	11.6	11.9	12.4	10.4	10.8	11.0	10.8	11.0	11.0	11.1
Under 1 year	—	—	—	—	—	—	—	—	*	*	—	—
1–4 years	—	—	—	—	—	—	—	—	*	*	—	—
5–14 years	0.2	0.3	0.3	0.4	0.8	0.7	0.7	0.6	0.6	0.7	0.7	0.5
15–24 years	4.5	5.2	8.8	12.3	13.2	10.2	9.9	9.9	9.7	10.3	10.0	9.9
15–19 years	2.7	3.6	5.9	8.5	11.1	8.0	7.9	7.4	7.3	8.2	7.7	7.3
20–24 years	6.2	7.1	12.2	16.1	15.1	12.5	12.0	12.4	12.1	12.5	12.4	12.5
25–44 years	11.6	12.2	15.4	15.6	15.2	13.4	13.8	14.0	13.8	13.9	13.7	13.8
25–34 years	9.1	10.0	14.1	16.0	15.2	12.0	12.8	12.6	12.7	12.7	12.4	12.3
35–44 years	14.3	14.2	16.9	15.4	15.3	14.5	14.7	15.3	14.9	15.0	14.9	15.1
45–64 years	23.5	22.0	20.6	15.9	15.3	13.5	14.4	14.9	15.0	15.4	15.4	16.0
45–54 years	20.9	20.7	20.0	15.9	14.8	14.4	15.2	15.7	15.9	16.6	16.5	17.2
55–64 years	26.8	23.7	21.4	15.9	16.0	12.1	13.1	13.6	13.8	13.8	13.9	14.5
65 years and over	30.0	24.5	20.8	17.6	20.5	15.2	15.3	15.6	14.6	14.3	14.7	14.2
65–74 years	29.6	23.0	20.8	16.9	17.9	12.5	13.3	13.5	12.7	12.3	12.6	12.6
75–84 years	31.1	27.9	21.2	19.1	24.9	17.6	17.4	17.7	16.4	16.3	16.9	15.9
85 years and over	28.8	26.0	19.0	19.2	22.2	19.6	17.5	18.0	16.9	16.4	16.9	15.9
Male												
All ages, age-adjusted[d]	21.2	20.0	19.8	19.9	21.5	17.7	18.2	18.4	18.0	18.0	18.0	18.0
All ages, crude	17.8	16.5	16.8	18.6	20.4	17.1	17.6	17.9	17.6	17.7	17.7	17.8
Under 1 year	—	—	—	—	—	—	—	—	*	*	—	—
1–4 years	—	—	—	—	—	—	—	—	*	*	—	—
5–14 years	0.3	0.4	0.5	0.6	1.1	1.2	1.0	0.9	0.9	0.9	1.0	0.7
15–24 years	6.5	8.2	13.5	20.2	22.0	17.1	16.6	16.5	16.0	16.8	16.2	16.2
15–19 years	3.5	5.6	8.8	13.8	18.1	13.0	12.9	12.2	11.6	12.6	12.1	11.5
20–24 years	9.3	11.5	19.3	26.8	25.7	21.4	20.5	20.8	20.2	20.8	20.2	20.8
25–44 years	17.2	17.9	20.9	24.0	24.4	21.3	22.1	22.2	21.9	21.7	21.6	21.5
25–34 years	13.4	14.7	19.8	25.0	24.8	19.6	21.0	20.5	20.6	20.4	19.9	19.7
35–44 years	21.3	21.0	22.1	22.5	23.9	22.8	23.1	23.7	23.2	23.0	23.1	23.2
45–64 years	37.1	34.4	30.0	23.7	24.3	21.3	22.5	23.5	23.5	23.7	24.0	24.8
45–54 years	32.0	31.6	27.9	22.9	23.2	22.4	23.4	24.4	24.4	24.8	25.2	26.2
55–64 years	43.6	38.1	32.7	24.5	25.7	19.4	21.1	22.2	22.3	22.1	22.2	22.7
65 years and over	52.8	44.0	38.4	35.0	41.6	31.1	31.5	31.8	29.8	29.0	29.5	28.5
65–74 years	50.5	39.6	36.0	30.4	32.2	22.7	24.6	24.7	23.4	22.6	22.7	22.7
75–84 years	58.3	52.5	42.8	42.3	56.1	38.6	37.8	38.1	35.1	34.8	35.8	33.3
85 years and over	58.3	57.4	42.4	50.6	65.9	57.5	51.1	50.7	47.8	45.0	45.0	43.2
Female												
All ages, age-adjusted[d]	5.6	5.6	7.4	5.7	4.8	4.0	4.0	4.2	4.2	4.5	4.4	4.5
All ages, crude	5.1	4.9	6.6	5.5	4.8	4.0	4.1	4.3	4.3	4.6	4.5	4.6
Under 1 year	—	—	—	—	—	—	—	—	*	*	*	*
1–4 years	—	—	—	—	—	—	—	—	*	*	*	*
5–14 years	0.1	0.1	0.2	0.2	0.4	0.3	0.3	0.3	0.3	0.5	0.3	0.3

TABLE 8.5

Death rates for suicide, by sex, race, Hispanic origin, and age, selected years 1950–2006 [CONTINUED]

[Data are based on death certificates]

Sex, race, Hispanic origin, and age	1950[a,b]	1960[a,b]	1970[b]	1980[b]	1990[b]	2000[c]	2001[c]	2002[c]	2003[c]	2004[c]	2005[c]	2006[c]
						Deaths per 100,000 resident population						
15–24 years	2.6	2.2	4.2	4.3	3.9	3.0	2.9	2.9	3.0	3.6	3.5	3.2
15–19 years	1.8	1.6	2.9	3.0	3.7	2.7	2.7	2.4	2.7	3.5	3.0	2.8
20–24 years	3.3	2.9	5.7	5.5	4.1	3.2	3.1	3.5	3.4	3.6	4.0	3.6
25–44 years	6.2	6.6	10.2	7.7	6.2	5.4	5.5	5.8	5.7	6.0	5.8	5.9
25–34 years	4.9	5.5	8.6	7.1	5.6	4.3	4.4	4.6	4.6	4.7	4.7	4.7
35–44 years	7.5	7.7	11.9	8.5	6.8	6.4	6.4	6.9	6.6	7.1	6.8	7.0
45–64 years	9.9	10.2	12.0	8.9	7.1	6.2	6.6	6.7	7.0	7.6	7.2	7.7
45–54 years	9.9	10.2	12.6	9.4	6.9	6.7	7.2	7.4	7.7	8.6	8.0	8.4
55–64 years	9.9	10.2	11.4	8.4	7.3	5.4	5.7	5.7	5.9	6.1	6.1	6.8
65 years and over	9.4	8.4	8.1	6.1	6.4	4.0	3.9	4.1	3.8	3.8	4.0	3.9
65–74 years	10.1	8.4	9.0	6.5	6.7	4.0	3.9	4.1	3.8	3.9	4.0	4.1
75–84 years	8.1	8.9	7.0	5.5	6.3	4.0	4.0	4.2	4.0	3.9	4.0	4.0
85 years and over	8.2	6.0	5.9	5.5	5.4	4.2	3.4	3.8	3.3	3.6	4.0	3.1
White male[e]												
All ages, age-adjusted[d]	22.3	21.1	20.8	20.9	22.8	19.1	19.6	20.0	19.6	19.6	19.6	19.6
All ages, crude	19.0	17.6	18.0	19.9	22.0	18.8	19.5	19.9	19.5	19.6	19.7	19.8
15–24 years	6.6	8.6	13.9	21.4	23.2	17.9	17.6	17.7	16.9	17.9	17.3	17.1
25–44 years	17.9	18.5	21.5	24.6	25.4	22.9	24.0	24.0	23.9	23.8	23.5	23.5
45–64 years	39.3	36.5	31.9	25.0	26.0	23.2	24.7	25.9	26.1	26.6	26.6	27.4
65 years and over	55.8	46.7	41.1	37.2	44.2	33.3	33.7	34.2	32.1	31.2	32.1	30.9
65–74 years	53.2	42.0	38.7	32.5	34.2	24.3	26.3	26.8	25.2	24.2	24.9	24.7
75–84 years	61.9	55.7	45.5	45.5	60.2	41.1	40.2	40.6	37.5	37.1	38.4	36.0
85 years and over	61.9	61.3	45.8	52.8	70.3	61.6	55.0	53.9	51.4	48.4	48.2	46.1
Black or African American male[e]												
All ages, age-adjusted[d]	7.5	8.4	10.0	11.4	12.8	10.0	9.8	9.8	9.4	9.6	9.2	9.4
All ages, crude	6.3	6.4	8.0	10.3	12.0	9.4	9.2	9.1	8.8	9.0	8.7	8.8
15–24 years	4.9	4.1	10.5	12.3	15.1	14.2	13.0	11.3	12.1	12.2	11.5	10.6
25–44 years	9.8	12.6	16.1	19.2	19.6	14.3	14.4	15.1	14.3	13.7	13.7	14.3
45–64 years	12.7	13.0	12.4	11.8	13.1	9.9	9.7	9.6	9.0	10.1	9.4	9.9
65 years and over	9.0	9.9	8.7	11.4	14.9	11.5	11.5	11.7	9.2	11.3	10.2	10.4
65–74 years	10.0	11.3	8.7	11.1	14.7	11.1	10.7	9.7	8.3	9.8	8.4	8.8
75–84 years[f]	*	*	*	10.5	14.4	12.1	13.5	13.8	11.3	15.0	12.8	11.6
85 years and over	—	*	*	*	*	*	*	*	*	*	*	*
American Indian or Alaska Native male[e]												
All ages, age-adjusted[d]	—	—	—	19.3	20.1	16.0	17.4	16.4	16.6	18.7	18.9	18.3
All ages, crude	—	—	—	20.9	20.9	15.9	17.0	16.8	17.1	19.5	19.8	19.3
15–24 years	—	—	—	45.3	49.1	26.2	24.7	27.9	27.2	30.7	32.7	35.9
25–44 years	—	—	—	31.2	27.8	24.5	27.6	26.8	30.1	30.8	29.4	26.0
45–64 years	—	—	—	*	*	15.4	17.0	14.1	9.5	16.0	16.8	18.0
65 years and over	—	—	—	*	*	*	*	*	*	*	*	*

TABLE 8.5

Death rates for suicide, by sex, race, Hispanic origin, and age, selected years 1950–2006 [CONTINUED]

[Data are based on death certificates]

Sex, race, Hispanic origin, and race	1950[a,b]	1960[a,b]	1970[b]	1980[b]	1990[b]	2000[c]	2001[c]	2002[c]	2003[c]	2004[c]	2005[c]	2006[c]
					Deaths per 100,000 resident population							
Asian or Pacific Islander male[e]												
All ages, age-adjusted[d]	—	—	—	10.7	9.6	8.6	8.4	8.0	8.5	8.4	7.3	7.9
All ages, crude	—	—	—	8.8	8.7	7.9	7.7	7.6	8.0	7.9	7.2	8.0
15–24 years	—	—	—	10.8	13.5	9.1	9.1	8.7	9.0	9.3	7.2	12.0
25–44 years	—	—	—	11.0	10.6	9.9	9.3	9.3	9.2	8.4	9.5	9.2
45–64 years	—	—	—	13.0	9.7	9.7	8.2	9.1	10.0	11.1	8.9	9.7
65 years and over	—	—	—	18.6	16.8	15.4	18.3	14.4	17.5	15.1	11.0	10.6
Hispanic or Latino male[e,g]												
All ages, age-adjusted[d]	—	—	—	—	13.7	10.3	10.1	9.9	9.7	9.8	9.4	8.8
All ages, crude	—	—	—	—	11.4	8.4	8.3	8.3	8.3	8.6	8.3	7.9
15–24 years	—	—	—	—	14.7	10.9	9.5	10.6	11.2	12.8	12.1	11.6
25–44 years	—	—	—	—	16.2	11.2	11.8	10.9	10.9	11.0	11.2	10.8
45–64 years	—	—	—	—	16.1	12.0	11.4	11.9	12.0	11.8	10.7	10.3
65 years and over	—	—	—	—	23.4	19.5	18.5	17.5	15.6	15.9	14.1	12.1
White, not Hispanic or Latino male[e]												
All ages, age-adjusted[d]	—	—	—	—	23.5	20.2	21.0	21.4	21.0	21.0	21.2	21.4
All ages, crude	—	—	—	—	23.1	20.4	21.4	21.9	21.6	21.6	22.0	22.3
15–24 years	—	—	—	—	24.4	19.5	19.6	19.3	18.2	19.0	18.4	18.5
25–44 years	—	—	—	—	26.4	25.1	26.4	26.9	26.8	26.8	26.6	26.9
45–64 years	—	—	—	—	26.8	24.0	25.9	27.2	27.4	27.4	28.2	29.3
65 years and over	—	—	—	—	45.4	33.9	34.4	35.1	33.1	32.1	33.2	32.3
White female[e]												
All ages, age-adjusted[d]	6.0	5.9	7.9	6.1	5.2	4.3	4.5	4.7	4.6	5.0	4.9	5.1
All ages, crude	5.5	5.3	7.1	5.9	5.3	4.4	4.6	4.8	4.7	5.1	5.0	5.2
15–24 years	2.7	2.3	4.2	4.6	4.2	3.1	3.1	3.1	3.1	3.8	3.7	3.4
25–44 years	6.6	7.0	11.0	8.1	6.6	6.0	6.2	6.6	6.4	6.6	6.5	6.8
45–64 years	10.6	10.9	13.0	9.6	7.7	6.9	7.3	7.5	7.8	8.5	8.1	8.8
65 years and over	9.9	8.8	8.5	6.4	6.8	4.3	4.1	4.3	4.0	4.0	4.2	4.1
Black or African American female[e]												
All ages, age-adjusted[d]	1.8	2.0	2.9	2.4	2.4	1.8	1.8	1.6	1.9	1.8	1.9	1.4
All ages, crude	1.5	1.6	2.6	2.2	2.3	1.7	1.7	1.5	1.8	1.8	1.8	1.4
15–24 years	1.8	*	3.8	2.3	2.3	2.2	1.3	1.7	2.0	2.2	1.7	1.8
25–44 years	2.3	3.0	4.8	4.3	3.8	2.6	2.6	2.4	2.8	2.9	2.8	2.0
45–64 years	2.7	3.1	2.9	2.5	2.9	2.1	2.5	2.1	2.4	2.2	2.5	1.9
65 years and over	*	*	2.6	*	1.9	1.3	1.3	1.1	1.4	*	1.4	*
American Indian or Alaska Native female[e]												
All ages, age-adjusted[d]	—	—	—	4.7	3.6	3.8	4.0	4.1	3.5	5.9	4.6	5.1
All ages, crude	—	—	—	4.7	3.7	4.0	4.4	4.3	3.7	6.2	5.0	5.4
15–24 years	—	—	—	*	*	*	*	7.4	8.3	10.5	10.1	8.9
25–44 years	—	—	—	10.7	*	7.2	6.1	5.6	4.6	9.8	7.4	8.0
45–64 years	—	—	—	*	*	*	*	*	*	*	*	*
65 years and over	—	—	—	*	*	*	*	*	*	*	*	*

TABLE 8.5

Death rates for suicide, by sex, race, Hispanic origin, and age, selected years 1950–2006 [CONTINUED]

[Data are based on death certificates]

Sex, race, Hispanic origin, and race	1950[a,b]	1960[a,b]	1970[b]	1980[b]	1990[b]	2000[c]	2001[c]	2002[c]	2003[c]	2004[c]	2005[c]	2006[c]
						Deaths per 100,000 resident population						
Asian or Pacific Islander female[e]												
All ages, age-adjusted[d]	—	—	—	5.5	4.1	2.8	2.9	3.0	3.1	3.5	3.3	3.4
All ages, crude	—	—	—	4.7	3.4	2.7	2.8	2.9	3.1	3.4	3.2	3.3
15–24 years	—	—	—	*	3.9	2.7	3.6	*	3.4	2.8	3.7	4.0
25–44 years	—	—	—	5.4	3.8	3.3	2.9	3.3	3.4	4.1	3.4	3.3
45–64 years	—	—	—	7.9	5.0	3.2	3.8	3.8	4.3	4.5	3.8	4.2
65 years and over	—	—	—	*	8.5	5.2	4.9	6.8	4.6	6.4	6.8	6.9
Hispanic or Latina female[e, g]												
All ages, age-adjusted[d]	—	—	—	—	2.3	1.7	1.6	1.8	1.7	2.0	1.8	1.8
All ages, crude	—	—	—	—	2.2	1.5	1.5	1.6	1.5	1.8	1.7	1.7
15–24 years	—	—	—	—	3.1	2.0	2.3	2.1	2.2	2.5	2.7	2.6
25–44 years	—	—	—	—	3.1	2.1	2.0	2.0	2.0	2.3	2.2	2.3
45–64 years	—	—	—	—	2.5	2.5	2.3	2.5	2.4	3.1	2.1	2.4
65 years and over	—	—	—	—	*	*	*	1.9	*	1.8	2.0	1.7
White, not Hispanic or Latina female[g]												
All ages, age-adjusted[d]	—	—	—	—	5.4	4.7	4.9	5.1	5.0	5.4	5.3	5.6
All ages, crude	—	—	—	—	5.6	4.9	5.0	5.3	5.3	5.7	5.6	5.9
15–24 years	—	—	—	—	4.3	3.3	3.3	3.4	3.3	4.0	3.9	3.5
25–44 years	—	—	—	—	7.0	6.7	6.9	7.5	7.2	7.5	7.4	7.8
45–64 years	—	—	—	—	8.0	7.3	7.8	8.0	8.3	9.1	8.7	9.5
65 years and over	—	—	—	—	7.0	4.4	4.3	4.5	4.2	4.1	4.3	4.3

—Category not applicable.

*Rates based on fewer than 20 deaths are considered unreliable and are not shown.

—Data not available.

[a]Includes deaths of persons who were not residents of the 50 states and the District of Columbia (D.C.).

[b]Underlying cause of death was coded according to the Sixth Revision of the International Classification of Diseases (ICD) in 1950, Seventh Revision in 1960, Eighth Revision in 1970, and Ninth Revision in 1980–1998. Starting with 1999 data, cause of death is coded according to ICD-10.

[c]Starting with 1999 data, age-adjusted rates are calculated using the year 2000 standard population. Prior to 2003, age-adjusted rates were calculated using standard million proportions based on rounded population numbers. Starting with 2003 data, unrounded population numbers are used to calculate age-adjusted rates.

[d]Age-adjusted rates are calculated using the year 2000 standard population.

[e]The race groups, white, black, Asian or Pacific Islander, and American Indian or Alaska Native, include persons of Hispanic and non-Hispanic origin. Persons of Hispanic origin may be of any race. Death rates for the American Indian or Alaska Native and Asian or Pacific Islander populations are known to be underestimated. Race, for a discussion of sources of bias in death rates by race and Hispanic origin.

[f]In 1950, rate is for the age group 75 years and over.

[g]Prior to 1997, excludes data from states lacking an Hispanic-origin item on the death certificate.

Notes: Starting with Health, United States, 2003, rates for 1991–1999 were revised using intercensal population estimates based on the 2000 census. Rates for 2000 were revised based on 2000 census counts. Rates for 2001 and later years were computed using 2000-based postcensal estimates. Figures for 2001 include September 11–related deaths for which death certificates were filed as of October 24, 2002. Age groups were selected to minimize the presentation of unstable age-specific death rates based on small numbers of deaths and for consistency among comparison groups. In 2003, seven states reported multiple-race data. In 2004, 15 states and D.C. reported multiple-race data. In 2005, 21 states and D.C. reported multiple-race data. In 2006, 25 states and D.C. reported multiple-race data. The multiple-race data for these states were bridged to the single-race categories of the 1977 Office of Management and Budget standards for comparability with other states.

SOURCE: Adapted from "Table 43. Death Rates for Suicide, by Sex, Race, Hispanic Origin, and Age: United States, Selected Years 1950–2006," in *Health, United States, 2009, With Special Feature on Technology*, Centers for Disease Control and Prevention, National Center for Health Statistics, 2010, http://www.cdc.gov/nchs/data/hus/hus09.pdf (accessed March 9, 2009)

Who Commits Suicide?

Suicide occurs among men and women of all racial, occupational, religious, and social groups, as well as, with the exception of the very young, all age groups. Table 8.5 lists the suicide death rates by age, sex, and race/ethnicity for selected years from 1950 to 2006. The youngest group in which suicides were documented was ages 5 to 14, with 0.5 suicides reported in 2006 per 100,000 resident population. Of every 100,000 teens ages 15 to 19, there were 7.3 suicides in 2006, and among adults ages 20 to 24, there were 12.5 suicides per 100,000 population.

The number of completed suicides does not give an accurate picture of the problem, because for every completed suicide there are many unsuccessful suicide attempts. For example, during the 1990s death rates for suicide declined, but in some age groups the rate of suicide attempts actually increased. In "Suicide in the U.S.," the NIMH notes that suicide attempts outnumber completed suicides by about 12 to 25 attempts per every suicide. Depression, substance abuse, physical abuse, and sexual abuse are risk factors for attempted suicide by adolescents.

According to the Centers for Disease Control and Prevention's Web-Based Injury Statistics Query and Reporting System and National Center for Injury Prevention and Control ("Suicide," Summer 2009, http://www.cdc.gov/violenceprevention/pdf/Suicide-DataSheet-a.pdf), approximately four times as many men die by suicide than women do. This is despite the fact that women attempt suicide two to three times as often as men. Men make up about three-fourths of total suicides, and white males account for most of that number. Men use more deadly weapons than women—more than half (56%) shoot themselves. Poisoning is the most common method of suicide for women (40.3%).

In 2006 the suicide rate for white males (19.6 per 100,000 population) was higher than the rates of other races and ethnicities. (See Table 8.5.) It was more than double the rate of non-Hispanic African-American males (9.4 per 100,000). Native Americans and Alaskan Natives had a suicide rate almost as high as that of whites (18.3 per 100,000). The suicide rates among young (15 to 24 years old) white and African-American men have increased dramatically. For white men in this age group it rose from 6.6 per 100,000 in 1950 to 17.1 in 2006, and for African-American men it increased from 4.9 per 100,000 to 10.6 per 100,000.

Among older white males, the suicide rate in 2006 was far higher than for any other racial group. Non-Hispanic white males aged 65 and older had a death rate from suicide more than three times higher (32.3 per 100,000) than the rate for African-American males (10.4 per 100,000). (See Table 8.5.)

For white and African-American women, the suicide rates were far lower than those for men in all age groups. The death rate from suicide for white women was 5.1 per 100,000 in 2006, and for African-American women the rate was less than half of that at 1.4 per 100,000. (See Table 8.5.) Young white women aged 15 to 24 had a much lower suicide rate (3.4 per 100,000) than white men in the same age group (17.1 per 100,000). For African-American women of all ages, the rate was also much lower (1.4 per 100,000) than the African-American male rate (9.4 per 100,000).

Female suicide rates do not change as drastically as men's do as they age. For non-Hispanic white women age 65 and older, the rate was 4.3 per 100,000 in 2006, compared with the non-Hispanic white male rate of 32.3 per 100,000. (See Table 8.5.) One widely held theory about the high rates among white men older than age 65 years is that these men, who traditionally have been in positions of power, have great difficulty adjusting to a life they may consider useless or diminished.

Why Do People Commit Suicide?

People commit suicide for various reasons. Notes left by people who have killed themselves usually tell of life crises that they believed were unbearable. Many describe enduring chronic pain, losing loved ones, being unable to pay bills, or finding themselves incapable of living independently.

Some suicides are committed on an irrational, impulsive whim. Researchers observe that even among those most determined to commit suicide, the desire is not as much to die as it is to escape the life they are leading and to end the pain they are suffering. Whatever the cause of their despair, they are desperately crying out for help.

Follow-up studies on suicide survivors reveal their intense ambivalence about actually dying. Not all survivors are glad to be alive, but for most, the attempted suicide marked a definite turning point. It was an urgent and dramatic signal that their problems demanded serious and immediate attention. Most of the survivors said that what they really wanted was to change their life.

Suicide among the Terminally Ill

Not all suicides are categorized as the acts of people who are mentally ill. Some people consider suicides committed by people who are terminally ill as rational choices. They argue that people who are terminally ill have the right to die—that is, the right to control the manner of their death. Patients with terminal diseases often worry that they will suffer long and painful deaths and that they stand a good chance of losing everything: health, independence, jobs, insurance, homes, and contact with loved ones and friends.

Researchers find that factors with significant impact on the quality of life include security, family, love, pleasurable activity, and freedom from pain and suffering. Sufferers of debilitating disease may lose all of these. For some, suicide is a last recourse to relieve pain, suffering, insecurity, dependence, or hopelessness.

The right to die and to choose the time and manner of death remains a hotly debated topic throughout the world. In the United States, just two states—Oregon and Washington—have legalized physician-assisted dying. Since 1997 Oregon's Death with Dignity Act has allowed a terminally ill adult to request a prescription for a lethal dose of drugs. The legislation contains many restrictions intended to protect both patients and the physicians who prescribe the drugs. In an analysis of its application, "Oregon's Experience: Evaluating the Record" (*American Journal of Bioethics*, vol. 9, no. 3, 2009), Ronald A. Lindsay observes that none of the untoward consequences its staunchest opponents feared—specifically that it would affect "vulnerable groups disproportionately, that legal assisted dying could not be confined to the competent terminally ill who voluntarily request assistance, and that the practice would result in frequent abuses"—have materialized. Lindsay asserts that Oregon's experience "argues in favor of legalization of assistance in dying."

According to the Oregon Department of Human Services (http://www.oregon.gov/DHS/ph/pas/docs/year12.pdf) in March 2010, 460 people have died after taking the medication since the program began. In 2009, of the 95 people who received the prescriptions that year, 53 took the medication while 30 succumbed to their illness. The remaining 12 were still living. Statistically, most recipients of the medication are over 55 and have terminal cancer.

In March 2008 Washington became the second state to permit physician-assisted suicide. Like the Oregon legislation, the law aims to restrict the practice to minimize the potential for abuse. Patients must make two requests, more than two weeks apart, and one must be in writing. The patient must be of sound mind and not suffering from depression, and two physicians must approve the request for a lethal dose of drugs.

Suicide's Warning Signs

Researchers believe that most suicidal people convey their intentions to someone among their friends and family, either openly or indirectly. The people they signal are those who know them well and are in the best position to recognize the signs and give help. Comments such as "You'd be better off without me," "No one will have to worry about me much longer," or even a casual "I've had it" may be signals of upcoming attempts. Some people who are suicidal put their affairs in order. They draw up wills, give away prized possessions, or act as if they are preparing for a long trip. They may even talk about going away.

Often, the indicator is a distinct change in personality or behavior. A normally happy person may become increasingly depressed. A regular churchgoer may stop attending services, or an avid runner may quit exercising. These types of changes, if added to expressions of worthlessness or hopelessness, can indicate not only that the person is seriously depressed but also that he or she may have decided to commit suicide. Even though the vast majority of people who are depressed are not suicidal, most of the suicide-prone are depressed. Researchers and health care practitioners caution that suicide threats and attempts should not be discounted as harmless bids for attention. Anyone thinking, talking about, or planning suicide should receive immediate professional evaluation and treatment.

CHAPTER 9
COMPLEMENTARY AND ALTERNATIVE MEDICINE

The National Center for Complementary and Alternative Medicine (NCCAM; formerly the Office of Alternative Medicine, established in 1992) is 1 of the 27 institutes and centers of the National Institutes of Health (NIH). The center was created because consumers of complementary and alternative medicine (CAM) and health care practitioners wanted to know whether available alternative medical options were safe and effective. In "NCCAM Facts-at-a-Glance and Mission" (March 8, 2010, http://nccam.nih.gov/about/ataglance/), the NCCAM states that its mission is to: "Explore complementary and alternative healing practices in the context of rigorous science... Train complementary and alternative medicine researchers.... Disseminate authoritative information to the public and professionals." To determine a method's or product's effectiveness and safety, the organization uses a hierarchy of evidence. Studies indicate that data on the efficacy and safety of CAM therapies span a continuum ranging from anecdotes and case studies through encouraging information obtained from large, well-developed clinical trials. (See Figure 9.1.)

The NCCAM (October 26, 2009, http://nccam.nih.gov/health/whatiscam/overview.htm) defines alternative medicine as "a group of diverse medical and health care systems, practices, and products that are not generally considered to be part of conventional medicine." Even though there is some overlap between them, the NCCAM further distinguishes between complementary, alternative, and integrative medicine in the following manner:

- Alternative medicine is therapy or treatment that is used instead of conventional medical treatment. One example of alternative medicine is the treatment of depression with St. John's wort (*hypericum*), a botanical, herbal medicine, rather than with conventional antidepressant drugs.

- Complementary medicine is alternative therapy or treatment that is used along with conventional medi-

cine, not in place of it. An example of complementary medicine is the addition of relaxation techniques or movement awareness therapies (such as the Alexander Technique, Pilates, and the Feldenkrais Method) to the traditional approaches of physical and occupational therapy used to rehabilitate people who have had a stroke. Complementary medicine appears to offer health benefits, but there is generally no scientific evidence to support its utility.

- Integrative medicine is the combination of conventional medical treatment and CAM therapies that have been scientifically researched and have demonstrated that they are both safe and effective. An example of integrative medicine is teaching stress management and relaxation techniques to people with high blood pressure and heart disease along with the use of traditional approaches such as weight management, exercise, and prescription drugs to reduce the risks and complications of heart disease.

Despite the classification system outlined by the NCCAM, CAM continues to be known by a variety of names—nontraditional medicine, unorthodox medical practices, and holistic health care—and reflects a wide range of philosophies, including the need for or reliance on scientific evidence of effectiveness. Generally, alternative therapies tend to be untested and unproven, whereas complementary and integrative practices that are used in conjunction with mainstream medicine are often those with a substantial scientific basis of demonstrated safety and efficacy.

THE GROWING POPULARITY OF CAM

Many people have turned to CAM approaches out of frustration that mainstream medicine cannot meet all their expectations and needs. Some CAM users are interested in natural, as opposed to pharmaceutical, solutions to health problems, while others want to take charge of

FIGURE 9.1

Hierarchy of evidence

Study design

BIAS

- Randomized controlled trials

- Cohort studies and case control studies

- Case reports and case series, non-systematic observations

Expert opinion

SOURCE: "Slide 15. Hierarchy of Evidence," in *Rating the Evidence: Using GRADE to Develop Clinical Practice Guidelines*, Slide Presentation from the AHRQ 2009 Annual Conference (Text Version), Agency for Healthcare Research and Quality, Rockville, MD, December 2009, http://www.ahrq.gov/about/annualconf09/falck-ytter_schunemann.htm (accessed January 22, 2010)

FIGURE 9.2

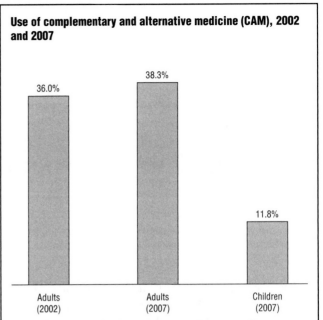

Use of complementary and alternative medicine (CAM), 2002 and 2007

SOURCE: "Figure 1. CAM Use by U.S. Adults and Children," in *The Use of Complementary and Alternative Medicine in the United States*, The National Center for Complementary and Alternative Medicine, National Institutes of Health, December 2008, http://nccam.nih.gov/news/camstats/2007/camuse.pdf (accessed January 22, 2010)

their health and are seeking self-care approaches to maintaining health and wellness. Helping this movement along is information technology, which is enabling easy access to sources of CAM information on the Internet and in print and electronic media, and advertising and marketing of new CAM products and methods. Citing data from the 2002 and 2007 National Health Interview Survey (NHIS), the NCCAM reports that in 2002, 36% of American adults used CAM approaches, and in 2007 about 38% of adults and 12% of children used some form of CAM. (See Figure 9.2.)

The CAM supplement to the 2007 NHIS (*Complementary and Alternative Medicine Use among Adults and Children: United States, 2007*, NCCAM, December 10, 2008, http://nccam.nih.gov/news/2008/nhsr12.pdf) contained questions about 36 types of CAM therapies, including those offered by providers—such as acupuncture, osteopathic manipulation, and chiropractic—as well as therapies that do not require a provider—such as the use of natural products (nutritional supplements and herbal remedies), special diets, and movement therapies. The survey did not ask about the use of folk remedies, such as eating chicken soup to relieve cold symptoms, or faith healing, such as praying for one's own or others' health.

CAM is used by people of all ages, although its use varies between age groups. In 2007 about 40% of adults ages 30 to 39, 40 to 49, and 60 to 69 said they used CAM, and more than 44% of adults ages 50 to 59 reported using CAM in the 12 months prior to the survey. (See Figure 9.3.) CAM use also varies by race and ethnicity. In 2007 more than half of Native American adults reported using CAM, compared with just 23.7% of Hispanic adults. (See Figure 9.4.)

In 2007 the most commonly used CAM therapies used by adults were natural products (17.7%) and mind body therapies—deep breathing (12.7%) and meditation (9.4%). (See Figure 9.5.) From 2002 to 2007 there were significant increases in the use of deep breathing, meditation, massage, and yoga. Among adults who reported using natural products in 2002, the most commonly used natural products were echinacea, traditionally used to treat or prevent colds, flu, and other infections; ginseng, traditionally used to support overall health and boost the immune system; and ginko biloba, traditionally used to treat a variety of conditions, including asthma, bronchitis, fatigue, and tinnitus (ringing or roaring sounds in the ears), and more recently used to enhance memory. (See Figure 9.6.) In 2007 the most frequently used natural product was fish oil/omega 3; found in certain plants and nuts as well as fatty fish, omega-3 fatty acids lower triglycerides and may reduce the risk of death, heart attack, dangerous abnormal heart rhythms, and strokes. The second most used natural product in 2007 was glucosamine (an amino sugar that the body produces and distributes in cartilage and other connective tissue that has been used to help prevent and treat arthritis and joint pain), followed by echinacea.

In 2007 half of the top 10 diseases or conditions for which CAM was used were musculoskeletal problems such as back, neck, and joint pain, arthritis, and other musculoskeletal complaints. (See Figure 9.7.) In 2002, 9.5% of people reported using CAM to treat head or chest

FIGURE 9.3

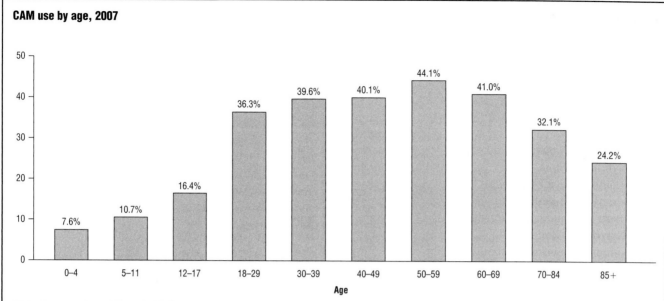

CAM use by age, 2007

CAM = Complementary and Alternative Medicine.

SOURCE: "Figure 2. CAM Use by Age—2007," in *The Use of Complementary and Alternative Medicine in the United States*, The National Center for Complementary and Alternative Medicine, National Institutes of Health, December 2008, http://nccam.nih.gov/news/camstats/2007/camuse.pdf (accessed January 22, 2010)

FIGURE 9.4

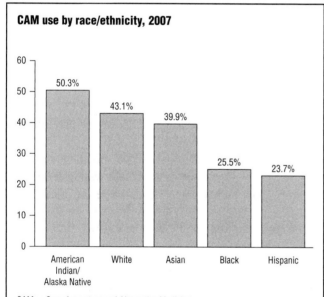

CAM use by race/ethnicity, 2007

CAM = Complementary and Alternative Medicine.

SOURCE: "Figure 3. CAM Use by Race/Ethnicity among Adults—2007," in *The Use of Complementary and Alternative Medicine in the United States*, The National Center for Complementary and Alternative Medicine, National Institutes of Health, December 2008, http://nccam.nih.gov/news/camstats/2007/camuse.pdf (accessed January 22, 2010)

colds; in 2007 just 2% used CAM to treat cold symptoms. This decline may be attributable to the fact that study results have been mixed in terms of echinacea's efficacy for the treatment of colds or flu, according to the NCCAM's "Herbs at a Glance: Echinacea" (December 7, 2009, http://nccam.nih.gov/health/echinacea/ataglance.htm).

Children's Use of CAM

The 2007 survey found that CAM use among children was higher among adolescents ages 12 to 17 (16.4%) than among younger children, and higher among white (12.8%) than African-American (5.9%) or Hispanic (7.9%) children. CAM use was significantly greater among children whose parents or other relatives used CAM (23.9%). (See Figure 9.8.) It also was higher, according to the survey, in families where the parents had more than a high school education (14.7%), in families that delayed seeking conventional medical care because of cost considerations (16.9%), and among children with 6 or more health conditions (23.8%). Like adults, CAM use among children most often relied on natural products, followed by chiropractic and osteopathic care, deep breathing, and yoga. (See Figure 9.9.)

The natural products children used most frequently in 2007 were echinacea and fish oil/omega 3. (See Figure 9.10.) The diseases or conditions for which children most frequently used CAM therapies were back/neck pain, head or chest colds, anxiety/stress, and other musculoskeletal complaints. (See Figure 9.11.)

Why Do People Seek CAM?

People turn to CAM for many different reasons. One of the most attractive features of CAM is an emphasis on the "whole person," rather than on simply the diseased organ or body part. CAM therapies and practitioners tend to consider patients as human beings rather than as simply physical bodies, and nearly all emphasize

FIGURE 9.5

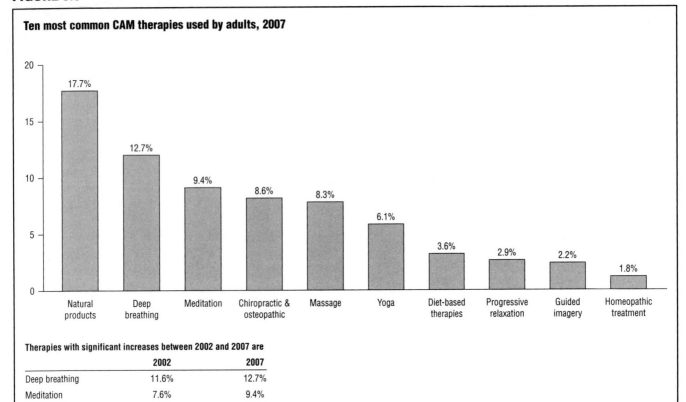

Ten most common CAM therapies used by adults, 2007

Therapies with significant increases between 2002 and 2007 are

	2002	2007
Deep breathing	11.6%	12.7%
Meditation	7.6%	9.4%
Massage	5.0%	8.3%
Yoga	5.1%	6.1%

CAM = Complementary and Alternative Medicine.

SOURCE: "Figure 4. 10 Most Common CAM Therapies among Adults—2007," in *The Use of Complementary and Alternative Medicine in the United States*, The National Center for Complementary and Alternative Medicine, National Institutes of Health, December 2008, http://nccam.nih.gov/news/camstats/ 2007/camuse.pdf (accessed January 22, 2010)

the mind-body connection and pay attention to emotional wellness and spirituality.

Some patients seek alternative therapies when conventional medicine fails to relieve their symptoms or when traditional treatment produces unpleasant side effects. In "Rethinking the Evidence Imperative: Why Patients Choose Complementary and Alternative Medicine" (*Leukemia & Lymphoma*, vol. 49, no. 2, February 2008), Isla Carboon details many of the reasons patients seek CAM. She observes that while CAM use has been linked to distrust of conventional medicine, there are many other motivations. Carboon observes that some cancer patients using CAM not only believe that it may benefit the course of their disease but also choose CAM as a way to regain control of their treatment. In some instances, they may see CAM as a last resort or a way to sustain hope when conventional treatment fails to reverse the course of disease or relieve symptoms.

Other CAM users cite bad experiences with conventional medical treatment, historically poor communication and interactions with physicians, the impersonality of

traditional medical care, and the desire for practitioner-patient partnerships characterized by shared decision making (rather than traditional physician-patient relationships in which physicians assume sole responsibility for decisions about patient care) for their interest in CAM.

People from All Walks of Life Use CAM

In addition to people who distrust or question conventional medical treatment, there are other groups that make frequent use of CAM. In "Complementary and Alternative Medicine Use, Spending, and Quality of Life in Early Stage Breast Cancer" (*Nursing Research*, vol. 59, no. 1, February 2010), Gwen Wyatt et al. observe that as much as 80% of women with breast cancer use CAM therapies to improve their quality of life during cancer treatment. Wyatt et al. find that biologically based therapies (primarily nutritional supplements) and mind-body therapies were used most often by a majority of the sample. By contrast, fewer women used therapies in the other three major CAM categories: manipulative and body based, energy, and alternative medical systems.

FIGURE 9.6

Ten most common natural products used by adults, 2002 and 2007

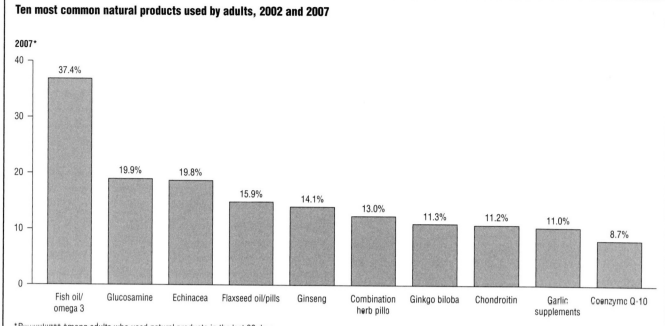

2007*

Fish oil/omega 3: 37.4%
Glucosamine: 19.9%
Echinacea: 19.8%
Flaxseed oil/pills: 15.9%
Ginseng: 14.1%
Combination herb pillo: 13.0%
Ginkgo biloba: 11.3%
Chondroitin: 11.2%
Garlic supplements: 11.0%
Coenzyme Q-10: 8.7%

*Percentages among adults who used natural products in the last 30 days.

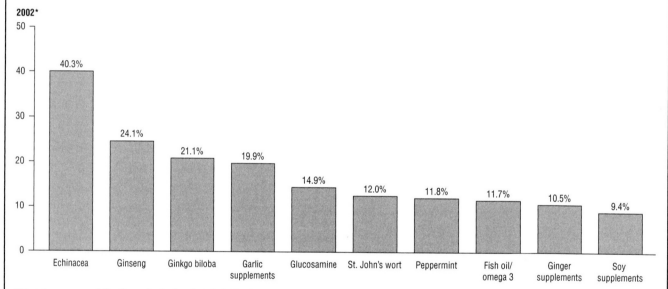

2002*

Echinacea: 40.3%
Ginseng: 24.1%
Ginkgo biloba: 21.1%
Garlic supplements: 19.9%
Glucosamine: 14.9%
St. John's wort: 12.0%
Peppermint: 11.8%
Fish oil/omega 3: 11.7%
Ginger supplements: 10.5%
Soy supplements: 9.4%

*Percentages among adults who used natural products in the last 12 months.

SOURCE: "Figure 5.10 Most Common Natural Products among Adults," in *The Use of Complementary and Alternative Medicine in the United States*, The National Center for Complementary and Alternative Medicine, National Institutes of Health, December 2008, http://nccam.nih.gov/news/camstats/2007/camuse.pdf (accessed January 22, 2010)

In "Complementary and Alternative Medical Therapy Utilization by People with Chronic Fatiguing Illnesses in the United States" (*BMC Complementary and Alternative Medicine*, vol. 7, no. 12, April 2007), James F. Jones et al. report on the use of alternative medicine by Americans suffering from chronic fatiguing (CF) illnesses. They find that 77% of CF sufferers reported using CAM. CAM use during the preceding 12 months was reported more frequently by women (56.8%) than men (44.2%) and increased significantly with increasing levels of educa-

tional attainment. People suffering from chronic fatigue were the most likely to have used body-based therapies such as chiropractic and massage and mind-based therapies such as prayer and relaxation techniques.

Tyler C. Smith et al. look at CAM use among U.S. military personnel in "Complementary and Alternative Medicine Use among US Navy and Marine Corps Personnel" (*BMC Complementary and Alternative Medicine*, vol. 7, no. 16, May 2007). They find that more than 37%

FIGURE 9.7

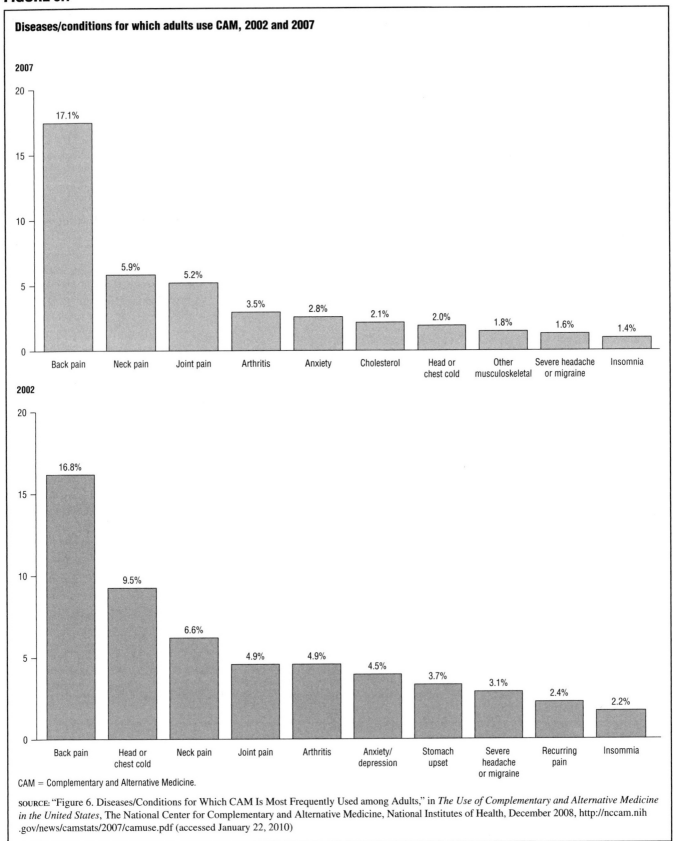

Diseases/conditions for which adults use CAM, 2002 and 2007

CAM = Complementary and Alternative Medicine.

SOURCE: "Figure 6. Diseases/Conditions for Which CAM Is Most Frequently Used among Adults," in *The Use of Complementary and Alternative Medicine in the United States*, The National Center for Complementary and Alternative Medicine, National Institutes of Health, December 2008, http://nccam.nih.gov/news/camstats/2007/camuse.pdf (accessed January 22, 2010)

of subjects reported using at least one CAM therapy during the past year. The most frequently reported CAM use was of herbal therapies (15.9%). Smith et al. conclude that CAM use among military personnel is comparable to that reported by previous studies of U.S. civilian populations.

FIGURE 9.8

Children using CAM, based on CAM use by parents or relatives, 2007

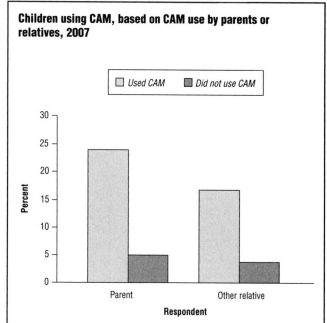

Notes: CAM is complementary and alternative medicine. Estimates are age adjusted using the projected 2000 U.S. population as the standard population.

SOURCE: Patricia M. Barnes, Barbara Bloom, and Richard L. Nahin, "Figure 3. Percentage of Children under 18 Years of Age Who Used Complementary and Alternative Medicine during the Past 12 Months, by Complementary and Alternative Medicine Use by Parent or Other Relative Respondent: United States, 2007," in "Complementary and Alternative Medicine Use among Adults and Children: United States, 2007," *National Health Statistics Report*, no. 12, National Center for Health Statistics, December 10, 2008, http://www.cdc.gov/nchs/data/nhsr/nhsr012.pdf (accessed January 22, 2010)

In "Complementary and Alternative Medicine Use for Treatment and Prevention of Late-Life Mood and Cognitive Disorders" (*Aging Health*, vol. 5, no. 1, February 2009), Helen Lavretsky notes that mood disorders (such as depression) and cognitive problems (such as mild memory impairment) associated with aging are among the most common reasons people turn to CAM therapies. These therapies are generally nutritional supplements such as St. John's wort, omega-3 fatty acids, and ginkgo biloba.

CAM Use in Traditional Medical Settings

In the 21st century, many CAM practices have joined the ranks of mainstream medicine. The Institute of Medicine finds in *Complementary and Alternative Medicine in the United States* (2005) that the integration of CAM and conventional medicine is occurring in many settings including hospitals, physicians' offices, and health maintenance organizations.

In "Hospital-Based Chiropractic Integration within a Large Private Hospital System in Minnesota: A 10-Year Example" (*Journal of Manipulative and Physiological Therapeutics*, vol. 32, no. 9, November 2009), Richard A. Branson observes that over the course of a decade, there was widespread support for integration of CAM practices into a large private hospital system. About three-quarters of physicians surveyed favored the integration of chiropractic services into the hospital system.

Another example of the acceptance of CAM use in traditional medical settings is the collaborative clinics that combine acupuncture and primary care at Oregon Health and Science University (OHSU) described by

FIGURE 9.9

10 most common therapies used by children, 2007

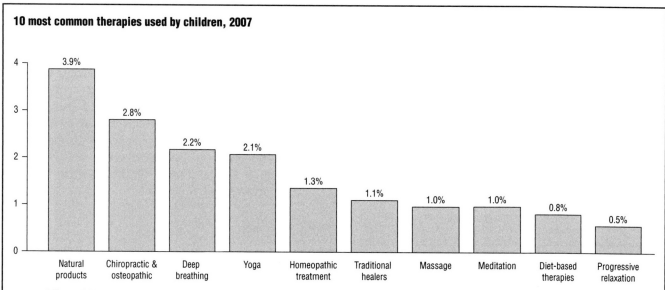

SOURCE: "Figure 7.10 Most Common Therapies among Children," in *The Use of Complementary and Alternative Medicine in the United States*, The National Center for Complementary and Alternative Medicine, National Institutes of Health, December 2008, http://nccam.nih.gov/news/camstats/2007/camuse.pdf (accessed January 22, 2010)

FIGURE 9.10

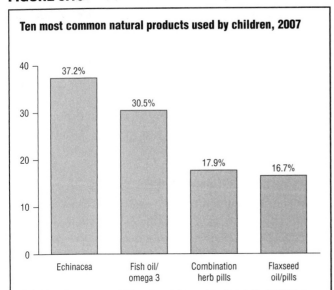

Ten most common natural products used by children, 2007

Note: Percentages among children who used natural products in the last 30 days.

SOURCE: "Figure 8. Most Common Natural Products among Children," in *The Use of Complementary and Alternative Medicine in the United States*, The National Center for Complementary and Alternative Medicine, National Institutes of Health, December 2008, http://nccam.nih.gov/news/camstats/2007/camuse.pdf (accessed January 22, 2010)

FIGURE 9.11

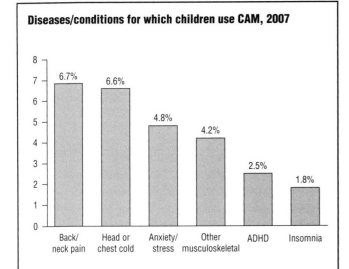

Diseases/conditions for which children use CAM, 2007

CAM = Complementary and Alternative Medicine.
ADHD = Attention Deficit Hyperactivity Disorder.

SOURCE: "Figure 9. Diseases/Conditions for Which CAM Is Most Frequently Used among Children," in *The Use of Complementary and Alternative Medicine in the United States*, The National Center for Complementary and Alternative Medicine, National Institutes of Health, December 2008, http://nccam.nih.gov/news/camstats/2007/camuse.pdf (accessed January 22, 2010)

Joanne Wu in "Integration of Acupuncture into Family Medicine Teaching Clinics" (*Journal of Alternative and Complementary Medicine*, vol. 15, no. 9, September 2009). More than three-quarters of the primary care physicians had referred patients to acupuncture; the majority of these patients were referred for pain relief.

TYPES OF CAM

The NCCAM categorizes CAM practices into four domains. There is some overlap between these CAM domains:

- Mind-body interventions—mind-body medicine is a range of practices that aims to use the power of the mind to influence symptoms of disease and healing. Increasingly, this type of alternative medicine has gained acceptance among medical professionals. Mind-body therapies—such as support groups for people suffering from a variety of medical problems; relaxation techniques; and art, dance, and music therapies—are now widely used by practitioners of conventional medicine. Less widely accepted mind-body techniques include meditation, breathing, hypnosis, and prayer.

- Biologically based therapies—this type of treatment uses organic (naturally occurring) substances such as herbs, food, and vitamins to treat symptoms of disease and improve health and wellness. Examples of biologically based therapies include dietary supplements, herbal remedies, and the hotly debated use of hormones such as human growth hormone and dehydroepiandrosterone (the most plentiful steroid hormone in the body) to combat disease and to slow aging.

- Manipulative and body-based practices—movement therapies, manipulative methods, and bodywork are another type of CAM. Examples of these methods are massage therapy, chiropractic, and osteopathic manipulation (also referred to as craniosacral manipulative therapy).

- Energy medicine—these techniques aim to influence energy fields that practitioners of this form of CAM believe exist in and around the body. Also called "biofield therapies," some are "touch" therapies and others do not involve direct contact with any part of the body. Reiki and Qi Gong are examples of biofield therapies. Other forms of energy therapies known as bioelectromagnetic-based therapies use magnetic energy, electromagnetic fields, pulsed fields, alternating current, or direct current fields to influence "energy flow."

The NCCAM also considers whole medical systems. Many of these alternative medical systems developed before conventional Western medicine or independent of it. Alternative medicine systems are based on different beliefs and philosophies and, as a result, approach both diagnosis and treatment of disease quite differently from traditional Western medicine. Examples of alternative medicine systems that began in Western cultures are homeopathy and naturopathic medicine. Alternative medicine systems that developed in other cultures include acupuncture, Ayurvedic medicine, and traditional Chinese medicine.

ALTERNATIVE MEDICINE SYSTEMS

Practically every culture has a medicine system; some developed more than one system, tradition, or philosophy to explain the causes of disease and suggest therapies to relieve symptoms. This section considers two alternative medicine systems that had their origins in Western culture (homeopathy and naturopathic medicine) and three that developed in non-Western cultures (acupuncture, Ayurvedic medicine, and traditional Chinese medicine).

Homeopathic Medicine

Homeopathic medicine (also called homeopathy) is based on the belief that "like cures like" and uses very diluted amounts of natural substances to encourage the body's own self-healing mechanisms. If taken in higher doses or stronger concentrations, the natural substances used by homeopathy to stimulate self-healing would likely produce the symptoms the diluted substances aim to relieve.

Homeopathy was developed by the German physician Samuel Hahnemann (1755–1843) in the 1790s. First experimenting on healthy subjects and himself, Hahnemann discovered that he could produce symptoms of particular diseases by injecting small doses of various herbal substances. This discovery inspired him to try another experiment: giving sick people extremely diluted formulations of substances that would produce the same symptoms they suffered from in an effort to evoke natural recovery and regeneration.

Hahnemann believed that homeopathic remedies—substances that caused symptoms similar to those caused by the disease but not diluted forms of the disease-causing agents—worked by activating the "vital force," the organizing energy system that governs health in a human being. There is no comparable belief in Western medicine, but the ideas of vital force bears some resemblance to the Ayurvedic concept of *prana* and to *qi* in Chinese medicine.

Homeopathy gained a foothold in the United States during the 1830s, when it appeared able to stem some epidemics, such as cholera (a devastating infectious disease that produces severe diarrhea), but by the 1900s it fell out of favor as traditional medical practice experienced greater success treating the diseases of the day. During the 1970s there was renewed interest in homeopathy in the United States, and by 2010 believers credited homeopathy with gentle, effective, and nontoxic treatment of many infections, emotional problems, and learning disorders.

Even though proponents assert that homeopathic medicine speeds healing, it cannot treat traumatic injuries, such as broken bones, or genetic diseases.

In "Homeopathic Medical Practice: Long-term Results of a Cohort Study with 3981 Patients" (*BMC Public Health*, vol. 5, November 3, 2005), Claudia M. Witt et al. conducted a study of nearly 4,000 patients diagnosed with a variety of chronic conditions such as allergic rhinitis (inflammation and swelling in the nose and sinuses due to allergy), headache, and atopic dermatitis (red, itchy, dry skin that results from exposure to an allergen or irritant). Witt et al. find that homeopathic treatment was beneficial and observe that the improvements in disease severity, symptoms, and quality of life were maintained throughout the 24 months following treatment.

More recently, Witt et al. looked at how patients receiving homeopathic treatment fared over the course of eight years of follow-up, in "How Healthy Are Chronically Ill Patients after Eight Years of Homeopathic Treatment?—Results from a Long Term Observational Study" (*BMC Public Health*, vol. 8, December 17, 2008). Witt et al. followed 3,709 patients and found that, in general, they had improved based on self-report of their complaints and quality of life measures. The greatest improvements were seen in younger patients, females, and those with greater disease severity at the onset of treatment.

Naturopathic Medicine

As its name suggests, naturopathic medicine, or naturopathy, uses naturally occurring substances to prevent, diagnose, and treat disease. This alternative medicine system, one of the oldest, has its origins in Native American culture and draws from Greek, Chinese, and Indian philosophies of health and illness.

Naturopathy was introduced in the United States by the German physician Benedict Lust (1872–1945), and its popularity rose, declined, and was rekindled in the same time period as homeopathy. Lust opened a school of naturopathic medicine in New York City. He and James Foster, a physician in Idaho using natural healing techniques, christened their blend of herbal medicine, manipulative therapies, homeopathy, nutrition, and psychology naturopathy.

The overarching principles of modern naturopathic medicine are "first, do no harm" and "nature has the power to heal." Naturopathy seeks to treat the whole person because disease is seen as arising from many causes rather than from a single cause. Naturopathic physicians are taught that "prevention is as important as cure" and to view creating and maintaining health as equally important as curing disease. They are instructed to identify and treat the causes of diseases rather than acting only to relieve symptoms. Naturopathy also requires practitioners to serve as teachers to encourage patients to assume personal responsibility for their health and actively participate in self-care.

Naturopathic physicians' treatment methods include nutritional counseling and the addition of dietary supplements, herbs, or vitamins to a patient's diet; hydrotherapy (water-based therapies, usually involving whirlpool or other baths); exercise; manipulation; massage; heat therapy; and electrical stimulation. They are trained to prescribe herbal medicines and homeopathic remedies, perform minor surgical procedures such as setting broken bones, and offer counseling services to help patients resolve emotional problems and modify their lifestyle to improve their health and wellness. Because naturopathy draws on Chinese and Indian medical techniques, naturopathic physicians often use Chinese herbs, acupuncture, and Ayurvedic medicine to treat disease.

The NCCAM reports that even though there is scant published research examining the efficacy of naturopathy as a system of treatment, some studies have been conducted to evaluate the individual therapies frequently recommended by naturopathic physicians. For example, diet and lifestyle changes have proved extremely valuable in treating heart disease and diabetes, and the use of acupuncture to treat pain has gained widespread acceptance. Ryan Bradley and Erica B. Odberg note in "Naturopathic Medicine and Type 2 Diabetes: A Retrospective Analysis from an Academic Clinic" (*Alternative Medicine Review*, vol. 155, no. 1, March 2006) that control of blood sugar and other vital statistics in patients receiving naturopathic care is comparable to published national averages. Bradley and Odberg assert that naturopathic physicians prescribe lifestyle changes that are supported by a high level of evidence of efficacy. In this study, 100% of patients received dietary counseling, 69% were taught stress reduction techniques, and 94% were prescribed exercise. Patients additionally received prescriptions for botanical and nutritional supplementation, often in combination with conventional medication, and there has been mounting evidence of their value in treatment.

Similarly, in "Naturopathic Care for Anxiety: A Randomized Controlled Trial ISRCTN78958974" (*PLOS One*, vol. 4, no. 8, August 31, 2009), Kieran Cooley et al. find that naturopathic care (NC) consisting of dietary counseling, deep breathing relaxation techniques, a standard multivitamin, and the herbal medicine ashwagandha (*Withania somnifera*), when compared with psychotherapy (PT) with deep breathing, was at least as effective in reducing moderate to severe anxiety. Cooley et al. conclude, "Both NC and PT led to significant improvements in patients' anxiety. Group comparison demonstrated a significant decrease in anxiety levels in the NC group over the PT group. Significant improvements in secondary quality of life measures were also observed in the NC group as compared to PT."

Acupuncture

Acupuncture is a Chinese practice that dates back more than 5,000 years. Even though Sir William Osler (1849–1919) called acupuncture the best available treatment for low back pain in the late 1800s, it was not widely used to treat pain in the United States until the 1970s. Chinese medicine describes acupuncture—the insertion of extremely thin, sterile needles into any of 360 specific points on the body—as a way to balance *qi* (also called *chi*), the body's vital life force that flows over the surface of the body and through internal organs. Traditional Western medicine explains the acknowledged effectiveness of acupuncture as the result of triggering the release of pain-relieving substances called endorphins, which occur naturally in the body, and neurotransmitters and neuropeptides, which influence brain chemistry.

There have been many studies on acupuncture's potential usefulness, but historically the results have been mixed due to complexities with study design and size. For example, a 2009 systematic review, "Evidence from the Cochrane Collaboration for Traditional Chinese Medicine Therapies" by Eric Manheimer et al. (*Journal of Alternative and Complementary Medicine*, vol. 15, no. 9, September 16, 2009), considered 26 studies of acupuncture and concluded that, while they suggested benefit, most studies were of poor quality. Nonetheless, there are many reports of acupuncture's effectiveness in reducing postoperative and chemotherapy nausea and vomiting as well as in the treatment of addiction, stroke rehabilitation, headache, menstrual cramps, tennis elbow, fibromyalgia, myofascial pain, osteoarthritis, low-back pain, carpal tunnel syndrome, and asthma. One NCCAM-funded study showed that acupuncture provides pain relief, improves function for people with osteoarthritis of the knee, and serves as an effective complement to traditional medical care. Another NCCAM-funded study (Michael Hollifield et al., "Acupuncture for Posttraumatic Stress Disorder: A Randomized Controlled Pilot Trial," *Journal of Nervous and Mental Disease*, vol. 195, no. 6, June 2007) indicated that acupuncture may help people with posttraumatic stress disorder, an anxiety disorder that can develop in response to a terrifying event or threat.

Ayurvedic Medicine

Ayurvedic medicine (also called Ayurveda, which means "science of life") is believed to be the oldest medical tradition and has been practiced in India and Asia for more than 5,000 years. With an emphasis on preventing disease and promoting wellness, its practitioners view emotional health and spiritual balance as vital for physical health and disease prevention. Ayurveda also considers diet, hygiene, sleep, lifestyle, and healthy relationships as powerful influences on health.

Practitioners aim to balance the three *doshas*—fundamental human qualities that they believe reside in varying concentrations in different parts of the human body. The *doshas* are thought to be disturbed by improper diet, sleep deprivation, travel, coffee, alcohol, or excessive exposure to the sun and are balanced with diet, exercise, detoxification (ritual cleansing of toxins), yoga, spiritual counseling, herbal medicine, breathing exercises, and chanting.

In "Utilization of Ayurveda in Health Care: An Approach for Prevention, Health Promotion, and Treatment of Disease. Part 1—Ayurveda, the Science of Life" (*Journal of Alternative and Complementary Medicine*, vol. 13, no. 9, November 2007), Hari Sharma et al. opine that while "Western allopathic medicine is excellent in handling acute medical crises, Ayurveda demonstrates an ability to manage chronic disorders that Western medicine has been unable to." Like other CAM, Ayurveda encourages patients to assume responsibility for their health and promotes self-care.

Traditional Chinese Medicine

Traditional Chinese medicine (TCM) combines nutrition, acupuncture, massage, herbal medicine, and Qi Gong (exercises to improve the flow of vital energy through the body) to help people achieve balance and unity of their mind, body, and spirit. TCM has been used for more than 3,000 years by about one-fourth of the world's population, and in the United States it has been embraced by naturopathic physicians, chiropractors, and other CAM practitioners.

One diagnostic technique that is noticeably different from Western medicine is the TCM approach to taking pulses. TCM practitioners take pulses at six different locations, including three points on each wrist, and pulses are described using 28 distinct qualities. Reading the pulses enables practitioners to evaluate *qi*.

TCM views balancing *qi* as central to health, wellness, and disease prevention and treatment. TCM also seeks to balance the feminine and masculine qualities of yin and yang using other techniques such as moxibustion (stimulating acupuncture points with heat) and cupping (increasing circulation by putting a heated jar on the skin of a body part).

Herbal medicine is the most commonly prescribed treatment; herbal preparations may be consumed as teas made from boiled fresh herbs or dried powders or in combined formulations known as patent medicines. More than 200 herbal preparations are used in TCM, and several, such as ginseng, ma huang, and ginger, have become popular in the United States. Ginseng is supposed to improve immunity and prevent illness; ma huang is a stimulant used to promote weight loss and relieve lung congestion; and ginger is prescribed to aid digestion,

relieve nausea, reduce osteoarthritic knee pain, and improve circulation.

Many modern pharmaceutical drugs are derived from TCM herbal medicines. For example, ma huang components are used to make ephedrine and pseudoephedrine. GBE, made from ginkgo biloba, is used to treat cerebral insufficiency (lack of blood flow to the brain).

Research to determine the effectiveness of TCM has focused on the efficacy of specific herbs and combinations of herbs. For example, tripterygium wilfordii Hook F (Chinese Thunder God vine) has been used to treat autoimmune and inflammatory disorders such as arthritis. In "Evidence of Effectiveness of Herbal Medicinal Products in the Treatment of Arthritis. Part 2: Rheumatoid Arthritis" (*Phytotherapy Research*, vol. 23, no. 12, December 2009), Melainie Cameron et al. report that three studies compared preparations of tripterygium wilfordii to placebos and returned favorable results in terms of their ability to relieve symptoms of arthritis.

MIND-BODY INTERVENTIONS

Mind-body interventions are practices based on the belief that the mind, body, and spirit are connected to one another and to environmental influences. The NCCAM observes in "What Is CAM?" (October 26, 2009, http://nccam.nih.gov/health/whatiscam/overview.htm) that some techniques that were formerly considered CAM, such as patient support groups and cognitive behavioral therapy, are now widely accepted and used by conventional medical practitioners. Mind-body medicine aims to improve physical, mental, and emotional well-being. According to Dr. Kenneth R. Pelletier (1946–), a clinical professor at the University of Arizona School of Medicine and author of *The Best Alternative Medicine* (2000), the guiding principles of mind-body medicine are:

- Stress and depression contribute to the development of, and hinder recovery from, chronic diseases because they create measurable hormonal imbalances.

- Psychoneuroimmunology explains how mental functioning provokes physical and biochemical changes that weaken immunity, lowering resistance to disease.

- Overall health improves when people are optimistic and have a positive outlook on life. Health and wellness are harmed by anger, depression, and chronic stress.

- The placebo effect (improved health and favorable physical changes in response to inactive medication such as a sugar pill) confirms the importance of mind-body medicine and is a valuable intervention.

- Social support from family, friends, coworkers, classmates, or organized self-help groups boosts the effectiveness of traditional and CAM therapies.

This section looks at two types of mind-body interventions: meditation and biofeedback. Other commonly used mind-body interventions include music and dance therapies, cognitive behavioral therapy, hypnosis, guided imagery and visualization, and a Chinese exercise discipline called Tai Chi Chuan.

Meditation

Historically, meditation has been used in religious training and practices and to enhance spiritual growth, but it is also a powerful self-care measure that may be used to relieve stress and promote healing. Transcendental meditation, an Indian practice that involves sitting and silently chanting a mantra (a word repeated to quiet the mind), aims to produce a healthy state of relaxation.

During the 1960s Herbert Benson (1935–) studied meditation, and he and his colleagues at Harvard University Medical School showed that people who meditate can reduce heart and respiration rates, lower blood levels of the hormone cortisol, and increase alpha waves (smooth, regular electrical oscillations in the human brain that occur when a person is awake and relaxed). Benson developed a relaxation technique loosely based on transcendental meditation that he dubbed the "relaxation response," and this technique quickly gained recognition in the United States and Europe.

There have been many studies performed to evaluate physical and psychological responses to meditation, and its benefits are universally accepted in the CAM and conventional medical communities. Research has focused on understanding how meditation works and the conditions it may help relieve.

In *Meditation Practices for Health: State of the Research* (June 2007, http://www.ahrq.gov/downloads/pub/evidence/pdf/meditation/medit.pdf), Maria B. Ospina et al. of the University of Alberta review research on a variety of meditation practices. An analysis of 813 research studies finds favorable therapeutic effects of meditation, such as:

- The ability to lower heart rate and blood pressure readings
- Reduced stress, anxiety, and pain
- Reduced intraocular pressure (pressure inside the eye)
- Reduction in cholesterol levels
- Increased breath holding time

Table 9.1 lists the conditions, diseases, and populations included in the research studies on meditation. It also distinguishes between observational and intervention studies about meditation practices. Most studies reviewed were conducted on healthy populations such as college students and healthy older adults living in the community. Some studies also considered people suffering from mental health problems, people with cardiovascular and circulatory problems, and people suffering from chronic pain.

In "Meditation: An Introduction" (October 26, 2009, http://nccam.nih.gov/health/meditation/overview.htm), the NCCAM states that meditation may exert its beneficial effects by reducing activity in the sympathetic nervous system (the system that mobilizes the body to respond in a "fight or flight" response when under stress) and increasing activity in the parasympathetic nervous system, which slows heart rate and breathing and dilates blood vessels to improve circulation.

Biofeedback

Biofeedback training is designed to help people learn to regulate body functions such as heart rate and blood pressure. Generally, sensitive monitoring devices are attached to the individual to measure and record a variety of physical responses such as skin temperature and electrical resistance, brain-wave activity, and respiration rate. There are also devices to monitor other functions such as bladder activity and acid in the stomach. By observing their own responses and following instructions given by highly trained technicians, most people are able to exert some degree of conscious control over these body functions. Biofeedback is especially effective for helping people learn to manage stress, and it has become a mainstream medical treatment for conditions such as high blood pressure, asthma, migraine headaches, and some types of urinary and fecal incontinence (inability to control bladder or bowel functions).

In "Treatment Preferences for CAM in Children with Chronic Pain" (*Evidence-Based Complementary and Alternative Medicine*, vol. 4, no. 3, 2007), a review of CAM practices used to treat children, Jennie C. I. Tsao et al. find that biofeedback is among the most preferred noninvasive therapies used to relieve pain and promote relaxation.

BIOLOGICALLY BASED THERAPIES

The principal treatments in biologically based therapies are herbal medicines and remedies, dietary supplements, and the use of hormones to combat disease and improve health. Because herbal medicines are used in a variety of other CAM practices, such as homeopathy, naturopathy, Ayurveda, and traditional Chinese medicine, this section describes a hotly contested biologically based therapy: the use of dietary supplements.

Dietary Supplements

Most CAM practitioners and many conventional medical practitioners agree that food sources are the best way to obtain nutrients. They also agree that it is difficult for many people to get sufficient quantities of specific

TABLE 9.1

Types of populations and conditions included in studies on meditation, through September 2005

Category of interest	Study condition	Intervention studies	Observational analytical studies	Total	Total studies per category
Circulatory and cardiovascular	Hypertension	35	2	37	61
	Other cardiovascular diseases	24	—	24	
Dental	Dental problems (NS)	1	—	1	2
	Periodontitis	—	1	1	
Dermatology	Psoriasis	3	—	3	3
Endocrine	Obesity	1	—	1	11
	Type II diabetes mellitus	10	—	10	
Gastrointestinal	Gastrointestinal disorders	1	—	1	3
	Irritable bowel syndrome	2	—	2	
Gynecology	Infertility	1	—	1	10
	Menopause	2	—	2	
	Postmenopause	1	3	4	
	Pregnancy	1	1	2	
	Premenstrual syndrome	1	—	1	
Healthy	College and university students	123	65	189	553
	Elderly	34	26	60	
	Healthy volunteers	90	160	250	
	Army and military	8	—	8	
	Prison inmates	7	3	10	
	Workers	25	3	28	
	Athletes	6	—	6	
	Smokers	3	—	3	
Immunologic	HIV	3	—	3	3
Sleep disorders	Insomnia	2	—	2	5
	Chronic insomnia	3	—	3	
Mental health disorders	Anger management	1	—	1	66
	Anxiety disorders	14	—	14	
	Binge eating disorder	3	—	3	
	Burnout	1	—	1	
	Depression	11	—	11	
	Miscellaneous psychiatric conditions	6	1	7	
	Mood disorders	3	—	3	
	Neurosis	1	—	1	
	Obsessive-compulsive disorder	1	—	1	
	Parents of children with behavior problems	1	—	1	
	Personality disorders	1	—	1	
	Postraumatic stress disorders	1	—	1	
	Psychosis	1	—	1	
	Schizophrenia	1	—	1	
	Schizophrenia AND antisocial personality disorders	1	—	1	
	Substance abuse	18	—	18	
Miscellaneous medical conditions	Heterogeneous patient population	10	—	10	11
	Chronic fatigue	1	—	1	
Musculoskeletal	Balance disorders	1	—	1	42
	Carpal tunnel syndrome	1	—	1	
	Multiple sclerosis	2	—	2	
	Muscular dystrophy	1	—	1	
	Chronic pain	10	1	11	
	Chronic rheumatic diseases	1	—	1	
	Fibromyalgia	10	—	10	
	Regional pain syndrome	1	—	1	
	Rheumatoid arthritis	6	—	6	
	Hyperkyphosis	1	—	1	
	Osteoarthritis	4	—	4	
	Osteoporosis	1	—	1	
	Postpolio syndrome	1	—	1	
	Total hip and knee replacement	1	—	1	
Neurological	Developmental disabilities	1	—	1	10
	Epilepsy	2	—	2	
	Migraine and tension headaches	3	—	3	
	Stroke	2	—	2	
	Traumatic brain injuries	2	—	2	

vitamins or minerals from their daily diet. For example, many researchers and nutritionists feel that the diets of most Americans do not contain enough chromium and that most women do not consume adequate amounts of iron. Furthermore, the CAM principle of treating each patient as an individual with unique physiologic and biochemical needs suggests that some individuals may need more of specific nutrients than others.

TABLE 9.1

Types of populations and conditions included in studies on meditation, through September 2005 [CONTINUED]

Category of interest	Study condition	Intervention studies	Observational analytical studies	Total	Total studies per category
Oncology	Cancer	12	—	12	12
Organ transplant	Organ transplantation	1	—	1	1
Renal	End-stage renal disease	1	—	1	1
Respiratory and pulmonary	Asthma	11	—	11	16
	COPD	1	—	1	
	Chronic airways obstruction	1	—	1	
	Chronic bronchitis	1	—	1	
	Pleural effusion	1	—	1	
	Pulmonary tuberculosis	1	—	1	
Vestibular	Tinnitus	2	—	2	3
	Vestibulopathy	1	—	1	
Total		**547**	**266**	**813**	**813**

COPD = chronic obstructive pulmonary disease; HIV = human immunodeficiency virus; NS = not specified.

SOURCE: Maria B. Ospina et al., "Table 21. Type of Populations and Conditions Included in Studies on Meditation," in *Meditation Practices for Health: State of the Research*, Agency for Healthcare Research and Quality, June 2007, http://www.ahrq.gov/downloads/pub/evidence/pdf/meditation/medit.pdf (accessed January 25, 2010)

Advocates of dietary supplements believe the recommended dietary allowances (RDAs) are too low for some vitamins and minerals, and they observe that it is difficult to obtain higher than the RDA of certain vitamins without also consuming an excess of fat and calories. An example of this dilemma is vitamin E, an antioxidant found in high-fat vegetable and seed oils. For men to get the RDA (15 international units [IU]) of vitamin E, they would have to, according to Pelletier in *The Best Alternative Medicine*, eat "248 slices of whole wheat bread, 16 dozen eggs, or 20 pounds of bacon." Several studies suggest that far higher doses—20 to 30 times greater than the RDA—may protect against heart disease or some cancers, but to obtain such doses from diet alone is impossible.

Whether to prescribe diets supplemented with vitamin E is just one of many questions about this particular issue. Another concern is the form of vitamin E available—supplements contain only alpha tocopherol instead of the variety of tocopherols available in foods. Is it better to take higher doses of one form of vitamin E at the risk of losing other perhaps equally valuable forms of vitamin E? Critics of dietary supplements use this question to support their view that people should attempt to obtain as many needed nutrients from food sources as possible, without relying on dietary supplements. Furthermore, there is no consensus about dosages higher than the RDA, although it is known that some vitamins and minerals, such as vitamins A and E and chromium, are toxic in high doses. For example, more than 400 IU of vitamin E taken daily may increase the risk of stroke, and high doses of vitamin E are generally not advised for people taking medications to reduce blood clotting.

Table 9.2 lists the characteristics and conditions that a dietary supplement must meet to conform with the legal

TABLE 9.2

About dietary supplements

Dietary supplements were defined in a law passed by Congress in 1994. A dietary supplement must meet all of the following conditions:

- It is a product (other than tobacco) that is intended to supplement the diet and that contains one or more of the following: vitamins, minerals, herbs or other botanicals, amino acids, or any combination of the above ingredients.
- It is intended to be taken in tablet, capsule, powder, softgel, gelcap, or liquid form.
- It is not represented for use as a conventional food or as a sole item of a meal or the diet.
- It is labeled as being a dietary supplement.

SOURCE: "About Dietary Supplements," in *Using Dietary Supplements Wisely*, National Institutes of Health, National Center for Complementary and Alternative Medicine, February 2009, http://nccam.nih.gov/health/supplements/wiseuse.htm#about (accessed January 25, 2010)

and regulatory requirements of the U.S. Food and Drug Administration (FDA). Unlike drugs, dietary supplements are considered foods; as a result, they go to market with far less testing and scrutiny and without FDA approval.

The legislation governing supplements, the Dietary Supplement Health and Education Act of 1994, also established the Office of Dietary Supplements (ODS) at the NIH. The mission of the ODS (2010, http://ods.od.nih.gov/About/about_ods.aspx) is "to strengthen knowledge and understanding of dietary supplements by evaluating scientific information, stimulating and supporting research, disseminating research results, and educating the public to foster an enhanced quality of life and health."

ARE DIETARY SUPPLEMENTS EFFECTIVE? Many dietary supplements have undergone rigorous testing to determine whether they are effective for the conditions they claim to address. However, some research questions the efficacy of several popular dietary supplements, and research continued in 2010 in an effort to resolve these questions. The combination of glucosamine (thought to play a role in cartilage formation) and chondroitin (which helps give cartilage elasticity, taken as a supplement to relieve arthritis pain) was found to be no more effective than a placebo. In "The Effect of Glucosamine and/or Chondroitin Sulfate on the Progression of Knee Osteoarthritis: A Report from the Glucosamine/Chondroitin Arthritis Intervention Trial" (*Arthritis & Rheumatism*, vol. 58, no. 10, October 2008), Allen D. Sawitzke et al. report the results of the NIH-sponsored Glucosamine/Chondroitin Arthritis Intervention Trial, which found that the combination of these supplements was no more effective than placebo in slowing the joint space loss and the loss of cartilage in the knees of people with osteoarthritis.

Another study, "Long-term Effects of Chondroitins 4 and 6 Sulfate on Knee Osteoarthritis: The Study on Osteoarthritis Progression Prevention, a Two-year, Randomized, Double-blind, Placebo-controlled Trial" (*Arthritis & Rheumatism*, vol. 60, no. 2, February 2009), arrives at a different conclusion. André Kahan et al. find that, among people with knee osteoarthritis, a supplement containing two forms of chondroitin sulfate (CS) did significantly reduce joint space loss and knee pain when compared with placebo. Kahan et al. conclude that "the long-term combined structure-modifying and symptom-modifying effects of CS suggest that it could be a disease-modifying agent in patients with knee [osteoarthritis]."

Similarly, in "Echinacea Species (Echinacea Angustifolia (DC.) Hell., Echinacea Pallida (Nutt.) Nutt., Echinacea Purpurea (L.) Moench): A Review of Their Chemistry, Pharmacology and Clinical Properties" (*Journal of Pharmacy and Pharmacology*, vol. 57, no. 8, August 2005), Joanne Barnes et al. reviewed research that assessed the safety and effectiveness of echinacea for the prevention and treatment of upper respiratory infections. Barnes et al. observe that several, but not all, clinical trials of echinacea preparations have reported effects better than those of a placebo. The investigators caution that the evidence of echinacea's effectiveness is not conclusive, because the studies are not comparable—they have included different patient groups and tested various different preparations and doses of echinacea. Klaus Linde et al. conducted a comprehensive review that assessed the available evidence from clinical trials investigating the effectiveness of echinacea extracts for the prevention and treatment of the common cold and reported their findings in "Echinacea for Preventing and Treating the Common Cold" (*Cochrane Library*, 2005). The results from Linde et al. were consistent with those of Barnes et al., suggesting that some echinacea preparations may be better than a placebo, for both treatment and prevention of colds, and may be more effective for treatment when taken at the onset of symptoms.

SOME DIETARY SUPPLEMENTS MAY BE HARMFUL. Because many dietary supplements are naturally occurring and available without a prescription, many consumers mistakenly believe that using them could not possibly be harmful. This is not the case, because dietary supplements have the potential to interact unfavorably with specific foods and drugs or even cause harm when taken on their own. The FDA has issued warnings and advised caution about the use of some dietary supplements. For example, in "Warning on Body Building Products Marketed as Containing Steroids or Steroid-Like Substances" (http://www.fda.gov/ForConsumers/ConsumerUpdates/ucm173739.htm), the FDA cautioned consumers on July 28, 2009, to stop using any body building products marketed as dietary supplements that may contain steroids or steroid-like substances because of their potential to cause serious liver injury, stroke, kidney failure, and pulmonary embolism (blockage of an artery in the lung).

MANIPULATIVE AND BODY-BASED METHODS

Manipulative therapies, such as osteopathic manipulation and chiropractic, and body-based methods (also known as bodywork), such as therapeutic massage, are CAM practices that have been tremendously popular during the last two decades. The CAM supplement to the 2007 NHIS finds that about 18 million adults and 700,000 children received massage therapy during the year prior to the survey. Enthusiasm for these CAM practices is at least in part attributed to their demonstrated ability to relieve aches and pains associated with musculoskeletal injuries and stress more effectively than treatment prescribed by conventional medical practitioners. As a result, these therapeutic modalities have made inroads into mainstream medicine.

Allison R. Mitchinson et al. confirm in "Acute Postoperative Pain Management Using Massage as an Adjuvant Therapy: A Randomized Trial" (*Archives of Surgery*, vol. 142, no. 12, December 2007) the efficacy of massage to relieve pain in patients who had undergone major surgery. The researchers conclude that "pharmacologic interventions alone may not address all of the factors involved in the experience of pain" and that "massage therapy improves pain management and postoperative anxiety among many patients who experience unrelieved postoperative pain."

In "Massage for Low Back Pain: An Updated Systematic Review within the Framework of the Cochrane Back Review Group" (*Spine*, vol. 34, no. 16, July 15, 2009), Andrea Furlan et al. reviewed 13 trials of massage for back pain. In two of the studies, massage proved more effective than a sham therapy, and eight studies compared massage with other back pain treatment. These studies found that in terms of pain relief, massage was comparable to exercise and that it was superior to treatments involving joint mobilization, relaxation therapy, physical therapy, acupuncture, and self-care education. Furlan et al. concluded, "Massage might be beneficial for patients with subacute and chronic nonspecific low back pain, especially when combined with exercises and education."

Chiropractic

The American Chiropractic Association (ACA; 2010, http://www.acatoday.org/level2_css.cfm?T1ID=13&T2ID=61&BT1ID=21&BT2ID=94) defines chiropractic as "a health care profession that focuses on disorders of the musculoskeletal system and the nervous system, and the effects of these disorders on general health. Chiropractic care is used most often to treat neuromusculoskeletal complaints, including but not limited to back pain, neck pain, pain in the joints of the arms or legs, and headaches." Doctors of chiropractic (also known as chiropractors) do not use or prescribe pharmaceutical drugs or perform surgery. Instead, they rely on adjustment and manipulation of the musculoskeletal system, particularly the spinal column.

Many chiropractors use nutritional therapy and prescribe dietary supplements, and some use a technique known as applied kinesiology to diagnose and treat disease. Applied kinesiology is based on the belief that every organ problem is associated with the weakness of a specific muscle. Chiropractors who use this technique claim they can accurately identify organ system dysfunction without any laboratory or other diagnostic tests.

Besides manipulation, chiropractors also use a variety of other therapies to support healing and relax muscles before they make manual adjustments. These treatments include the following:

- Heat and cold therapy to relieve pain, speed healing, and reduce swelling

- Hydrotherapy to relax muscles and stimulate blood circulation

- Immobilization such as casts, wraps, traction, and splints to protect injured areas

- Electrotherapy to deliver deep-tissue massage and boost circulation

- Ultrasound to relieve muscle spasms and reduce swelling

According to the ACA (2010, http://www.acatoday.org/pdf/Gen_Chiro_Info.pdf), chiropractic is the third-largest specialty group of health care professionals after medicine and dentistry. Visits to chiropractors are most often for treatment of low back pain, neck pain, and headaches. Critics of chiropractic are concerned about injuries resulting from powerful "high velocity" manual adjustments, and some physicians question chiropractors' abilities to establish medical diagnoses. Others worry that people seeking chiropractic care instead of traditional allopathic (conventional) medical care may be foregoing lifesaving diagnoses and treatment.

EFFECTIVENESS OF CHIROPRACTIC. In "Backgrounder" (November 2009, http://nccam.nih.gov/health/chiropractic/D403_BKG.pdf), a review of the relevant literature, the NCCAM notes that most patients seek chiropractic treatment for shoulder, neck, or back pain. The NCCAM's assessment of the available research is that spinal manipulation, which also may be performed by physical therapists, osteopaths, and some conventional medical doctors, may provide relief from low-back pain. Spinal manipulation appears to be safe and as effective as conventional treatments. In "Spinal Manipulation for Low-Back Pain" (April 2009, http://nccam.nih.gov/health/pain/spinemanipulation.htm), the NCCAM notes that research currently underway aims to find out whether the effects of spinal manipulation depend on the duration and frequency of treatment. Some studies report short-term relief—up to three months—from low-back pain, and some pain relief can last as long as one year.

ENERGY THERAPIES

Energy therapies that purport to influence energy fields in and around the body are among the CAM practices that arouse the most suspicion from the conventional medical community. Some skeptics attribute the health benefits reported by patients who have received energy therapies to the placebo effect (a perceived beneficial result that occurs from the therapy because of the patient's expectation that the therapy will help). Despite a widespread lack of understanding and acceptance from traditional health care practitioners, some hospitals and pioneering practitioners are incorporating energy therapies into their treatment programs.

Reiki

An ancient Japanese technique, Reiki is bioenergetic healing intended to restore physical, emotional, mental, and spiritual balance. The unique therapy takes its name from two Japanese words. *Rei* means higher power, wisdom, and all that exists, and *ki* is the life force, or the energy that runs through living things.

Based on the teachings of Mikao Usui (1865–1926), Reiki is a universal healing vibration that flows through the practitioner to the client. Practitioners act as a channel for Reiki energy, and as it passes through practitioners, it acts to strengthen and harmonize them simultaneously as it heals their clients.

There are more than a dozen styles of Reiki, each with its own subtle variations. Students studying with Usui Reiki masters receive a series of "attunements" and may progress through three levels or degrees of training. Level I connects the practitioner to the Reiki channel and initiates the flow of healing energy. Level II teaches distance or remote healing. Level III initiates the practitioner to the role of master and teacher.

Some practitioners use a variety of other therapies, including meditation, prayer, chanting, breathing, and movement education. Most often performed as hands-on bodywork, Reiki is believed by its therapists to convey energy to calm nerves, relax muscles, and ease pain without any physical touch. During the second level of training, practitioners learn to deliver Reiki energy remotely, over long distances.

There are many case studies describing the effectiveness of Reiki to reduce anxiety and relieve discomfort, but as of 2010 there were no published reports of rigorous research designed to determine its efficacy. In "A Systematic Review of the Therapeutic Effects of Reiki," published in the November 2009 issue of the *Journal of Complementary Medicine* (vol. 15, no. 11), Sondra vanderVaart et al. found all of the studies on Reiki lacking in rigor. Although 9 of 12 trials reported a significant therapeutic effect, the reviewers concluded, "The serious methodological and reporting limitations of limited existing Reiki studies preclude a definitive conclusion on its effectiveness. High-quality randomized controlled trials are needed to address the effectiveness of Reiki over placebo." NCCAM-funded research considers some of the as yet unanswered questions about Reiki, including:

- How does it work?
- Is Reiki a safe and effective treatment for fibromyalgia and other chronic pain?
- Can Reiki relieve anxiety and improve the well-being of patients with diseases such as cancer and the acquired immunodeficiency syndrome?
- Can Reiki help control blood sugar levels, improve heart function, or relieve nerve pain in people with Type 2 diabetes?

The effects of Reiki on nerve pain suffered by patients with diabetes was examined by Elena A. Gillespie, Brenda W. Gillespie, and Martin J. Stevens in "Painful Diabetic Neuropathy [PDN]: Impact of an Alternative Approach" (*Diabetes Care*, vol. 30, no. 4, April 2007). In a randomized, placebo-controlled trial, subjects were placed in one of three treatment groups—Reiki, mimic Reiki, or usual care—for 12 weeks. During the study period, patients were assessed for pain by using pain scores and walking distance. Both the Reiki and mimic Reiki groups showed improvements in pain and walking distance, compared with the usual care group; however, at the end of the study there were no significant differences between the groups. Gillespie, Gillespie, and Stevens conclude that "Reiki is no more effective than mimic-Reiki in decreasing pain perception and improving walking distance in subjects with PDN. However, the reduction of pain symptoms observed in both treatment groups is consistent with the concept that the formation of a 'sustained partnership' between the health care provider and the patient can have direct therapeutic benefits."

COMPLEMENTING TRADITIONAL MEDICINE. Clinics and hospitals across the United States offer Reiki to women in labor, surgical patients, and those suffering from pain, anxiety, sleep disorders, headaches, asthma, and eating disorders. According to the Center for Reiki Research (2010, http://www.centerforreikiresearch.org/), in 2010, 65 hospitals in the United States offered patients Reiki treatments.

In conventional medical settings, Reiki is usually presented as a method to reduce stress and promote relaxation, thereby enhancing the body's natural ability to heal itself. To gain credibility with traditional physicians and other mainstream professionals, Reiki therapists often downplay the spiritual benefits of the practice and avoid mentioning other CAM practices.

Even though its effectiveness has not been documented in scientific studies, Reiki has gained acceptance because it is viewed as a complement, rather than as an alternative, to traditional Western medicine. Considered safe by many health care practitioners, it is well received by patients who seem to respond favorably to the time and attention, as well as to the healing energy, offered by Reiki therapists.

IMPORTANT NAMES
AND ADDRESSES

Alzheimer's Association
225 N. Michigan Ave., 17th Fl.
Chicago, IL 60601-7633
(312) 335-8700
1-800-272-3900
URL: http://www.alz.org/

**American Academy of Child
and Adolescent Psychiatry**
3615 Wisconsin Ave. NW
Washington, DC 20016-3007
(202) 966-7300
FAX: (202) 966-2891
URL: http://www.aacap.org/

American Academy of Pediatrics
141 Northwest Point Blvd.
Elk Grove Village, IL 60007-1098
(847) 434-4000
FAX: (847) 434-8000
E-mail: kidsdocs@aap.org
URL: http://www.aap.org/

**American Association
of Suicidology**
5221 Wisconsin Ave. NW
Washington, DC 20015
(202) 237-2280
FAX: (202) 237-2282
E-mail: info@suicidology.org
URL: http://www.suicidology.org/

American Cancer Society
1599 Clifton Rd. NE
Atlanta, GA 30329-4251
(404) 320-3333
1-800-227-2345
URL: http://www.cancer.org/

American Chiropractic Association
1701 Clarendon Blvd.
Arlington, VA 22209
(703) 276-8800
FAX: (703) 243-2593
URL: http://www.acatoday.org/

**American College of Obstetricians
and Gynecologists**
PO Box 96920
Washington, DC 20090-6920
(202) 638-5577
URL: http://www.acog.org/

American Diabetes Association
1701 N. Beauregard St.
Alexandria, VA 22311
1-800-342-2383
E-mail: askada@diabetes.org
URL: http://www.diabetes.org/

**American Heart Association
National Center**
7272 Greenville Ave.
Dallas, TX 75231
1-800-242-8721
URL: http://www.americanheart.org/

American Lung Association
1301 Pennsylvania Ave. NW
Washington, DC 20004
(202) 785-3355
1-800-548-8252
FAX: (202) 452-1805
URL: http://www.lungusa.org/

American Parkinson Disease Association
135 Parkinson Ave.
Staten Island, NY 10305
(718) 981-8001
1-800-223-2732
FAX: (718) 981-4399
E-mail: apda@apdaparkinson.org
URL: http://www.apdaparkinson.org/

American Psychiatric Association
1000 Wilson Blvd., Ste. 1825
Arlington, VA 22209-3901
(703) 907-7300
1-888-357-7924
E-mail: apa@psych.org
URL: http://www.psych.org/

**American Psychological
Association**
750 First St. NE
Washington, DC 20002-4242
(202) 336-5500
1-800-374-2721
URL: http://www.apa.org/

Arthritis Foundation
PO Box 7669
Atlanta, GA 30357-0669
1-800-283-7800
URL: http://www.arthritis.org/

Autism Society of America
4340 East-West Hwy., Ste. 350
Bethesda, MD 20814
(301) 657-0881
1-800-328-8476
URL: http://www.autism-society.org/

**Centers for Disease Control
and Prevention**
1600 Clifton Rd.
Atlanta, GA 30333
(404) 498-1515
1-800-232-4636
E-mail: cdcinfo@cdc.gov
URL: http://www.cdc.gov/

Cystic Fibrosis Foundation
6931 Arlington Rd., 2nd Fl.
Bethesda, MD 20814
(301) 951-4422
1-800-344-4823
FAX: (301) 951-6378
E-mail: info@cff.org
URL: http://www.cff.org/

Epilepsy Foundation
8301 Professional Pl.
Landover, MD 20785
1-800-332-1000
URL: http://www.epilepsyfoundation.org/

**Huntington's Disease Society
of America**
505 Eighth Ave., Ste. 902
New York, NY 10018
(212) 242-1968
1-800-345-4372
FAX: (212) 239-3430
E-mail: hdsainfo@hdsa.org
URL: http://www.hdsa.org/

**March of Dimes Birth Defects
Foundation**
1275 Mamaroneck Ave.
White Plains, NY 10605
(914) 997-4488
URL: http://www.modimes.org/

**Muscular Dystrophy Association
National Headquarters**
3300 E. Sunrise Dr.
Tucson, AZ 85718
1-800-572-1717
E-mail: mda@mdausa.org
URL: http://www.mdausa.org/

**National Center for Complementary
and Alternative Medicine
National Institutes of Health**
9000 Rockville Pike
Bethesda, MD 20892
(301) 519-3153
1-888-644-6226

FAX: (866) 464-3616
E-mail: info@nccam.nih.gov
URL: http://www.nccam.nih.gov/

**National Center for Health Statistics
U.S. Department of Health
and Human Services**
3311 Toledo Rd.
Hyattsville, MD 20782
1-800-232-4636
E-mail: cdcinfo@cdc.gov
URL: http://www.cdc.gov/nchs/

National Fibromyalgia Association
2121 S. Towne Centre Pl., Ste. 300
Anaheim, CA 92806
(714) 921-0150
URL: http://www.fmaware.org/

National Mental Health Association
2000 N. Beauregard St., Sixth Fl.
Alexandria, VA 22311
(703) 684-7722
1-800-969-6642
FAX: (703) 684-5968
URL: http://www.nmha.org/

National Multiple Sclerosis Society
733 Third Ave., 3rd Fl.
New York, NY 10017
1-800-344-4867
URL: http://www.nmss.org/

National Osteoporosis Foundation
1150 17th St. NW, Ste. 850
Washington, DC 20036
(202) 223-2226
1-800-231-4222
URL: http://www.nof.org/

**National Tay-Sachs and Allied
Diseases Association**
2001 Beacon St., Ste. 204
Boston, MA 02135
1-800-906-8723
FAX: (617) 277-0134
E-mail: info@ntsad.org
URL: http://www.ntsad.org/

**Sickle Cell Disease Association
of America, Inc.**
231 E. Baltimore St., Ste. 800
Baltimore, MD 21202
(410) 528-1555
1-800-421-8453
FAX: (410) 528-1495
E-mail: scdaa@sicklecelldisease.org
URL: http://www.sicklecelldisease.org/

United Network for Organ Sharing
700 N. Fourth St.
Richmond, VA 23219
(804) 782-4800
FAX: (804) 782-4817
URL: http://www.unos.org/

RESOURCES

The Centers for Disease Control and Prevention (CDC) tracks nationwide health trends and reports its findings in several periodicals, especially in the *Advance Data* series, the annual *HIV/AIDS Surveillance Reports*, and the *Morbidity and Mortality Weekly Reports*. The CDC's National Center for Injury Prevention and Control provides data about deaths and disability caused by accidents and violence. The National Center for Health Statistics (NCHS) provides a complete statistical overview of the nation's health in its annual *Health, United States*. The NCHS periodicals *National Vital Statistics Reports* and *Vital and Health Statistics* detail U.S. birth and death data and trends.

The National Health Interview Surveys offer information about the lifestyles, health behaviors, and health risks of Americans. The CDC publishes *Health Risks in the United States: Behavioral Risk Factor Surveillance System*—the results of surveys in each state asking adults questions about a wide range of behaviors affecting their health. The National Health and Nutrition Examination Survey (NHANES) conducted by NIMH and the NCHS also helps to characterize the health and well-being of Americans. Working with other agencies and professional organizations, the CDC helped produce *Healthy People 2010*, which served as a blueprint for improving the health of Americans during the first decade of the 21st century, and *Healthy People 2020*, which details goals and objectives for the coming decade.

Mental health and illness in the United States were detailed in the landmark report *Mental Health: A Report of the Surgeon General* (1999) and in follow-up reports, including *Mental Health: Culture, Race and Ethnicity* (2001) and *Achieving the Promise: Transforming Mental Health Care in America* (2003). In addition, the Center for Mental Health Services reports data describing the nation's mental health status and services in its periodic *Mental Health, United States*. The National Institute of Mental Health (NIMH is one of the National Institutes of Health) provides detailed information about mental health research and treatment of mental illness The Harvard School of Medicine *National Comorbidity Survey* (2007) and the NIMH publication *The Numbers Count: Mental Disorders in America* (2008) provide estimates of the incidence and prevalence of mental disorders.

The National Institutes of Health provides definitions, epidemiological data, and research findings about a comprehensive range of medical and public health subjects. The National Center for Complementary and Alternative Medicine defines and describes a range of alternative, complementary, and integrative medical practices. The National Institute of Environmental Health Sciences provides information about environmental hazards and behaviors that jeopardize health.

Medical, public health, and nursing journals offer a wealth of disease-specific information and research findings. The studies cited in this edition are drawn from a wide range of professional publications, including the *Annals of Internal Medicine*, *Archives of General Psychiatry*, *Circulation*, *Journal of the American Medical Association*, *Lancet*, *New England Journal of Medicine*, and *Public Health Reports*.

The American Cancer Society's *Cancer Facts and Figures 2009* (2009) provided valuable data, as did the Alzheimer's Association, the American Diabetes Association, the American Heart Association, the American Lung Association, and the National Osteoporosis Foundation, all of which are excellent resources for information about the epidemiology of diseases, treatments, and clinical trials. Many other professional associations, voluntary medical organizations, and foundations dedicated to research, education, and advocacy related to other specific medical conditions and disabling diseases proved useful sources for up-to-date information in this edition.

INDEX

Page references in italics refer to photographs. References with the letter t following them indicate the presence of a table. The letter f indicates a figure. If more than one table or figure appears on a particular page, the exact item number for the table or figure being referenced is provided.

A

A2M-2 gene, 120
Abdominal examination, 55
Abortion, 72
Accidents, as cause of death, 29–30
Acetylcholine, 118, 121–122
Achieving the Promise: Transforming Mental Health Care in America (President's New Freedom Commission on Mental Health), 45
Acikel, Sadik, 11
ACIP (Advisory Committee on Immunization Practices), 136–137
ACMG (American College of Medical Genetics), 66
Acquired immunodeficiency syndrome. *See* Human immunodeficiency virus/ acquired immunodeficiency syndrome
ACS. *See* American Cancer Society
Activity
    limitation of, caused by chronic health conditions among older adults, by age, 109(*f*5.11)
    limitation of, caused by chronic health conditions among working-age adults, by age, 109(*f*5.10)
    limited by arthritis, 112
    limited by asthma, 102
    limited by chronic diseases, 108–109
Acupuncture, 184
"Acupuncture for Posttraumatic Stress Disorder: A Randomized Controlled Pilot Trial" (Hollifield), 184
"Acute and Chronic Otitis Media" (Morris & Leach), 127

"Acute Postoperative Pain Management Using Massage as an Adjuvant Therapy: A Randomized Trial" (Mitchinson et al.), 189
Acute Stroke Management (Jauch et al.), 89
AD. *See* Alzheimer's disease
ADD (attention deficit disorder), 163–164
ADDL (amyloid-beta-derived diffusible ligand), 121
ADDM: Autism and Developmental Disabilities Monitoring Network (CDC), 155
Addresses/names, of organizations, 193–194
ADHD. *See* Attention deficit hyperactivity disorder
Adolescents
    with ADD/ADHD, 163–164
    anxiety among, 162–163
    bipolar disorder and, 159–160
    birthrates among, 6
    depression and, 159
    diabetes in, 43
    with disruptive disorders, 164–165
    eating disorders among, 165
    immunization schedule, recommended childhood/adolescent, by vaccine/age, 36*f*
    mental health, adolescent intervention programs, 45–46, 46(*t*2.7)
    with mental health disorders, 60
    mental illness among, 152
    screening for depression, 40
    suicide prevention, 46–47
    who had depressive episode, 153(*f*8.3)
    See also Youth violence prevention
Adults
    with ADD/ADHD, 163
    genetic testing in, 70–71
    with psychological distress in past 30 days, 153(*f*8.4)

    with psychological distress in past 30 days, by age group/sex, 154(*f*8.5)
    with psychological distress in past 30 days, by race/ethnicity, 154(*f*8.6)
    psychological distress of, 152–154
Advisory Committee on Immunization Practices (ACIP), 136–137
"Aerobic Capacity, Strength, Flexibility, and Activity Level in Unimpaired Extremely Low Birth Weight (≤800 g) Survivors at 17 Years of Age Compared with Term-Born Control Subjects" (Rogers), 14–15
African-Americans
    asthma among, 102
    cancer and, 92
    heart disease and, 82
    hypertension and, 90
    males, life expectancy of, 19
    SCD risk of, 75
Age
    activity, limitation of, caused by chronic health conditions among older adults, by age, 109(*f*5.11)
    activity, limitation of, caused by chronic health conditions among working-age adults, by age, 109(*f*5.10)
    Alzheimer's disease and, 119
    asthma and, 102
    CAM use by, 176, 177(*f*9.3)
    cancer and, 90
    death rates for cancer by sex, age, ethnicity, race, 95*t*–99*t*
    diabetes prevalence and, 104, 108(*f*5.8)
    flu vaccinations for older adults, 134–135
    heart disease in women and, 84–85
    as heart disease risk factor, 82
    mammogram use and, 92
    osteoporosis and, 114
    Pap test and, 42, 94*t*
    Parkinson's disease and, 118

physical activity and, 83
prostate cancer and, 101–102
YPPL and, 23, 29–30
Agency for Healthcare Research and Quality, 89–90
Agoraphobia, 161–162
AHA. *See* American Heart Association
Ahmed, Shahana, 64–65
AIDS. *See* Human immunodeficiency virus/acquired immunodeficiency syndrome
AIDS Epidemic Update 2009 (Joint United Nations Programme on HIV/AIDS and WHO), 141
AIDS-defining events, 143
AIM (awareness, intervention, and methodology), 46, 46(*t*2.8)
Air Force Suicide Prevention Program, 48–49
Air pollutants
asthma from, 102, 103
chronic bronchitis from, 104
Akdemir, Ramazan, 11
Alcohol, 91
Alleles, 63–64
Allen, Karen, 50
Allergens, 102–103
Alpha-1-antitrypsin deficiency, 73
"Alpha-2 Macroglobulin Is Genetically Associated with Alzheimer Disease" (Blacker et al.), 120
Alternative medicine
acupuncture, 184
Ayurvedic medicine, 184–185
definition of, 175
homeopathic medicine, 183
naturopathic medicine, 183–184
overview of, 182–183
traditional Chinese medicine, 185
See also Complementary and alternative medicine
Alzheimer, Alois, 119–120
Alzheimer's Association
contact information, 193
on number of Americans with AD, 119
Alzheimer's disease (AD)
causes of, symptoms of, 120
description of, 119–120
impact on caregivers' health/well-being, 122–123
testing/treatments for, 121–122
American Academy of Child and Adolescent Psychiatry, 164, 193
American Academy of Pediatrics, 70–71, 193
American Association of Suicidology, 193
American Cancer Society (ACS)
on breast cancer, 100–101
breast/cervical cancers, screening/early detection of, 40–41
on cancer incidence, 90

cervical cancer screening guidelines and, 42
on colon/rectal cancer, 93–94
contact information, 193
on prostate cancer, 101–102
on warning signs of cancer, 92
"The American Cancer Society Great American Health Check" (ACS), 92
"American Cancer Society Responds to Changes to USPSTF Mammography Guidelines" (ACS), 40
American Chiropractic Association, 190, 193
American College of Medical Genetics (ACMG), 66
American College of Obstetrics and Gynecologists, 41–42, 193
American College of Radiology/American Roentgen Ray Society, 40
American College of Surgeons Oncology Group, 100
American Diabetes Association, 193
American Heart Association (AHA)
contact information, 193
on heart attack warning signals, 79
on stroke, 88
on women and heart disease, 84
American Lung Association, 103, 193
American Medical Association, 56
American Parkinson Disease Association, 193
American Psychiatric Association (APA)
contact information, 193
DSM-IV, 59–60, 155, 156
American Psychological Association, 193
"America's Children: Key National Indicators of Well-Being, 2009" (Federal Interagency Forum on Child and Family Statistics), 163
Amir, Nader, 162
Amniocentesis
description of, 59
for Huntington's disease diagnosis, 74
prenatal diagnostics with, 69
AMP (Attention Modification Program), 162
Amputation, 44
Amyloid plaques, 120
Amyloid protein, 120
Amyloid-beta-derived diffusible ligand (ADDL), 121
Anabolic agents, 115
Anencephaly, 16, 59
"Anencephaly" (NIH), 16
Angina pectoris, 79
Angioplasty, 81
Animals, health benefits of, 50
Annual physicals, value of, 56
Anorexia nervosa, 165–166
Anthrax, 148–149
Antibiotics
educating physicians/patients about use of, 129, 132

resistant strains of bacteria and, 126–128
Anticonvulsant drugs, 160
"Antidepressant Drug Effects and Depression Severity" (Fournier), 158
Antidepressants
side effects of, 158*t*
for treatment of depression, 157–158
Anti-inflammatory drugs, 122
Antipsychotic drugs, 160
Antiresorptive agents, 115
Antiretroviral drugs, 143–145
Anxiety
naturopathic medicine for, 184
Reiki to reduce, 191
Anxiety disorders
agoraphobia, 161–162
among children/adolescents, 162–163
drugs used to treat, 168(*t*8.4)
obsessive-compulsive disorder, 162
overview of, 160–161
panic disorder, 161
phobia treatment programs, 162
phobias, 161
types of, 155
APA. *See* American Psychiatric Association
"APOE Genotype Predicts When—Not Whether—One Is Predisposed to Develop Alzheimer Disease" (Meyer et al.), 120
Apolipoprotein E (apoE), 120
Applied kinesiology, 190
Aromatase inhibitors, 101
Arthritis
drug treatment, setbacks in, 113–114
prevalence of, 112, 112*t*
research, 112–113
SLE, 111–112
types of, 111
Arthritis Foundation
on arthritis prevalence, 112
contact information, 193
on types of arthritis, 111
Arthritis: Meeting the Challenge—At a Glance 2009 (CDC), 112
"Arthritis Related Statistics" (National Center for Chronic Disease Prevention), 112
ASDs. *See* Autism spectrum disorders
Ashkenazi descent, 77
"Asian flu," 135
Asperger, Hans, 156
Asperger's disorder, 156
Assessment interview, 59
"Association of Autism with Polymorphisms in the Paired-Like Homeodomain Transcription Factor 1 (*PITX1*) on Chromosome 5q31: A Candidate Gene Analysis" (Philippi), 156
Asthma
causes of, 102–103

prevalence of current, among persons of all ages, by age group, race/ethnicity, 103(ƒ5.5)

prevalence of current, among persons of all ages, by age group, sex, 103(ƒ5.6)

Attention deficit disorder (ADD), 163–164

Attention deficit hyperactivity disorder (ADHD)
in children/adolescents, 60
drugs used to treat, 168(t8.3)
overview of, 163–164

Attention Modification Program (AMP), 162

"Attention Training in Individuals with Generalized Social Phobia: A Randomized Controlled Trial" (Amir), 162

Atypical autism, 156

Auscultation, 54

Autism and Developmental Disabilities Monitoring (ADDM) Network, 155

Autism Society of America, 193

Autism spectrum disorders (ASDs)
Asperger's disorder, 156
changes in prevalence, 156ƒ
overview of, 155–156
Rett's disorder, 156–157

Autonomic nerves, 55ƒ, 56

Autopsy, 121

Avian influenza, 135–136

Awareness, intervention, and methodology (AIM), 46, 46(t2.8)

Ayanian, John Z., 56

Ayurvedic medicine, 184–185

Azidothymidine, 143

Aztreonam, 73

Aztreonam for Inhalation Solution (NDA 50-814) for Improvement of Respiratory Symptoms in Cystic Fibrosis Patients (FDA), 73

B

B gene, 114–115

Back, 55

Back to Sleep campaign, 18

"Backgrounder" (NCCAM), 190

Bacteria, resistant strains of, 126–129, 132

Balci, Mustafa Mucahit, 11

Balloon angioplasty, 80

Barker, Sandra B., 50

Barnard, Christiaan, 81–82

Barnes, Joanne, 189

Becker, Dorothy, 107

Beidel, Deborah C., 162

"Beliefs about Eating and Eating Disorders" (Wilson), 165

Belik, Shay-Lee, 47–48

Bellamy, Richard, 149

"The Benefits of Human-Companion Animal Interaction: A Review" (Barker & Wolen), 50

Benign tumors, 90

Benson, Herbert, 186

The Best Alternative Medicine (Pelletier), 185, 188

Best Practices of Youth Violence Prevention: A Sourcebook for Community Action (Thornton et al.), 37–38

Beta-amyloid protein, 121, 122

Beta-secretase, 122

Bextra, 113

"Big Win for Merck in Vioxx 2" (Smith), 114

Bio-barcode assay, 121

Biofeedback, 186

Biologic terrorism, 148–149

Biological markers, 40, 121

Biologically based therapies
description of, 182
dietary supplements, 186–189, 188t

Biopsy
for cervical/breast cancer, 43
sentinel lymph node biopsy, 100

Bipolar disorder, 159–160

Birmingham, Wendy, 49

Birth defects, 15–17

"Birth Defects" (CDC), 15

Birth Defects and Development Disabilities Prevention Act, 17

Birth Defects Prevention Act, 17

"Birth Weight and the Risk of Testicular Cancer: A Meta-Analysis" (Michos, Xue, & Michels), 14

"Birth Weight as a Risk Factor for Breast Cancer: A Meta-Analysis of 18 Epidemiological Studies" (Xu), 11, 14

Birthrates
fertility rate vs., 2
by mother's age/race/Hispanic origin 1950–2006, 3t–6t
by mother's age/race/Hispanic origin 1970–2005, 8t
U.S., 2, 6

Births
birth weight effects on disease risk, 11, 14–17
live in U.S., 2
prenatal care/prematurity/LBW, 6–8, 11
U.S. birthrates, 2, 6

"Births: Final Data for 2006" (Martin), 2

Bittner, Daniel M., 122

Black, Sandra E., 122

Blacker, Deborah, 120

Blascovich, Jim, 50

Blood cholesterol, 44

"Blood Folate Levels: The Latest NHANES Results" (McDowell), 17

Blood glucose
diabetes prevention and, 43–44
in diabetics, 104
fasting blood glucose test, 57

heart disease and, 84
See also Diabetes

Blood pressure
high blood pressure in adults age 20/ older, 83t–84t
marriage and, 49
measurement of in physical exam, 54
screening for hypertension, 39
See also High blood pressure

Blood tests, 59

Blood thinners, 88

Bones
arthritis and, 111
bone marrow transplant, 76
osteoporosis, 114–116, 115t
x-ray to measure bone density, 58

Bradley, Ryan, 184

Brain
Alzheimer's disease and, 119–123
Parkinson's disease and, 118–119
stroke and, 86 89

Branson, Richard A., 181

BRCA1 gene, 100–101

BRCA2 gene, 100–101

Breast and Cervical Cancer Mortality Prevention Act, 42

Breast cancer
breast exam for, 55, 58
CAM therapies for, 178
chemoprevention for, 70
deaths from, 86
genetic research on, 100–101
incidence of, 94
NBCCEDP, number of women served in, 42ƒ
recommended screening for, 41t
screening and early detection of, 40–43
screening guidelines for, 40, 92
treatment of, 100

Breast Cancer Facts and Figures 2009–2010 (American Cancer Society), 40–41

Bronchitis, chronic, 103–104

Bulik, Cynthia M., 166

Bulimia nervosa, 166

Bush, George W., 119

Butte, Nancy F., 15

Bypass surgery, 80–81

C

CABG (coronary artery bypass graft) surgery, 80–81

Calcium, 57, 115

CAM. See Complementary and alternative medicine

Cambodia, avian influenza in, 135

Cameron, Melainie, 185

Campo, Julián, 143

"Can a Costly Intervention Be Cost-Effective?: An Analysis of Violence Prevention" (Foster), 165

"Can a Nationwide Media Campaign Affect Antibiotic Use?" (Hemo et al.), 129, 132

"Canadian Alzheimer's Disease Caregiver Survey: Baby-Boomer Caregivers and Burden of Care" (Black et al.), 122

Cancer
    African-Americans and, 92
    breast cancer, 94, 100–101
    breast cancer, recommended screening for, 41*t*
    breast/cervical cancers, screening/early detection of, 40–43
    CAM use for, 178
    causes, who gets, who survives, 90–91
    colon/rectal cancer, 93–94
    death rates for cancer by sex, age, ethnicity, race, 95*t*–99*t*
    death rates for leading causes of death for all ages, 89*f*
    gender and, 92
    genetic inheritance and, 72
    lung cancer, 92–93
    mammography use by selected age groups, 93*t*
    National Breast and Cervical Cancer Early Detection Program, number of women served in, 42*f*
    overview of, 90
    Pap smear use by selected age groups, 94*t*
    prostate cancer, 101–102
    skin cancer, 101
    warning signs of, 92

Cancer Facts and Figures, 2009 (American Cancer Society)
    on African-Americans and cancer, 92
    on breast cancer treatment, 100
    on cancer incidence, 90
    on prostate cancer, 101–102
    on skin cancer, 101

Cancer Incidence and Mortality Rates— United States, 2004 (National Cancer Institute), 101

Capillary refill time, 55

Carboon, Isla, 178

Cardiovascular diseases
    bypass surgery, 80–81
    catheter-based interventions, 81–82
    cigarette smoking among men, women, high school students, and mothers during pregnancy, 82*f*
    death rates for leading causes of death for all ages, 89*f*
    health conditions/risk factors, 87*t*
    heart attack, angina pectoris, 79–80
    high blood pressure, 89–90
    high blood pressure in adults age 20/ older, 83*t*–84*t*
    high cholesterol levels in adults age 20/ older, 85*t*–86*t*
    obesity, prevalence of, among adults aged 20 years/older, 88*f*
    overview of, 79
    risk factors for heart disease, 82–84
    stroke, 86–89
    treatments for heart disease, 80
    women and heart disease, 84–86

"Cardiovascular Reactivity and the Presence of Pets, Friends, and Spouses: The Truth about Cats and Dogs" (Allen, Blascovich, & Mendes), 50

Cardiovascular system, physical exam of, 55

Caregivers, 122–123

Carrier identification, 68

Catheter-based interventions, 81–82

Causes
    of Alzheimer's disease, 120
    of multiple sclerosis, 117
    of youth violence, 37
    See also Risk factors

"Causes of Cancer in the World: Comparative Risk Assessment of Nine Behavioral and Environmental Risk Factors" (Danaei et al.), 91

CBT. *See* Cognitive behavioral therapy

CD (conduct disorder), 164–165

CDC. *See* Centers for Disease Control and Prevention

Celebrex, 113–114

Celecoxib, 113–114

Center for Reiki Research, 191

Centers for Disease Control and Prevention (CDC)
    ADDM Network, 155
    on antibiotic resistance, 129
    antibiotic resistance campaign of, 129
    on arthritis, 112
    on asthma, 102
    on birth defects, 15
    on chronic diseases, 79
    on cigarette smoking, 82, 82*f*
    contact information, 193
    on Down syndrome, 69
    H1N1 flu and, 136–138
    on HIV/AIDS, 141–143
    on immunizations, 132–134
    on infectious diseases, notifiable, 125–126, 126*t*
    on life expectancy, 19
    on Lyme disease, 145, 146
    on MRSA, 129
    on muscular dystrophy, 74
    on pandemic influenza, 135
    on physical exercise, 83
    on Prevention Research Centers, 49
    on SARS, 146–148
    on screening for colorectal cancer, 94
    on sickle cell disease, 75
    on SLE, 111–112
    on stroke, 88
    on suicide, 173
    on suicide prevention, 47
    on tuberculosis, 139–141
    on youth violence prevention, 37–38

Central nerves, 55*f*, 56

"Cerebrospinal Fluid Biomarker Signature in Alzheimer's Disease Neuroimaging Initiative Subjects" (Shaw et al.), 121

Cerebrovascular disease. *See* Stroke (cerebrovascular disease)

Cervical cancer
    cases of, deaths from, 41
    from HPV, 91
    NBCCEDP, number of women served in, 42*f*
    Pap smear use by selected age groups, 94*t*
    pelvic exam for, 55
    screening guidelines for, 41–43

CF (cystic fibrosis), 70, 73

Chandler, Carrol H., 48

"Changing the Way Diabetes Is Treated" (National Diabetes Education Program), 44

Chemoprevention, 70

Chemotherapy
    acupuncture to reduce nausea, 184
    for breast cancer, 100, 101
    for colorectal cancer, 94
    for prostate cancer, 102

Chest, physical examination of, 54–55

Chicken pox (varicella), 125, 134

Children
    with ADD/ADHD, 163–164
    anxiety among, 162–163
    arthritis in, 112
    asthma in, 102
    with bipolar disorder, 159–160
    CAM, diseases/conditions for which children use, 182(*f*9.11)
    CAM therapies used by children, ten most common, 181(*f*9.9)
    CAM use by, 177
    CAM use by, based on CAM use by parents or relatives, 181(*f*9.8)
    cancer survivors, 91
    deaths, causes of, 23, 29
    deaths from cancer, 90
    depression and, 159
    diabesity, double diabetes in, 107–108
    with disruptive disorders, 164–165
    with emotional/behavioral difficulties, 152(*f*8.2)
    flu vaccine, response to, 134
    genetic testing in, 70–71
    immunization schedule, recommended childhood/adolescent, by vaccine/age, 36*f*
    with mental health disorders, 60

mental illness among, numbers of, 152

natural products used by, 182(*f*9.10)

psychoactive medication, prescribing for, 167–168

Type 1 diabetes mellitus prevention, 43

Chinese medicine

    acupuncture, 184

    traditional, 185

Chiropractic, 181, 190

Chlamydia, 125

Cholesterol

    high cholesterol levels in adults age 20/older, 85*t*–86*t*

    as risk factor for heart disease, 82–83

Cholinesterase inhibitors, 121–122

Chondroitin, 189

Chorea, 73

Chorionic villus sampling (CVS)

    description of, 58–59

    for Huntington's disease diagnosis, 74

    prenatal diagnostics with, 69

Chow, Vivian W., 122

Christine, C. W., 119

Chromosomal disorders, 64–65

Chromosome 21, 6, 69

Chronic bronchitis, 103–104

Chronic diseases

    activity, limitation of, caused by chronic health conditions among older adults, by age, 109(*f*5.11)

    activity, limitation of, caused by chronic health conditions among working-age adults, by age, 109(*f*5.10)

    asthma, prevalence of current, among persons of all ages, by age group, race/ethnicity, 103(*f*5.5)

    asthma, prevalence of current, among persons of all ages, by age group, sex, 103(*f*5.6)

    cancer, 90–94, 100–102

    cardiovascular diseases, 79–90

    cigarette smoking among men, women, high school students, and mothers during pregnancy, 82*f*

    death, ten leading causes of/death rates of, 80*f*

    death rates for cancer by sex, age, ethnicity, race, 95*t*–99*t*

    death rates for leading causes of death for all ages, 89*f*

    diabetes, 104108

    diabetes, prevalence of diagnosed, among adults aged 18 years/over, 107*f*

    diabetes, prevalence of diagnosed, among adults aged 18 years/over, by age group, sex, 108(*f*5.8)

    diabetes, prevalence of diagnosed, among adults aged 18 years/over, by race/ethnicity, 108(*f*5.9)

    health conditions/risk factors, 87*t*

high blood pressure in adults age 20/older, 83*t*–84*t*

high cholesterol levels in adults age 20/older, 85*t*–86*t*

limit activity, 108–109

mammography use by selected age groups, 93*t*

obesity, prevalence of among adults aged 20 years/older, 88*f*

Pap smear use by selected age groups, 94*t*

primary prevention of, 37

respiratory diseases, frequency of, among persons 18/older, 105*t*–106*t*

respiratory diseases, lung health, 102–104

"Chronic Diseases and Health Promotion" (CDC), 79

Chronic fatiguing illnesses, 179

Chronic obstructive pulmonary disease (COPD), 103–104

Cigarette smoking. *See* Tobacco

Clinical trial, 100

Clinton, Bill, 17

Cognitive behavioral therapy (CBT)

    description of, 158

    in treatment of eating disorders, 166

    in treatment of panic disorder, 161

    in treatment of phobias, 162

Collins, Francis S., 119

Colon cancer, 93–94

Colonoscopy, 58

"Colorectal Cancer Control Program (CRCCP)" (CDC), 94

Columbia University, TeenScreen program, 45–46, 46(*t*2.7)

Communicable diseases, 39

"Complementary and Alternative Medical Therapy Utilization by People with Chronic Fatiguing Illnesses in the United States" (Jones et al.), 179

Complementary and alternative medicine (CAM)

    acupuncture, 184

    Ayurvedic medicine, 184–185

    biologically based therapies, 186–189

    children using CAM, based on use by parents or relatives, 181(*f*9.8)

    children's use of, 177

    dietary supplements, information about, 188*t*

    diseases/conditions for which adults use, 180*f*

    diseases/conditions for which children use CAM, 182(*f*9.11)

    energy therapies, 190–191

    hierarchy of evidence, 176(*f*9.1)

    homeopathic medicine, 183

    manipulative therapies, body-based methods, 189–190

    meditation, types of populations/conditions included in studies on, 187*t*–188*t*

mind-body interventions, 185–186

natural products used by adults, ten most common, 179*f*

natural products used by children, ten most common, 182(*f*9.10)

naturopathic medicine, 183–184

overview of, 175

people who use, 178–181

popularity of, 175–177

reasons people turn to, 177–178

therapies used by adults, ten most common, 178*f*

therapies used by children, ten most common, 181(*f*9.9)

traditional Chinese medicine, 185

types of, 182–183

use by age, 177(*f*9.3)

use by race/ethnicity, 177(*f*9.4)

use in traditional medical settings, 181–182

use of, 176(*f*9.2)

Complementary and Alternative Medicine in the United States (Institute of Medicine), 181

"Complementary and Alternative Medicine Use, Spending, and Quality of Life in Early Stage Breast Cancer" (Wyatt et al.), 178

Complementary and Alternative Medicine Use among Adults and Children: United States, 2007 (NCCAM), 176

"Complementary and Alternative Medicine Use among US Navy and Marine Corps Personnel" (Smith et al.), 179–180

"Complementary and Alternative Medicine Use for Treatment and Prevention of Late-Life Mood and Cognitive Disorders" (Lavretsky), 181

Complementary medicine, 175

"Composition of Gestational Weight Gain Impacts Maternal Fat Retention and Infant Birth Weight" (Butte), 15

Computed tomography (CT) scan, 58

COMT inhibitors, 118

Conduct disorder (CD), 164–165

"Conduct Disorders" (American Academy of Child and Adolescent Psychiatry), 164

Contact information, 193–194

Contagious diseases. *See* Infectious diseases

"The Contribution of Human Synovial Stem Cells to Skeletal Muscle Regeneration" (Meng), 74

Cooley, Kieran, 184

COPD (chronic obstructive pulmonary disease), 103–104

Corbett, Elizabeth L., 139

Coriolanus (Shakespeare), 125

Cornwell, Erin York, 50

Coronary artery bypass graft (CABG) surgery, 80–81

Couillard, Philippe, 88–89

Counseling, 48

COX-2 inhibitors, 113–114
Cranial nerves
    description of, 56
    nervous system diagram, 55*f*
Crude birth rates
    by mother's age/race/Hispanic origin 1950–2006, 3*t*–6*t*
    by mother's age/race/Hispanic origin 1970–2005, 8*t*
    trends in, 2
CT (computed tomography) scan, 58
"Current SARS Situation" (CDC), 147–148
Cutler, David M., 19
CVS. *See* Chorionic villus sampling
Cystic fibrosis (CF), 70, 73
Cystic Fibrosis Foundation, 193

D

Danaei, Goodarz, 91
Dardarin, 118
"Data and Statistics" (CDC), 139
Dating violence, prevention of, 38
Death rates. *See* Mortality rates
Death with Dignity Act (Oregon), 174
Deaths
    from Alzheimer's disease, 119
    from breast/cervical cancers, 41
    from cancer, 90, 92
    from cardiovascular diseases, 79
    causes/numbers of by sex/race/Hispanic origin, 20*t*–23*t*
    from colon/rectal cancer, 93
    from COPD, 103
    from diabetes, 108
    from diabetes/heart disease, 84
    from H1N1 flu, 136*f*, 138
    from HIV/AIDS, 142, 145
    from infectious diseases, 125
    leading causes/numbers of, by age, 29*t*–30*t*
    leading causes of/death rates of, 80*f*
    from pandemic influenzas, 135
    from skin cancer, 101
    from stroke, 88
    from tuberculosis, 139
    YPLL before age 75 by sex/race, 24*t*–28*t*
Deaths: Final Data for 2006 (NCHS), 119
Degenerative diseases
    Alzheimer's disease, 119–123
    arthritis, 111–114, 112*t*
    multiple sclerosis, 116–117
    osteoporosis, 114–116
    osteoporosis, causes of bone loss/ fractures in, 115*f*
    osteoporosis pyramid for prevention/ treatment, 116*f*
    Parkinson's disease, 117–119
DeLeo, Frank R., 129
Dental disease, 44

Deoxyribonucleic acid. *See* DNA
Depression
    causes of, 157
    children with, 159
    defining, 157
    mind-body interventions and, 185
    percent of population suffering from, 155
    screening guidelines for, 40
    suicide and, 174
    symptoms of, 157*t*
    treatment of, 157–158
Depression (NIMH), 158
"Depression Care in the United States: Too Little for Too Few" (González), 154–155
"Developmental Defects and Childhood Cancer" (Slavin & Wiesner), 71
Developmental disorders, 155–157
Di Mario, Carlo, 81
Diabesity, 106–107
Diabesity: The Obesity-Diabetes Epidemic That Threatens America—And What We Must Do to Stop It (Kaufman), 107
Diabetes
    causes of, 105–106
    deaths from, 108
    diabesity, double diabetes, 106–108
    fasting blood glucose test, 57
    heart disease and, 84
    naturopathic medicine and, 184
    obesity and, 19
    prevalence of, 104
    prevalence of diagnosed, among adults aged 18 years/over, 107*f*
    prevalence of diagnosed, among adults aged 18 years/over, by age group, sex, 108(*f*5.8)
    prevalence of diagnosed, among adults aged 18 years/over, by race/ethnicity, 108(*f*5.9)
    tertiary prevention of, 43–44
    warning signs of, 104
Diabetic ketoacidosis, 44
Diabetic neuropathy, 43, 44
Diabetic retinopathy, 43, 44
Diagnosis of disease
    Alzheimer's disease, 121
    definition of diagnosis, 53
    diagnostic testing, 56–59
    lung cancer, 93
    medical histories, 53–54
    mental illness, 59–61
    multiple sclerosis, 117
    nervous system, 55*f*
    physical examination, 54–56
Diagnostic and Statistical Manual of Mental Disorders (DSM-IV) (American Psychiatric Association)
    on Asperger's disorder, 156
    criteria for mental illness, 59–60

    on mental disorders, 155
Diagnostic testing
    for Alzheimer's disease, 121
    CVS, 69
    description of, 56
    for diabetes, 104
    for diagnosis of disease, 56–59
    diagnostic imaging techniques, 57–58
    diagnostic procedures, 58
    genetic testing, 65
    laboratory tests, 57
    for multiple sclerosis, 117
    PGD, 68
    prenatal, 58–59
    reliability/validity of, 56–57
Diastolic blood pressure, 54
Diet
    for hypertension control, 90
    naturopathic medicine and, 184
    for osteoporosis, 114, 115
    as risk factor for cancer, 91
Dietary Supplement Health and Education Act of 1994, 188
Dietary supplements
    CAM beliefs about, 186–188
    effectiveness of, 188–189
    information about, 188*t*
Dieting, 165
"The Difference between Latent TB Infection and Active TB Disease" (CDC), 139
Diphtheria, 132
Disability, 112
Disease
    birth weight influences on risk of, 11, 14–15
    CAM, diseases/conditions for which adults use, 180*f*
    CAM, diseases/conditions for which children use, 182(*f*9.11)
    genetic testing for, 65
    inherited diseases, 72–77
    See also Chronic diseases; Diagnosis of disease; Infectious diseases; Prevention of disease
Disease-modifying antirheumatic drugs (DMARDs), 113
Disorders, genetic, 64–65
Disruptive disorders, 164–165
"The Dissolution of the Oedipus Complex" (Freud), 63
DMARDs (disease-modifying antirheumatic drugs), 113
DMD (Duchenne muscular dystrophy), 68, 74
DNA (deoxyribonucleic acid)
    arthritis and, 113
    description of, 63
    gene tests, 66*t*
    See also Genetics

Dominant genes, 64

Donegan, Sarah, 149

Donepezil, 122

Donnelly, John, 47

Dopamine, 118, 160

A Dose of Sanity: Mind, Medicine, and Misdiagnosis (Walker), 53

Doshas, 185

Double diabetes, 107–108

"Double Diabetes: A Mixture of Type 1 and Type 2 Diabetes in Youth" (Pozzilli & Guglielmi), 107–108

Double-contrast barium enema, 94

Down syndrome
    prevalence of, 69(t4.3)
    testing for, 69

"Down Syndrome Cases at Birth Increased" (CDC), 69

Drugli, May B., 165

Drugs
    for ADHD, 168(t8.3)
    for AIDS, 143–145
    for Alzheimer's disease, 121–122
    anticonvulsants, 160
    antipsychotics, 160
    for anxiety disorders, 168(t8.4)
    for arthritis, 113–114
    for avian influenza, 135
    for breast cancer, 101
    for H1N1 flu, 138
    lithium, 160
    for MS treatment, 117
    for osteoporosis treatment, 115
    for Parkinson's disease, 118
    for phobias, 162
    psychoactive, prescribing to children, 167–168
    for SLE treatment, 112
    for stroke treatment, 88

Duchenne muscular dystrophy (DMD), 68, 74

"Dynamic Mapping of Cortical Development before and after the Onset of Pediatric Bipolar Illness" (Gogtay), 159

Dysthymic disorder (dysthymia), 157, 159

E

Early Release of Selected Estimates Based on Data from the January–June 2009 National Health Interview Survey (NCHS), 84

"Eating Behavior among Women with Anorexia Nervosa" (Sysko), 167

Eating disorders
    anorexia nervosa, 165–166
    bulimia nervosa, 166
    treatment of, 166–167

Eating Disorders (NIMH), 165

Eating Disorders Coalition for Research, Policy, and Action, 167

Echinacea
    effectiveness of, 177, 189
    use of by adults, 176

"Echinacea for Preventing and Treating the Common Cold" (Linde et al.), 189

"Echinacea Species (Echinacea Angustifolia (DC.) Hell., Echinacea Pallida (Nutt.) Nutt., Echinacea Purpurea (L.) Moench): A Review of Their Chemistry, Pharmacology and Clinical Properties" (Barnes et al.), 189

ECT (electroconvulsive therapy), 158

Education
    on antibiotics use, 129, 132
    on diabetes, 44
    for health promotion, 35

"The Effect of Glucosamine and/or Chondroitin Sulfate on the Progression of Knee Osteoarthritis: A Report from the Glucosamine/Chondroitin Arthritis Intervention Trial" (Sawitzke et al.), 189

"Effectiveness of Influenza Vaccine in the Community-Dwelling Elderly" (Nichol et al.), 135

"Effects of Percutaneous Coronary Interventions in Silent Ischemia after Myocardial Infarction" (Erne et al.), 81

"Eight-Year Experience with Minimally Invasive Cardiothoracic Surgery" (Iribarne et al.), 81

Electrocardiogram, 58

Electroconvulsive therapy (ECT), 158

Electrode implants, 119

"Eliminate Disparities in Lupus" (CDC), 111–112

ELISA (enzyme-linked immunosorbent assay) test, 57

"Emerging Infectious Diseases: A 10-Year Perspective from the National Institute of Allergy and Infectious Diseases" (Fauci et al.), 145

Emotional wellness, 1

Emphysema, 104

Employment, 49

Enema, double-contrast barium, 94

Energy therapies
    description of, 182
    Reiki, 190–191

Environmental Protection Agency, 93

Enzyme-linked immunosorbent assay (ELISA) test, 57

Epidemic, of influenza, 134

Epidemiologist, 2

"Epidemiology of Treatment Failure: A Focus on Recent Trends" (Hull et al.), 145

Epilepsy Foundation, 193

Erasmus, Desiderius, 35

Erne, Paul, 81

Estrogen, 101

"Ethical and Policy Issues in Newborn Screening" (Ross), 71

Ethics, 71–72

Evaluation, of prevention program, 38

"Evidence from the Cochrane Collaboration for Traditional Chinese Medicine Therapies" (Manheimer et al.), 184

Evidence, hierarchy of, 175, 176(f9.1)

"Evidence of Effectiveness of Herbal Medicinal Products in the Treatment of Arthritis. Part 2: Rheumatoid Arthritis" (Cameron et al.), 185

Examination. *See* Physical examination

Exercise
    heart disease and, 83–84
    for osteoporosis treatment, 115, 116
    See also Activity

"Exercise Effects on Bone Mineral Density: Relationships to Change in Fitness and Fatness" (Stewart et al.), 116

Extrapulmonary TB, 139

Eye examination, 54

F

Fagerlin, Angela, 70

False-negative/false-positive results, 57

Family systems therapy, 167

Family-based therapy, 167

"Fast Facts on Osteoporosis" (National Osteoporosis Foundation), 114

Fasting blood glucose test, 57, 104

Fauci, Anthony S., 145, 148–149

FDA. *See* U.S. Food and Drug Administration

Federal Interagency Forum on Child and Family Statistics, 163

Females
    arthritis among, 111
    breast cancer screening guidelines, 40
    breast/cervical cancers, screening/early detection of, 40–43
    breast/pelvic examination, 55
    eating disorders among, 165
    heart disease and, 84–86
    mammogram/Pap test for, 92
    multiple sclerosis and, 117
    osteoporosis and, 114, 116
    Pap smear use by selected age groups, 94t
    relationships, health connection for, 49
    suicide rates among, 173
    unmarried, birth rates of, 2, 6
    See also Births; Pregnancy

Fertility rates
    birth rate *vs.*, 2
    by mother's age/race/Hispanic origin 1950–2006, 3t–6t
    by mother's age/race/Hispanic origin 1970–2005, 8t
    in U.S., 2, 6

Fetus, 58–59

Fibromyalgia, 111

"Finding Alzheimer's before a Mind Fails" (Grady), 121

Fish oil/omega 3, 176

Fitzpatrick, Tanya R., 49

"Five- to Six-Year Outcome and Its Prediction for Children with ODD/CD Treated with Parent Training" (Drugli), 165

Flexible sigmoidoscopy test, 58, 94

Flu. *See* Influenza

Flynn, Laurie, 46

Folic acid, 16–17

"Folic Acid" (March of Dimes), 17

Food. *See* Diet

"Forecasting the Effects of Obesity and Smoking on U.S. Life Expectancy" (Stewart, Cutler, & Rosen), 19

Foster, E. Michael, 165

Foster, James, 183

Fournier, Jay C., 158

Fox, Maggie, 135

Fox, Nick C., 121

Fractures, 114, 115*t*

Frank, Samuel, 74

Freitag, Christine M., 156

"Frequently Asked Questions about SARS" (CDC), 146

Freud, Sigmund, 63

Frieden, Thomas R., 1

Friedmann, Erika, 50

Frye, Cheryl A., 49

Furlan, Andrea, 189–190

G

Galantamine, 122

Gallant, Joel E., 145

Gamble, Carrol L., 149

Gamma-secretase, 122

GDNF (glial cell line–derived neurotrophic factor), 118–119

Gender

arthritis and, 111–112

asthma and, 102

cancer and, 92

death rates for cancer by sex, age, ethnicity, race, 95*t*–99*t*

diabetes and, 104, 108(*f*5.8)

heart disease and, 82, 84–86

HIV/AIDS and, 142

mental health disorders and, 60

multiple sclerosis and, 117

osteoporosis and, 114

relationships and health by, 49

YPPL and, 23

Gene therapy, 118–119

Genes

associated with autism, 156

as cause of ADHD, 163

"Genes and Human Disease: Monogenic Diseases" (WHO), 75

"Genetic Conditions: Cystic Fibrosis" (Genetics Home Reference), 73

"Genetic Conditions: Huntington Disease" (Genetics Home Reference), 73

"Genetic Disease Testing Leads Some Adults Not to Have Kids" (Marchione), 71

Genetic Information Nondiscrimination Act (GINA), 72

"Genetic Testing in Children and Young People" (Parker), 71

Genetics

Alzheimer's disease and, 120

breast cancer research, 100–101

DNA-based gene tests, 66*t*

Down syndrome, prevalence of, 69(*t*4.3)

genetic disorders, 64–65

genetic inheritance, 63–64

genetic testing, 65–66, 68

inherited diseases, 72–77

multiple sclerosis and, 117

newborn screening program, decision-making process for, 67*f*

osteoporosis and, 114–115

overview of, 63

Parkinson's disease and, 118

prenatal tests, 69(*t*4.2)

recessive disorder when both parents carry gene, chances of inheriting, 68*f*

sickle cell anemia, 75*f*

sickle cell trait, inheritance of, 76*f*

SLE and, 112

testing, ethical considerations, 71–72

testing and human reproduction, 68–69

testing in children/adults, 70–71

X-linked recessive inheritance, 65*f*

"Genetics" (U.S. Library of Medicine), 64

"Genetics: Breast Cancer as an Exemplar" (Hamilton), 71

Genetics Home Reference, 73

"The Genetics of Autistic Disorders and Its Clinical Relevance: A Review of the Literature" (Freitag), 156

"Genomewide Association Study for Onset Age in Parkinson Disease" (Latourelle), 118

"Genomic and Epigenetic Evidence for Oxytocin Receptor Deficiency in Autism" (Gregory), 156

Genomics, 63–64

Georganopoulou, Dimitra G., 121

Giardiasis, 126

Gillespie, Brenda W., 191

Gillespie, Elena A., 191

GINA (Genetic Information Nondiscrimination Act), 72

Ginger, 185

Ginkgo biloba, 176, 181, 185

Ginseng, 176, 185

Glatiramer acetate, 117

Glial cell line–derived neurotrophic factor (GDNF), 118–119

"The Global Burden of Cancer: Priorities for Prevention" (Thun), 91

Glucosamine

effectiveness of, 189

use of by adults, 176

Glucose, 43–44

See also Blood glucose

Goals

of *Healthy People 2020*, 50–51, 51*f*

of secondary prevention, 38–39

of youth violence prevention, 38(*t*2.3)

Goate, Alison, 120

Gogtay, Nitin, 159

Goldsmith, Sara K., 45

Gonorrhea, 125

González, Hector M., 155

Goodwin, Frederick K., 159

Gould, Madelyn S., 45–46

Gout, 111

Grady, Denise, 121

Graham, David J., 113

Gregory, Simon G., 156

Group therapy, 167

"The Growing Burden of Tuberculosis: Global Trends and Interactions with the HIV Epidemic" (Corbett et al.), 139

Guglielmi, Chiara, 107–108

Guillemot, Didier, 129

"Gulf War Servicemen and Servicewomen: The Long Road Home and the Role of Health Care Professionals to Enhance the Troops' Health and Healing" (McFee), 47

H

H1N1 influenza (swine flu)

flu activity by state, week ending January 2, 2010, 138*f*

flu activity by state, week ending October 17, 2009, 137*f*

hospitalizations/deaths from, 136*f*

outbreak of, 136–137

preventive measures, 137–138

"H5N1 Bird Flu Virus Mutations Facilitate Human Infection" (Reuters Health Information), 135

H5N1 flu, 135–136

Haemophilus influenza type b, 132

Hahnemann, Samuel, 183

Hamilton, Rebekah, 71

Hardie, Kate, 88

Harrison's Principles of Internal Medicine, 53, 57

HD (Huntington's disease), 73–74

Head, 54

"Health, Marriage, and Longer Life for Men" (RAND Corporation), 49

Health, of AD caregivers, 122–123

Health, United States, 2008 (NCHS), 108–109

Health, United States, 2009 (NCHS)
    on arthritis, 112
    on chronic conditions limiting activity, 109
    cigarette smoking among men, women, high school students, and mothers during pregnancy, 82, 82*f*
    on death rates, 23
    on deaths from cancer, 90
    on deaths from COPD, 103
    on deaths from diabetes, 108
    on life expectancy, 19
    on prenatal care, 7
    on stroke, 88
Health Care and Education Reconciliation Act of 2010, 30–31
Health care reform, 30–31
Health care settings
    MDROs in, prevention/control recommendations, 130*t*–131*t*
    MRSA in, 129
"Health Effects of Exposure to Secondhand Smoke" (Environmental Protection Agency), 93
Health in the United States, 2009 (CDC), 83
Health promotion, 35
Health Resources and Services Administration (HRSA) Organ Procurement and Transplantation Network, 82
Health/wellness
    birthrates/fertility rates, 2, 6–8, 11, 14–17
    crude birth/fertility/birth rates by mother's age/race/Hispanic origin 1950–2006, 3*t*–6*t*
    crude birth/fertility/birth rates by mother's age/race/Hispanic origin 1970–2005, 8*t*
    death, leading causes of/numbers of, by age, 29*t*–30*t*
    deaths, causes/numbers of, by sex/race/Hispanic origin, 20*t*–23*t*
    definition of, 1–2
    health care reform, 30–31
    health of U.S., 2
    infant mortality, 17–18
    infant mortality rates, international rankings of, 18*t*
    infant/neonatal/postnatal mortality rates, 17(*f*1.3)
    LBW births by mother's age, 16*f*
    LBW births by race/ethnicity/state, 14*t*–15*t*
    LBW live births, 12*t*–13*t*
    life expectancy, 18–19
    life expectancy at birth/age 65, by race/sex, 19*f*
    mortality, 20–23, 29–30
    persons who said health was excellent/very good, 31*f*
    persons who said health was excellent/very good, by age/sex, 32(*f*1.7)

persons who said health was excellent/very good, by race/ethnicity, 33*f*
    pregnancy, weight gain recommendations during, 16*t*
    prenatal care, early, 9*t*–10*t*
    self-assessed health status, 31
    self-assessed health status, by sex, 32(*f*1.6)
    spina bifida, rates of, 17(*f*1.2)
    YPLL before age 75 by sex/race, 24*t*–28*t*
Healthy People 2020 (HHS), 50–51, 51*f*
"Healthy Youth! Health Topics: Asthma" (CDC), 102
Heart
    cardiovascular system, examination of, 55
    electrocardiogram for assessment of, 58
    high blood pressure and, 89–90
Heart attack
    from arthritis drugs, 113–114
    description of, 79
    immediate care for, 79–80
    warning signals of, 79
    for women, 84–86
"Heart Attack Symptoms and Warning Signs" (American Heart Association), 79
Heart disease
    bypass surgery, 80–81
    catheter-based interventions, 81–82
    cigarette smoking among men, women, high school students, and mothers during pregnancy, 82*f*
    as complication of diabetes, 43
    death rates for leading causes of death for all ages, 89*f*
    diabetes complications, prevention of, 44
    genetic inheritance and, 72
    heart attack, 79–80
    high blood pressure in adults age 20/older, 83*t*–84*t*
    pets and, 50
    risk factors for, 82–84
    rofecoxib, 113
    screening guidelines for, 40
    treatments for, 80
    women and, 84–86
    See also Cardiovascular diseases
"Heart Disease and Stroke Statistics—2008 Update: A Report from the American Heart Association Statistics Committee and Stroke Statistics Subcommittee" (Rosamond et al.), 84–86
"Heart Disease and Stroke Statistics—2010 Update" (Lloyd-Jones et al.)
    on bypass surgery, 81
    on life expectancy, 79
    on risk factors for heart disease, 82
    on stroke, 88, 89
Heart transplants, 81–82
Hemo, Beatriz, 129, 132
Heparin, 88
Hepatitis A, 133

Hepatitis B, 91, 133
HER2 gene, 101
Herbal medicine, Chinese, 185
"Herbs at Glance" (NCCAM), 177
"Herceptin: Novel Therapy Targets HER2-Positive Breast Cancer" (Mayo Clinic), 101
Heredity. *See* Genetics
Hexosaminidase A (hex-A), 77
HHS. *See* U.S. Department of Health and Human Services
High blood pressure
    in adults age 20/older, 83*t*–84*t*
    as complication of diabetes, 43
    overview of, 89–90
    prevalence of, 90
    as risk factor for heart disease, 82
    screening for, 39
High serum cholesterol, 82–83
Highly active antiretroviral therapy, 145
HIV. *See* Human immunodeficiency virus/acquired immunodeficiency syndrome
HIV/AIDS Surveillance Report: Cases of HIV Infection and AIDS in the United States and Dependent Areas, 2007 (CDC), 141–142
Hollifield, Michael, 184
Holt-Lunstad, Julianne, 49
"Homeopathic Medical Practice: Long-term Results of a Cohort Study with 3981 Patients" (Witt et al.), 183
Homeopathic medicine, 183
Homosexuality, 60
"Hong Kong flu," 135
Hormone replacement therapy (HRT), 115
Hormone therapy
    for breast cancer, 100
    for prostate cancer, 102
    for SLE treatment, 112
Hospital
    chiropractic services in, 181
    Reiki in, 191
"Hospital-Based Chiropractic Integration within a Large Private Hospital System in Minnesota: A 10-Year Example" (Branson), 181
Hospitalizations
    H1N1 hospitalizations/deaths, 136*f*
    from influenza, 134–135
"How Healthy Are Chronically Ill Patients after Eight Years of Homeopathic Treatment?—Results from a Long Term Observational Study" (Witt et al.), 183
"How to Recognize When to Ask for Help" (U.S. Department of Veterans Affairs), 47, 48
HPV. *See* Human papillomavirus
HRSA (Health Resources and Services Administration) Organ Procurement and Transplantation Network, 82
HRT (hormone replacement therapy), 115

Huang, Elbert S., 107
Hudson, James I., 166
Hull, Mark W., 145
Human immunodeficiency virus/acquired
    immunodeficiency syndrome (HIV/AIDS)
    AIDS, estimated numbers of cases/rates
        of, by race/ethnicity, age, sex, 143*t*
    AIDS cases, estimated numbers of, by
        year of diagnosis, characteristics of
        persons, 144*t*
    ELISA test for, 57
    number of cases of, 125
    opportunistic infections, 143
    transmission of, 142–143
    treatment of, 143–145
    in U.S., 141–142
    worldwide, 141
Human papillomavirus (HPV)
    immunization, 133
    as risk for cervical cancer, 91
    vaccine for, 42
"The Human-Companion Animal Bond:
    How Humans Benefit" (Friedmann &
    Son), 50
Huntington Study Group TETRA-HD, 74
Huntington's disease (HD), 73–74
Huntington's Disease Society of America, 194
Hyaline membrane, 8
Hyperosmolar coma, 44
Hypertension. *See* High blood pressure
"Hypertension Awareness, Treatment, and
    Control—Continued Disparities in
    Adults: United States, 2005–2006"
    (Ostchega et al.), 90

I

Identification, carrier, 68
Imaging studies
    for Alzheimer's disease testing, 121
    CT/MRI scans, 58
    for MS diagnosis, 117
    x-rays/ultrasound, 57–58
Immune system
    arthritis treatment and, 112–113
    multiple sclerosis and, 117
    opportunistic infections with HIV/AIDS,
        143
    tuberculosis and, 139
Immunization
    for H1N1 flu, 136–137
    influenza vaccines, 134–135
    for Lyme disease, 145–146
    for prevention of infectious diseases,
        132–134
    as primary prevention, 35–36, 37
    schedule, recommended childhood/
        adolescent, by vaccine/age, 36*f*
    schedule, recommended for adults, by
        vaccine, age group, 132*f*
Implants, electrode, 119

Indinavir, 145
"Induced Pluripotent Stem Cell Lines
    Derived from Human Somatic Cells"
    (Yu et al.), 119
Infant mortality
    rates, 17(*f*1.3)
    in U.S., 17–18
Infants, genetic screening of, 66
Infection
    increased risk of from diabetes, 44
    with influenza, 134
    opportunistic, HIV/AIDS and, 143
Infectious diseases
    AIDS, estimated numbers of cases/rates
        of, by race/ethnicity, age, sex, 143*t*
    AIDS cases, estimated numbers of, by
        year of diagnosis, characteristics of
        persons, 144*t*
    bacteria, resistant strains of, 126–129, 132
    biologic terrorism, 148–149
    flu activity by state, week ending
        January 2, 2010, 138*f*
    flu activity by state, week ending
        October 17, 2009, 137*f*
    H1N1 hospitalizations/deaths, 136*f*
    HIV/AIDS, 141–145
    immunization for prevention of,
        132–134
    immunization schedule, recommended
        for adults, by vaccine, age group, 132*f*
    influenza, 134–138
    Lyme disease, 145–146
    Lyme disease, reported cases of, 146*f*
    Lyme disease cases, geographic
        distribution of, 147*f*
    MDROs in health care settings,
        prevention/control recommendations,
        130*t*–131*t*
    most frequently reported, 125–126
    nationally notifiable infectious diseases, 125*t*
    notifiable diseases, reported cases of, by
        month, 127*t*–128*t*
    overview of, 125
    primary prevention of, 35–36
    severe acute respiratory syndrome,
        146–148
    TB, latent TB infection/TB disease, 139*t*
    TB, multidrug-resistant, in persons with
        no previous TB, by origin of birth, 141*t*
    TB, multidrug-resistant, in persons with
        previous history of TB, by origin of
        birth, 142*t*
    TB cases, reported, 139*f*
    TB cases in foreign-born persons,
        140(*f*7.7)
    TB cases in U.S.-born vs. foreign-born
        people, 140(*f*7.8)
    tuberculosis, 138–141
    vaccines recommended for some adults
        based on medical/other indications, 133*f*
    West Nile virus, 146, 148*f*

Inflammation, 111
"Influence of Companion Animals on the
    Physical and Psychological Health of
    Older People: An Analysis of a One-Year
    Longitudinal Study" (Raina et al.), 50
Influenza
    description of, 134
    flu activity by state, week ending
        January 2, 2010, 138*f*
    flu activity by state, week ending
        October 17, 2009, 137*f*
    H1N1 hospitalizations/deaths, 136*f*
    immunization, 133
    pandemic, 135–138
    vaccines, 134–135
"Influenza Vaccination in the Elderly:
    Seeking New Correlates of Protection and
    Improved Vaccines" (McElhaney), 134
Inheritance, genetic, 63–64
Inherited diseases
    cystic fibrosis, 73
    Huntington's disease, 73–74
    muscular dystrophy, 74
    overview of, 72–73
    sickle-cell disease, 74–76
    Tay-Sachs disease, 76–77
Injuries, unintentional, 89*f*
Insomnia, 122–123
"Insomnia in Caregivers of Persons with
    Dementia: Who Is at Risk and What Can
    Be Done about It?" (McCurry et al.),
    122–123
Institute of Medicine, 181
Insulin
    double diabetes and, 107
    tertiary prevention of diabetes, 43–44
Insurance, health
    genetic testing and, 72
    health care reform and, 30–31
"Integration of Acupuncture into Family
    Medicine Teaching Clinics" (Wu), 182
"Integration of Diagnostic and
    Communication Technologies" (Malik),
    60–61
Integrative medicine, 175
Intellectual wellness, 1
Intentional epidemics, 148–149
Interleukin Genetics, 115
*International Classification of Diseases:
    Classification of Mental and
    Behavioural Disorders (ICD-10)*
    (WHO), 59
Interpersonal psychotherapy (IPT), 167
Interventions
    adolescent mental health intervention
        programs, 45–46
    developing/testing, 37
    youth violence, possible settings for
        interventions to prevent, 38(*t*2.2)
IPT (interpersonal psychotherapy), 167
Iribarne, Alexander, 81

"Is There Something Unique about Marriage? The Relative Impact of Marital Status, Relationship Quality, and Network Social Support on Ambulatory Blood Pressure and Mental Health" (Holt-Lunstad, Birmingham, & Jones), 49

Israel, 129–130

J

Jamison, Kay Redfield, 159
Jauch, Edward C., 89
Jenney, Meriel, 91
Jensen, Peter, 164
Jews, 77, 118
Joint United Nations Programme on HIV/ AIDS, 141
Joints. *See* Arthritis
Jones, Brandon Q., 49
Jones, James F., 179

K

Kahan, André, 189
Kaljser, Magnus, 11
Kanner, Leo, 155
Kaufman, Francine R., 107
Kidney disease, 43–44
Kobayashi, Scott D., 129
Koch, Robert, 141

L

Laboratory tests, 57
Lang, Undine E., 160
Latent TB, 139, 139t
"The Latest Osteoporosis Research" (*Arthritis Today*), 115
Latourelle, Jeanne C., 118
Lavretsky, Helen, 181
Lawsuits, 114
LBW. *See* Low birth weight
LDL (low-density lipoproteins), 44
L-dopa (levodopa), 118
Le Grange, Daniel, 167
Leach, Amanda J., 127
"Learning about Cystic Fibrosis" (NHGRI), 73
Leavitt, Michael O., 135
Lee, Carol H., 40
Legislation and international treaties
    Birth Defects and Development Disabilities Prevention Act, 17
    Birth Defects Prevention Act, 17
    Breast and Cervical Cancer Mortality Prevention Act, 42
    Death with Dignity Act (Oregon), 174
    Dietary Supplement Health and Education Act of 1994, 188
    Genetic Information Nondiscrimination Act, 72
    Health Care and Education Reconciliation Act of 2010, 30–31

Patient Protection and Affordable Care Act, 30–31
Lesage, Suzanne, 118
Leucine-rich repeat kinase 2 (LRRK2), 118
Levitt, Gill, 91
Levodopa (L-dopa), 118
Life expectancy
    at birth/age 65 by race/sex, 19f
    cardiovascular diseases and, 79
    overview of, 18–19
    in U.S., 18–19
"Life Expectancy at All Time High; Death Rates Reach New Low, New Report Shows" (CDC), 19
Lifestyle
    for disease prevention, 35
    for hypertension control, 90
    naturopathic medicine and, 184
    See also Diet; Exercise
"Limitations on Physical Performance and Daily Activities among Long-Term Survivors of Childhood Cancer" (Ness et al.), 91
Linde, Klaus, 189
Lindsay, Ronald A., 174
Lipids, 57
"List of Vaccine-Preventable Diseases" (CDC), 132–134
Lithium, 160
Liver, 55
Lloyd-Jones, Donald
    on bypass surgery, 81
    on cardiovascular diseases, 79
    on risk factors for heart disease, 82
    on stroke, 88, 89
Loeb, Susan J., 86
"Long-Term Effects of Chondroitins 4 and 6 Sulfate on Knee Osteoarthritis: The Study on Osteoarthritis Progression Prevention, a Two-year, Randomized, Double-blind, Placebo-controlled Trial" (Kahan et al.), 189
"Long-Term Outcomes after Breast Conservation Therapy for Early Stage Breast Cancer in a Community Setting" (McClosky et al.), 100
"Low Birth Weight and Increased Cardiovascular Risk: Fetal Programming" (Balci, Acikel, & Akdemir), 11
Low birth weight (LBW)
    births by mother's age, 16f
    births by race/ethnicity/state, 14t–15t
    live births, 12t–13t
    overview of, 7–8
    risk of disease and, 11, 14–15
Low-density lipoproteins (LDL), 44
LRRK2 (leucine-rich repeat kinase 2), 118
"LRRK2 G2019S as a Cause of Parkinson's Disease in Ashkenazi Jews" (Ozelius), 118

"LRRK2 G2019S as a Cause of Parkinson's Disease in North African Arabs" (Lesage et al.), 118
Lumpectomy, 100
Lung cancer
    death rate for, 90–91
    incidence rate/deaths from, 92
    risk factors for, 93
Lungs
    asthma, 102–103
    asthma, prevalence of current, among persons of all ages, by age group, race/ ethnicity, 103(f5.5)
    asthma, prevalence of current, among persons of all ages, by age group, sex, 103(f5.6)
    chronic obstructive pulmonary disease, 103–104
    cigarette smoking among men, women, high school students, and mothers during pregnancy, 82f
    influenza and, 134
    physical examination, 54–55
    respiratory diseases, frequency of, among persons 18/older, 105t–106t
    tuberculosis in, 139
Lust, Benedict, 183
Lyme disease
    cases, geographic distribution of, 147f
    description of, 145
    number of cases of, 125
    reported cases of, 146f
    vaccine for, 145–146
Lynch, Joseph P., 127–128

M

Ma huang, 185
Magnetic resonance imaging (MRI) scan, 58, 117
"Major Depressive Disorder in Children and Adolescents" (USPSTF), 40
Males
    eating disorders among, 165
    HIV/AIDS and, 142
    LBW and testicular cancer, 14
    life expectancy of, 19
    osteoporosis and, 114
    prostate cancer, 101–102
    relationships, health connection for, 49
    suicide rates among, 173
Malignant melanoma, 101
Malignant tumors, 90
Malik, Nafees N., 60–61
"Mammogram Math" (Paulos), 40
Mammography
    use by selected age groups, 93t
    USPSTF breast cancer screening guidelines, 40, 92
    x-ray technology for, 58

Management of Multidrug-Resistant Organisms in Healthcare Settings, 2006 (Siegel et al.), 129

"Managing Asthma in Primary Care: Putting New Guideline Recommendations into Context" (Wechsler), 103

Manheimer, Eric, 184

Manic depression. *See* Bipolar disorder

Manic-Depressive Illness (Goodwin & Jamison), 159

Manipulative therapies, body-based methods, 182, 189–190

MAO-B inhibitors, 118

March, John S., 158

March of Dimes Foundation
    contact information, 194
    on folic acid, 17
    on newborn screening, 66
    on prenatal care, 7
    on spina bifida, 16

Marchione, Marilynn, 71

Marikangas, Kathleen
    on children suffering anxiety/panic disorder, 162
    on children suffering from ADHD, 163
    on children suffering mental illness, 152

Marriage, health benefits of, 49

Martin, Joyce A.
    "Births: Final Data for 2006," 2, 6
    on prenatal care, 7

Martino, Davide, 163

"Massage for Low Back Pain: An Updated Systematic Review within the Framework of the Cochrane Back Review Group" (Furlan et al.), 189–190

Massage therapy, 189–190

Mastectomy, 100

Mathews, T. J., 16

Mayo Clinic, 101

Mazziotta, John C., 121

McClosky, Susan A., 100

McCurry, Susan M., 122–123

McDowell, Margaret A., 17

McElhaney, Janet E., 134

McFee, Robin B., 47

MD (muscular dystrophy), 74

MDROs. *See* Multidrug-resistant organisms

Measles, 133

"Measuring Social Isolation among Older Adults Using Multiple Indicators from the NSHAP Study" (Cornwell & Waite), 50

Medical histories, 53–54

Medication, psychoactive, 167–168

Meditation
    effects of, 186
    types of populations/conditions included in studies on, 187t–188t
    use of by adults, 176

"Meditation: An Introduction" (NCCAM), 186

Meditation Practices for Health: State of the Research (Ospina et al.), 186

Mehrotra, Ateev, 56

Memantine, 122

Men. *See* Males

Mendelian disorders, 64

Mendes, Wendy B., 50

Meng, Jinhong, 74

Meningitis, 133

Menopause, 84

Mental health
    adolescent intervention programs, 45–46
    Columbia University teen mental health screening program, 46(t2.7)
    disorders, 151
    primary prevention, 35
    problems, 151
    programs, types of, 45
    screening for depression, 40
    secondary prevention example, 39
    suicide prevention, 46–47
    suicide risk, warning signs for, 48t
    suicide risk factors, protective factors, national prevention strategy, 46(t2.8)

Mental Health: A Report of the Surgeon General (Office of the Surgeon General)
    definition of mental illness, 151
    on mental illness diagnosis, 60
    on suicide as serious public health problem, 46

Mental illness
    ADD/ADHD, 163–164
    ADHD, drugs used to treat, 168(t8.3)
    adolescents who had depressive episode, 153(f8.3)
    adults with psychological distress in past 30 days, 153(f8.4)
    adults with psychological distress in past 30 days, by age group/sex, 154(f8.5)
    adults with psychological distress in past 30 days, by race/ethnicity, 154(f8.6)
    antidepressants, side effects of, 158t
    anxiety disorders, 160–163
    anxiety disorders, drugs used to treat, 168(t8.4)
    autism spectrum disorder, changes in prevalence of, 156f
    autism spectrum disorders, 155–157
    bipolar disorder, 159–160
    children with emotional/behavioral difficulties, 152(f8.2)
    death rates for suicide, by sex/race/ Hispanic origin/age, 169t–172t
    depression, 157–159
    diagnosis of, 59–61
    disruptive disorders, 164–165
    eating disorders, 165–167
    genetic inheritance and, 72
    mental distress, Americans reporting frequent, 152(f8.1)
    numbers affected by, 151–155
    overview of, 151
    psychoactive medication, prescribing for children, 167–168
    schizophrenia, 160
    suicide, 168, 173–174
    symptoms of depression, 157t
    types of, 155

"Mental Illness Exacts Heavy Toll, Beginning in Youth" (NIMH), 60

Mentoring activities, 38, 38(t2.4)

Merck, 113, 114

Merikangas, Kathleen Ries, 60

Metcalfe, Kelly A., 101

Methicillin-resistant *Staphylococcus aureus* (MRSA), 129

Mexican-Americans, hypertension and, 90

Meyer, Marion R., 120

Mind-body interventions
    biofeedback, 186
    description of, 182
    guiding principles of, 185
    meditation, 186, 187t–188t
    use of by adults, 176

Mitchinson, Allison R., 189

Mitochondrial disorders, 64–65

Mitoxantrone, 117

"Modeling an Anti-Amyloid Combination Therapy for Alzheimer's Disease" (Chow et al.), 122

"Molecular Mechanisms of Schizophrenia" (Lang), 160

Monogenic disorders, 64

Moreno, Carmen, 159

Morris, John C., 121

Morris, Peter S., 127

Mortality
    age differences, 23, 29–30
    infant, in U.S., 17–18
    racial/gender differences, 23
    YPLL, 20–23

Mortality rates
    for cancer by sex, age, ethnicity, race, 95t–99t
    death, ten leading causes of/death rates of, 80f
    for heart disease, 85–86
    infant, international rankings, 18t
    infant/neonatal/postnatal, 17(f1.3)
    for leading causes of death for all ages, 89f
    for SLE, 112
    for suicide, 168
    for suicide, by sex/race/Hispanic origin/ age, 169t–172t

Mosca, Lori, 86

Mosquitoes, 146

Mothers. *See* Births; Pregnancy

MRI (magnetic resonance imaging) scan, 58, 117

MRSA (methicillin-resistant *Staphylococcus aureus*), 129
MS (multiple sclerosis), 116–117
Multidrug-resistant organisms (MDROs)
in health care settings, prevention/control recommendations, 130*t*–131*t*
methicillin-resistant *Staphylococcus aureus*, 129
Streptococcus pneumoniae, 127–128
Multidrug-resistant TB
in persons with no previous TB, by origin of birth, 141*t*
in persons with previous history of TB, by origin of birth, 142*t*
in U.S., 140–141
Multifactorial disorders, 64–65
Multiple sclerosis (MS), 116–117
Mumps, 133
Muscular dystrophy (MD), 74
Muscular Dystrophy Association, 194
Mycobacterium tuberculosis
discovery of, 141
TB caused by, 138
Myelin sheath, 116, 117
Myocardial infarction. *See* Heart attack
"Myocardial Infarction in Women: Promoting Symptom Recognition, Early Diagnosis, and Risk Assessment" (Zbierajewski-Eischeid & Loeb), 86
Myotonic dystrophy, 70, 74

N

Names/addresses, of organizations, 193–194
"Nanoparticle-Based Detection in Cerebral Spinal Fluid of a Soluble Pathogenic Biomarker for Alzheimer's Disease" (Georganopoulou et al.), 121
Naproxen, 113–114
National Asthma Education and Prevention Program, 103
National Breast and Cervical Cancer Early Detection Program (NBCCEDP), 42–43, 42*f*
National Cancer Institute, 101, 113
National Center for Biotechnology Information, 120
National Center for Chronic Disease Prevention, 112, 151
National Center for Complementary and Alternative Medicine (NCCAM)
on chiropractic, 190
contact information, 194
on mind-body interventions, 185
mission of, 175
on naturopathic medicine, 184
on types of CAM, 182
on use of CAM, 176
National Center for Health Statistics (NCHS)
on Alzheimer's disease, 119
on asthma, 102

on chronic conditions limiting activity, 108–109
contact information, 194
on death rates, 23
on deaths from diabetes, 108
on life expectancy, 19
on obesity, 84
on prenatal care, 7
on stroke, 88
National Comorbidity Survey (Harvard School of Medicine), 151–152
National Diabetes Education Program (NDEP), 44
The National Diabetes Education Program: Ten Years of Progress 1997–2007 (NDEP), 44
"National Diabetes Statistics, 2007" (National Institute of Diabetes and Digestive and Kidney Diseases)
on deaths from diabetes, 108
on diabetes, 43
on diabetes and heart disease, 84
on preventing complications of diabetes, 44
National Electronic Telecommunications System for Surveillance (NETSS), 125
National Fibromyalgia Association, 111, 194
National Health and Nutrition Examination Survey (NHANES)
on ADHD among children, 163, 164
on anxiety among children/adolescents, 162
on psychological distress, 152–154
National Heart Lung and Blood Institute (NHLBI), 75, 79, 103
National Human Genome Research Institute (NHGRI), 73
National Institute of Allergy and Infectious Diseases (NIAID), 147, 148–149
National Institute of Arthritis and Musculoskeletal and Skin Diseases (NIAMS), 114
National Institute of Diabetes and Digestive and Kidney Diseases (NIDDK)
on deaths from diabetes, 108
on diabetes, 43
on diabetes and heart disease, 84
on preventing complications of diabetes, 44
National Institute of Mental Health (NIMH)
on ADHD, 163
on agoraphobia, 162
on anxiety disorder, 161
on bipolar disorder, 159
on bulimia nervosa, 166
on depression, 157, 158
on eating disorders, 165
on mental disorders, 151, 155
on mental illness, 167, 168
on mental illness diagnosis, 60
on panic disorder, 161
on schizophrenia, 160
on social phobias, 161

on suicide, 168, 173
National Institute of Neurological Disorders and Stroke (NINDS), 74
National Institute on Aging, 120
National Institutes of Health (NIH)
on anencephaly, 16
on diabetes, 43
on physical examination, 54
on suicide prevention, 46–47
National Library of Medicine's Genetics Home Reference, 73
National Mental Health Association, 194
National Multiple Sclerosis Society
contact information, 194
on prevalence of MS, 116–117
National Osteoporosis Foundation (NOF), 114, 194
National Parkinson Foundation, 117–118
National Social Life, Health, and Aging Project (NSHAP), 50
"National Study of Women's Awareness, Preventive Action, and Barriers to Cardiovascular Health" (Mosca), 86
National Suicide Prevention Lifeline, 48
National Surgical Adjuvant Breast and Bowel Project, 100
National Tay-Sachs and Allied Diseases Association, 194
"National Trends in the Outpatient Diagnosis and Treatment of Bipolar Disorder in Youth" (Moreno et al.), 159
National Wellness Institute, 1
Native Americans and Alaskan Natives, 176
Natural products
use of by adults, 176
used by adults, ten most common, 179*f*
used by children, 177
used by children, ten most common, 182(*f*9.10)
"Naturopathic Care for Anxiety: A Randomized Controlled Trial ISRCTN78958974" (Cooley et al.), 184
Naturopathic medicine, 183–184
"Naturopathic Medicine and Type 2 Diabetes: A Retrospective Analysis from an Academic Clinic" (Bradley & Odberg), 184
NBCCEDP (National Breast and Cervical Cancer Early Detection Program), 42–43, 42*f*
NCCAM. *See* National Center for Complementary and Alternative Medicine
"NCCAM Facts-at-a-Glance and Mission" (NCCAM), 175
NCHS. *See* National Center for Health Statistics
NDEP (National Diabetes Education Program), 44
Neck, examination of, 54

"The Need for Outreach in Preventing Suicide among Young Veterans" (Sareen & Belik), 47

Neergaard, Lauran, 107

Neonatal mortality rates, 17(*f*1.3)

Neonatal technology, 17–18

Nervous system
illustration of, 55*f*
multiple sclerosis and, 116–117
neurologic exam, 55–56
stroke and, 86–88

Ness, Kirsten, 91

NETSS (National Electronic Telecommunications System for Surveillance), 125

Neural tube defects (NTDs), 16, 59

Neurofibrillary tangles, 120

Neurologic examination, 55–56

Neurological disorders, 72

"Neurosteroids' Effects and Mechanisms for Social, Cognitive, Emotional, and Physical Functions" (Frye), 49

"New Cervical Cancer Screening Guidelines Released" (Young), 42

New Jersey, Vioxx case in, 114

"New Research to Help Youth with Mental Disorders Transition to Adulthood" (NIMH), 60

"New Survey Results Show Huge Burden of Diabetes" (NIH), 43

Newborn screening program
conditions included in decision-making process, 67*f*
genetic screening, 66

Newborn Screening: Toward a Uniform Screening Panel and System (ACMG), 66

"Newly Discovered Breast Cancer Susceptibility Loci on 3p24 and 17q23.2" (Ahmed), 64–65

NHANES. *See* National Health and Nutrition Examination Survey

NHGRI (National Human Genome Research Institute), 73

NHLBI (National Heart Lung and Blood Institute), 75, 79, 103

NHLBI Fact Book, Fiscal Year 2008 (National Heart Lung and Blood Institute), 79

NIAID (National Institute of Allergy and Infectious Diseases), 147, 148–149

"NIAID Renews Funding for National Emerging Infectious Diseases Research Network" (NIAID), 149

NIAMS (National Institute of Arthritis and Musculoskeletal and Skin Diseases), 114

Nichol, Kristin L., 135

NIDDK. *See* National Institute of Diabetes and Digestive and Kidney Diseases

NIH. *See* National Institutes of Health

NIMH. *See* National Institute of Mental Health

NINDS (National Institute of Neurological Disorders and Stroke), 74

"NINDS Huntington's Disease Information Page" (NINDS), 74

NOF. *See* National Osteoporosis Foundation

Nonsteroidal anti-inflammatory drugs (NSAIDs)
for arthritis, 113
COX-2 inhibitors, 113–114
for SLE treatment, 112

Notifiable diseases
list of, 125–126
nationally notifiable infectious diseases, 126*t*
reported cases of, 127*t*–128*t*

NSAIDs. *See* Nonsteroidal anti-inflammatory drugs

NSHAP (National Social Life, Health, and Aging Project), 50

NTDs (neural tube defects), 16, 59

The Numbers Count: Mental Disorders in America (NIMH), 60, 151, 155

O

Obama, Barack
health care reform and, 30
stem cell research and, 119

Obesity
diabesity, 106–107
double diabetes and, 107
heart disease and, 84
mortality rates and, 19
prevalence of, among adults aged 20 years/older, 88*f*

Obsessive-compulsive disorder (OCD), 162

Occupational wellness, 1

OCD (obsessive-compulsive disorder), 162

Odberg, Erica B., 184

ODD (oppositional defiant disorder), 164

ODS (Office of Dietary Supplements), 188

Office of Dietary Supplements (ODS), 188

OGTT (oral glucose tolerance test), 104

OHSU (Oregon Health and Science University), 181–182

OIs (opportunistic infections), 143

Older adults
activity, limitation of, caused by chronic health conditions among older adults, by age, 109(*f*5.11)
flu vaccinations for, 134–135

"Older Americans and Cardiovascular Diseases—Statistics" (American Heart Association), 88

Olfsen, Mark, 160

"A One Year Trial of Methylphenidate in the Treatment of ADHD" (Wender), 164

"Oophorectomy for Breast Cancer Prevention in Women with BRCA1 or BRCA2 Mutations" (Metcalfe), 101

Operations. *See* Surgery

Opportunistic infections (OIs), 143

Oppositional defiant disorder (ODD), 164

Oral glucose tolerance test (OGTT), 104

"Oral Transmission of HIV, Reality or Fiction? An Update" (Campo et al.), 143

Oregon, Death with Dignity Act, 174

Oregon Health and Science University (OHSU), 181–182

"Oregon's Experience: Evaluating the Record" (Lindsay), 174

Oseltamivir, 138

Osler, William, 184

Ospina, Maria B., 186

Ostchega, Yechiam, 90

Osteoarthritis
description of, 111
dietary supplements and, 189

Osteoporosis
causes of bone loss/fractures in, 115*f*
description of, treatment of, 114–115
exercise for, 116
pyramid for prevention/treatment, 116*f*

Osteoporosis Overview (NIAMS), 114

Otoscope, 54

"Overview of Healthcare-associated MRSA" (CDC), 129

Oxytocin, 156

Ozelius, Laurie J., 118

P

Pain
acupuncture for, 184
biofeedback for, 186
massage for pain relief, 189–190
Reiki and, 191

"Painful Diabetic Neuropathy [PDN]: Impact of an Alternative Approach" (Gillespie, Gillespie, & Stevens), 191

PANDAS (pediatric autoimmune neuropsychiatric disorders associated with streptococcal) infections, 163

"The PANDAS Subgroup of Tic Disorders and Childhood-Onset Obsessive-Compulsive Disorder" (Martino), 163

"Pandemic Flu: Key Facts" (CDC), 135

Pandemic influenza
avian influenza, 135–136
H1N1 flu, 136–137, 136*f*
preventive measures, 137–138

Pandemic Planning Update VI (Leavitt), 135

"Panel Presentations on Issues Impacting the Strategic Plan" (CDC), 142

Panic disorder, 161

Pap test (Papanicolaou test)
cervical cancer screening guidelines, 41–42
number of women screened, 92
in pelvic examination, 55
use by selected age groups, 94*t*

Parents. *See* Births; Pregnancy
  adolescent mental health intervention
    programs and, 45
  children using CAM, based on CAM use
    by parents or relatives, 181(*f*9.8)
Parker, Michael, 71
Parkinsonism, 117–118
Parkinson's disease
  description of, 117–118
  experimental therapies, 118–119
  genetic link, 118
Patient Protection and Affordable Care Act
  (PPACA), 30–31
Paulos, John Allen, 40
Pavlik, Valory N., 122
PCI (percutaneous coronary intervention), 81
PDD-NOS (pervasive developmental
  disorder not otherwise specified), 156
PDN (painful diabetic neuropathy), 191
Peak flow meter, 54
Pediatric autoimmune neuropsychiatric
  disorders associated with streptococcal
  (PANDAS) infections, 163
Pelletier, Kenneth R., 185, 188
Pelvic examination, 55
Penicillin-resistant pneumococcus, 128, 129
"Perceived Barriers to Mental Health
  Service Utilization in the United States,
  Ontario, and the Netherlands" (Sareen),
  154–155
Percussion, 54, 55
Percutaneous coronary intervention (PCI), 81
"Percutaneous Coronary Intervention
  Following Thrombolysis: For Whom and
  When?" (Taglieri & Di Mario), 81
"Perinatal Risk Factors for Ischemic Heart
  Disease" (Kaijser), 11
Peripheral nerves, 55*f*, 56
Periumbilical blood sampling (PUBS), 69
Personal life, 49–51
Personal responsibility, 35
Pertussis, 133
Pervasive developmental disorder not
  otherwise specified (PDD-NOS), 156
Pervasive developmental disorders,
  155–157
PET (positron emission tomography) scan, 58
Petitti, Diana, 40
Pets, health benefits of, 50
Pfizer, 113, 114
PGD (preimplantation genetic diagnosis), 68
Phenotypes, 63–64
Philippi, Anne, 156
Phobias, 161–162
Physical activity. *See* Activity; Exercise
"Physical Activity Guidelines for
  Americans" (HHS), 83
Physical examination
  areas of, 54–56
  nervous system, 55*f*
  vital signs, 54

Physician-assisted dying, 174
Physiological symptoms, 53–54
PIs (protease inhibitors), 143–145
Pittsburgh Compound B, 121
Placebo effect
  dietary supplements vs., 189
  energy therapies and, 190
  mind-body interventions and, 185
Pneumococcal bacteria
  description of, effects of, 126–128
  immunization, 134
  penicillin-resistant, 129
  vaccine, 128
Pneumoconiosis, 102
Pneumocystis carinii pneumonia, 143
Pneumonia
  with influenza, 134
  opportunistic infections with HIV/
    AIDS, 143
Poliomyelitis (polio), 134
Polygenic disorders, 64–65
Population-based programs, for mental
  health prevention, 45
Positron emission tomography (PET) scan, 58
Postnatal mortality rates, 17(*f*1.3)
"The Power of Biomedical Research"
  (Fauci), 148–149
Pozilli, Paolo, 107–108
PPACA (Patient Protection and Affordable
  Care Act), 30–31
"Predicting Recurrent Stroke after Minor
  Stroke and Transient Ischemic Attack"
  (Couillard et al.), 88–89
Predictive genetic testing, 70
Pregnancy
  cigarette smoking among men, women,
    high school students, and mothers
    during pregnancy, 82*f*
  mother's weight gain, effect on LBW, 15
  prenatal care, 6–7
  prenatal diagnostic testing, 58–59
  problems from diabetes, 44
  weight gain recommendations during, 16*t*
  See also Births
Prehypertension, 89–90
"Prehypertension Accounts for a
  Substantial Number of Hospitalizations,
  Nursing Home Admissions, and
  Premature Deaths" (Agency for
  Healthcare Research and Quality), 89–90
Preimplantation genetic diagnosis (PGD), 68
Prematurity, 7–8
Prenatal care
  early, 9*t*–10*t*
  overview of, 6–7
Prenatal tests
  genetic testing, 68–69
  types of, 69(*t*4.2)
Prescription drugs. *See* Drugs

President's New Freedom Commission on
  Mental Health, 45
"Prevalence, Heritability, and Prospective
  Risk Factors for Anorexia Nervosa"
  (Bulik), 166
"The Prevalence and Correlates of Eating
  Disorders in the National Comorbidity
  Survey Replication" (Hudson), 166
"Prevalence and Treatment of Mental
  Disorders among US Children in the
  2001–2004 NHANES" (Merikangas et
  al.), 60, 152, 162
"Prevalence of Autism Spectrum
  Disorders—Autism and Developmental
  Disabilities Monitoring Network, United
  States, 2006" (Rice), 155
"Prevalence of Duchenne/Becker Muscular
  Dystrophy among Males Aged 5–24
  Years—Four States, 2007" (CDC), 74
"Preventing Suicide: Program Activities
  Guide" (CDC), 47
Prevention
  Ayurvedic medicine and, 184–185
  of birth defects, 16–17
  of H1N1 flu, 137–138
  immunization for, 132–134
  of MDROs in health care settings,
    130*t*–131*t*
Prevention of disease
  breast cancer, recommended screening
    for, 41*t*
  Columbia University teen mental health
    screening program, 46(*t*2.7)
  Healthy People 2020 goals, action plan
    to achieve, 51*f*
  immunization schedule, recommended
    childhood/adolescent, by vaccine/
    age, 36*f*
  mental health prevention programs, 45–46
  mentoring activities, 38(*t*2.4)
  NBCCEDP, number of women served
    in, 42*f*
  overview of, 35
  preventive services, recommended, 39*t*
  primary prevention, 35–38
  research/goals, 49
  secondary prevention, 38–43
  suicide, active military/veterans at risk
    for, 47–49
  suicide prevention, 46–47
  suicide risk, warning signs for, 48*t*
  suicide risk factors, protective factors,
    national prevention strategy, 46(*t*2.8)
  tertiary prevention, 43–44
  work, social activities, personal
    relationships as key to, 49–51
  youth violence, possible settings for
    interventions, 38(*t*2.2)
  youth violence, potential participant
    groups for interventions to prevent, 37*t*
  youth violence prevention, goal/
    objectives of goal, 38(*t*2.3)

Prevention Research Centers, 49
"Prevention Research Centers—Building the Scientific Research Base with Community Partners: At a Glance 2010" (CDC), 49
"Preventive Health Examinations and Preventive Gynecological Examinations in the United States" (Mehrotra, Zaslavsky, & Ayanian), 56
Primary prevention
    description of, 35–37
    immunization schedule, recommended childhood/adolescent, by vaccine/age, 36f
    mentoring activities, 38(t2.4)
    research/goals for, 49
    of youth violence, 37–38
    youth violence, possible settings for interventions to prevent, 38(t2.2)
    youth violence, potential participant groups for interventions to prevent, 37t
    youth violence prevention, goal/objectives of goal, 38(t2.3)
"Projecting the Future Diabetes Population Size and Related Costs for the U.S." (Huang et al.), 107
Prosorba therapy, 113
Prostate cancer
    detection of, 101–102
    prostate specific antigen, 57
    treatment of, 102
Prostatectomy, 102
Prostate-specific antigen (PSA) screening, 101–102
Protease inhibitors (PIs), 143–145
PSA (prostate-specific antigen) screening, 101–102
Psychoactive medication, 167–168
Psychological distress, 152–154
Psychotherapy, 158
PUBS (periumbilical blood sampling), 69
Pulse rate
    cardiovascular system, examination of, 55
    measurement of, 54
    in TCM approach, 185

Q

Qi (chi), 184, 185
Qi Gong, 185
"The Quality of Dyadic Relationships, Leisure Activities, and Health among Older Women" (Fitzpatrick), 49
"Questions & Answers: 200 H1N1 Flu ('Swine Flu') and You" (CDC), 136
"Quick Facts: Prenatal Care Overview" (March of Dimes), 7

R

Race/ethnicity
    asthma and, 102
    CAM use by, 176, 177(f9.4)
    cancer among African-Americans, 92
    death rates for cancer by sex, age, ethnicity, race, 95t–99t
    diabetes and, 104, 108(f5.9)
    heart disease and, 82, 85–86
    HIV/AIDS and, 142
    hypertension and, 90
    mental health disorders and, 60
    obesity and, 84
    suicide and, 173
    YPPL and, 23
Radiation
    for breast cancer, 100
    from diagnostic imaging techniques, 57
    for prostate cancer, 102
Raina, Parminder, 50
RAND Corporation, 49
"A Randomized Controlled Comparison of Family-Based Treatment and Supportive Psychotherapy for Adolescent Bulimia Nervosa" (le Grange), 167
"Randomized Phase II Trial of First-Line Trastuzumab Plus Docetaxel and Capecitabine Compared with Trastuzumab Plus Docetaxel in HER2-Positive Metastatic Breast Cancer" (Wardley et al.), 101
Rapid plasma reagin test, 57
Rasmussen, Kathleen M., 15
RDAs (recommended dietary allowances), 188
Reactive depression, 159
Recessive disorder, 68f
Recessive genes, 64
Recommended dietary allowances (RDAs), 188
Rectal cancer, 93–94
Reducing Suicide: A National Imperative (Goldsmith et al.), 45
"Reduction of Antibiotic Use in the Community Reduces the Rate of Colonization with Penicillin G-Nonsusceptible Streptococcus Pneumoniae" (Guillemot et al.), 129
Reflexes, 56
Rehabilitation, for stroke survivors, 88–89
Reiki, 190–191
"Rejuvenating the Immune System in Rheumatoid Arthritis" (Weyand), 113
"Relation between Pet Ownership and Heart Rate Variability in Patients with Healed Myocardial Infarcts" (Friedmann et al.), 50
Relationships, 49–50
Relaxation response, 186
"Reported Tuberculosis in the United States, 2008" (CDC), 139–140
Reproduction, human, 68–69
Research
    on Alzheimer's disease, 119–120
    on arthritis, 112–113
    on osteoporosis, 114–115
    on prevention of disease, 49
    stem cell research for PD, 119
    for suicide prevention, 47
Respiration, 54
Respiratory diseases
    asthma, 102–103
    asthma, prevalence of current, among persons of all ages, by age group, race/ethnicity, 103(f5.5)
    asthma, prevalence of current, among persons of all ages, by age group, sex, 103(f5.6)
    chronic obstructive pulmonary diseases, 103–104
    cigarette smoking among men, women, high school students, and mothers during pregnancy, 82f
    death rates for leading causes of death for all ages, 89f
    frequency of, among persons 18/older, 105t–106t
"Rethinking the Evidence Imperative: Why Patients Choose Complementary and Alternative Medicine" (Carboon), 178
Rett's disorder, 156–157
Reuters Health Information, 135
Rheumatic diseases. See Arthritis
Rheumatoid arthritis, 111, 113
Rice, Catherine, 155
"Rising Military Suicides" (Donnelly), 47
Risk factors
    for asthma, 102
    for breast cancer, 100
    for cancer, 91
    cigarette smoking among men, women, high school students, and mothers during pregnancy, 82f
    for colon/rectal cancer, 94
    for heart disease, 82–84
    for lung cancer, 93
"Risk of Acute Myocardial Infarction and Sudden Cardiac Death in Patients Treated with COX-2 Selective and Non-selective NSAIDs" (Graham et al.), 113
Ritonavir, 145
Rivastigmine, 122
Rofecoxib, 113–114
Rogers, Marilyn, 14–15
Rosamond, Wayne, 84–86
Rosen, Allison, B., 19
Ross, Lainie Friedman, 71
Rubella (German measles), 134

S

Sachs, Bernard, 77
"Safety and Tolerability of Putaminal AADC Gene Therapy for Parkinson's Disease" (Christine et al.), 119
Salmonellosis, 125
Saquinavir, 145
Sareen, Jitender, 47–48, 154–155

SARS (severe acute respiratory syndrome), 146–148

Sawitzke, Allen D., 189

SCD. *See* Sickle-cell disease

Schizophrenia, 160

"Schizophrenia" (NIMH), 160

School
- mental health, adolescent intervention programs, 45–46
- youth violence prevention at, 37–38

"School-Based Mental Health Checkups Lead to High Rates of Follow-up Care for Teens" (Flynn), 46

"A School-Based Program to Prevent Adolescent Dating Violence: A Cluster Randomized Trial" (Wolfe et al.), 38

"The Science behind the Human Genome Project" (Human Genome Project), 63

Screening
- adolescent mental health intervention programs, 45–46
- breast cancer, recommended screening for, 41*t*
- for breast/cervical cancers, 40–43
- for cancer, 92
- for colon/rectal cancer, 94
- Columbia University teen mental health screening program, 46(*t*2.7)
- diagnostic testing, 56–59
- genetic, for infant abnormalities, 66, 68
- guidelines for heart disease, depression, breast cancer, 40
- mammography use by selected age groups, 93*t*
- NBCCEDP, number of women served in, 42*f*
- for prostate cancer, 101–102
- recommended preventive services, 39, 39*t*

"Screening for Depression in Adults" (USPSTF), 40

Secondary prevention
- breast/cervical cancers, screening/early detection of, 40–43
- definition of, 35
- goals of, 38–39
- recommended preventive services, 39*t*
- USPSTF screening guidelines for heart disease, depression, breast cancer, 40

Secondhand smoking, 93

"Segregation of a Missense Mutation in the Amyloid Precursor Protein Gene with Familial Alzheimer's Disease" (Goate et al.), 120

Selective programs, for mental health prevention, 45

Selective serotonin reuptake inhibitors (SSRIs), 158, 163

Self-assessed health
- overview of, 30, 31
- persons who said health was excellent/very good, 31*f*
- persons who said health was excellent/very good, by age/sex, 32(*f*1.7)

persons who said health was excellent/very good, by race/ethnicity, 33*f*

status by sex, 32(*f*1.6)

Sensitivity, of diagnostic testing, 57

Sensory system test, 56

Sentinel lymph node (SLN) biopsy, 100

Separation anxiety disorder, 162–163

"Service Use by At-Risk Youths after School-Based Suicide Screening" (Gould et al.), 45–46

"SET-C Versus Fluoxetine in the Treatment of Childhood Social Phobia" (Beidel), 162

Severe acute respiratory syndrome (SARS), 146–148

Sexually transmitted diseases (STDs), 125
- *See also* Acquired immunodeficiency syndrome/human immunodeficiency virus (AIDS/HIV)

Shakespeare, William, 125

Sharma, Hari, 185

Shaw, Leslie M., 121

Shigellosis, 125

"Short-term Adapted Physical Activity Program Improves Bone Quality in Osteopenic/Osteoporotic Postmenopausal Women" (Tolomio et al.), 116

Shumway, Norman, 82

"Sickle Cell Disease: 10 Things You Need to Know" (CDC), 75

Sickle Cell Disease Association of America, Inc., 194

Sickle-cell disease (SCD)
- anemia, 75*f*
- cure for, 75–76
- inheritance of trait, 76*f*
- overview of, 74–75

Side effects
- of AIDS drugs, 145
- of antidepressants, 158*t*
- of bipolar disorder drugs, 160

Siegel, Jane D., 129

"Signs and Symptoms of Cancer" (American Cancer Society), 92

Single-gene disorders, 64

Situationally predisposed panic attacks, 161

Skin cancer
- overview of, 101
- primary prevention for, 35

Slavin, Thomas P., 71

SLE (systemic lupus erythematosus), 111–112

SLN (sentinel lymph node) biopsy, 100

Smith, Aaron, 114

Smith, Tyler C., 179–180

Smoking. *See* Tobacco

Social activities, 49–50

Social condition, mental illness as, 60

Social phobias, 161

Social services, for youth violence prevention, 38

Social supports
- health benefits of, 49–50
- mind-body interventions and, 185

Social wellness
- definition of, 1
- mental illness and, 151

Son, Heesook, 50

"Spanish flu," 135

Specificity, of diagnostic testing, 57

Sphygmomanometer, 54, 89

Spina bifida
- common neural tube defect, 59
- description of, 16
- rates of, 17(*f*1.2)

"Spina Bifida" (March of Dimes), 16

Spinal manipulation, 190

"Spinal Manipulation for Low-Back Pain" (NCCAM), 190

Spiritual wellness, 1

Spleen examination, 55

SSRIs (selective serotonin reuptake inhibitors), 158, 163

Staph infections, MRSA, 129

Staphylococcus aureus, 129

States
- flu activity by state, week ending January 2, 2010, 138*f*
- flu activity by state, week ending October 17, 2009, 137*f*
- Lyme disease cases, geographic distribution of, 147*f*
- newborn screening programs in, 66, 68
- West Nile virus activity, geographic distribution of, 148*f*

"States Expand Newborn Screening for Life-Threatening Disorders" (March of Dimes), 66

Statistical information
- activity, limitation of, caused by chronic health conditions among older adults, by age, 109(*f*5.11)
- activity, limitation of, caused by chronic health conditions among working-age adults, by age, 109(*f*5.10)
- AIDS, estimated numbers of cases/rates of, by race/ethnicity, age, sex, 143*t*
- AIDS cases, estimated numbers of, by year of diagnosis, characteristics of persons, 144*t*
- arthritis, projected prevalence of physician-diagnosed, among adults aged 18/older, 112*t*
- asthma, prevalence of current, among persons of all ages, by age group, race/ethnicity, 103(*f*5.5)
- asthma, prevalence of current, among persons of all ages, by age group, sex, 103(*f*5.6)
- autism spectrum disorder, changes in prevalence of, 156*f*
- CAM, diseases/conditions for which adults use, 180*f*

CAM, use of, 176(*f*9.2)

CAM therapies used by adults, 178*f*

CAM therapies used by children, 181(*f*9.9)

CAM use by age, 177(*f*9.3)

CAM use by race/ethnicity, 177(*f*9.4)

children using CAM, based on use by parents or relatives, 181(*f*9.8)

children with emotional/behavioral difficulties, 152(*f*8.2)

cigarette smoking among men, women, high school students, mothers during pregnancy, 82*f*

crude birth rates/fertility rates, birth rates, by mother's age/race/Hispanic origin 1950–2006, 3*t*–6*t*

crude birth/fertility/birth rates by mother's age/race/Hispanic origin 1970–2005, 8*t*

death, leading causes of, numbers of, by age, 29*t*–30*t*

death, ten leading causes of/death rates of, 80*f*

death rates for cancer by sex, age, ethnicity, race, 95*t*–99*t*

death rates for leading causes of death for all ages, 89*f*

deaths, causes/numbers of, by sex/race/Hispanic origin, 20*t*–23*t*

depressive episode, adolescents who had, 153(*f*8.3)

diabetes, prevalence of diagnosed, among adults aged 18 years/over, 107*f*

diabetes, prevalence of diagnosed, among adults aged 18 years/over, by age group, sex, 108(*f*5.8)

diabetes, prevalence of diagnosed, among adults aged 18 years/over, by race/ethnicity, 108(*f*5.9)

diseases/conditions for which children use CAM, 182(*f*9.11)

Down syndrome, prevalence of, 69(*t*4.3)

flu activity by state, week ending January 2, 2010, 138*f*

flu activity by state, week ending October 17, 2009, 137*f*

H1N1 hospitalizations/deaths, 136*f*

health conditions/risk factors, 87*t*

high blood pressure in adults age 20/older, 83*t*–84*t*

high cholesterol levels in adults age 20/older, 85*t*–86*t*

infant mortality rates, international rankings of, 18*t*

infant/neonatal/postnatal mortality rates, 17(*f*1.3)

LBW births by mother's age, 16*f*

LBW births by race/ethnicity/state, 14*t*–15*t*

LBW live births, 12*t*–13*t*

life expectancy at birth/age 65, by race/sex, 19*f*

Lyme disease, reported cases of, 146*f*

Lyme disease cases, geographic distribution of, 147*f*

mammography use by selected age groups, 93*t*

meditation, types of populations/conditions included in studies on, 187*t*–188*t*

mental distress, Americans reporting frequent, 152(*f*8.1)

natural products used by adults, 179*f*

natural products used by children, 182(*f*9.10)

notifiable diseases, reported cases of, 127*t*–128*t*

obesity, prevalence of, among adults aged 20 years/older, 88*f*

Pap smear use by selected age groups, 94*t*

persons who said health was excellent/very good, 31*f*

persons who said health was excellent/very good by age/sex, 32(*f*1.7)

persons who said health was excellent/very good by race/ethnicity, 33*f*

pregnancy, weight gain recommendations during, 16*t*

prenatal care, early, 9*t*–10*t*

psychological distress, adults with, in past 30 days, 153(*f*8.4)

psychological distress, adults with, in past 30 days, by age group/sex, 154(*f*8.5)

psychological distress, adults with, in past 30 days, by race/ethnicity, 154(*f*8.6)

respiratory diseases, frequency of, among persons 18/older, 105*t*–106*t*

self-assessed health status by sex, 32(*f*1.6)

spina bifida, rates of, 17(*f*1.2)

TB, multidrug-resistant, in persons with no previous TB, by origin of birth, 141*t*

TB, multidrug-resistant, in persons with previous history of TB, by origin of birth, 142*t*

TB cases, reported, 139*f*

TB cases in foreign-born persons, 140(*f*7.7)

TB cases in U.S.-born vs. foreign-born people, 140(*f*7.8)

West Nile virus activity, geographic distribution of, 148*f*

YPLL before age 75 by sex/race, 24*t*–28*t*

Stem cell research, 119

Stents, 80, 81

Stethoscope, 54, 55

Stevens, Martin J., 191

Stewart, Kerry J., 116

Stewart, Susan T., 19

Stigma, social, 151

Stomach cancer, 90–91

Stool occult blood test, 57

Stool test, 94

Streptococcus pneumoniae, 127–128

"Streptococcus Pneumoniae: Does Antimicrobial Resistance Matter?" (Lynch & Zhanel), 127–128

Stress
   meditation and, 186
   mind-body interventions and, 185
   work stress and health, 49

Stroke (cerebrovascular disease)
   as complication of diabetes, 43
   death rates for leading causes of death for all ages, 89*f*
   deaths from, 79, 88
   effects of, 86–88
   prevention of diabetes complications, 44
   rehabilitation for survivors, 88–89
   women and, 85

Sudden infant death syndrome, 17–18

Suicide
   active military/veterans at risk for, 47–49
   adolescent mental health intervention programs and, 45–46
   among terminally ill, 173–174
   Columbia University teen mental health screening program, 46(*t*2.7)
   death rates, by sex/race/Hispanic origin/age, 169*t*–172*t*
   overview of, 168
   persons at risk, 173
   prevention, 46–47
   reasons for, 173
   risk factors, protective factors, national prevention strategy, 46(*t*2.8)
   risk, warning signs for, 48*t*
   warning signs, 174

"Suicide Facts at a Glance" (NIH), 46–47

"Suicide in the U.S." (NIMH), 173

"Suicide in the U.S.: Statistics and Prevention" (NIMH), 168

"Suicide Prevention: A Leadership Challenge for All" (Chandler), 48

Summary Health Statistics for U.S. Children: National Health Interview Survey, 2008 (NCHS), 102

Surgery
   for breast cancer, 100
   bypass surgery, 80–81
   coronary artery bypass graft surgery, 80–81
   heart transplants, 81–82
   for prostate cancer, 102

Surveillance, 37, 48

Survival rate
   for breast cancer, 100
   for prostate cancer, 102

Survivors
   of cancer, 90–91
   of stroke, 88–89

"Survivors of Childhood Cancer" (Jenney & Levitt), 91

Swine flu. *See* H1N1 influenza (swine flu)

Symptomatic genetic testing, 70
Symptoms
    of Alzheimer's disease, 120
    of cancer, 92
    of depression, 157t
    of diabetes, 104
    of H1N1 flu, 136
    of influenza, 134
    in medical history, 53–54
    of multiple sclerosis, 116
    of Parkinson's disease, 118
    of SARS, 146–147
    of SLE (systemic lupus erythematosus),
        112
    of suicide, 174
Syphilis, 125
Sysko, Robin, 167
"A Systematic Review of the Therapeutic
    Effects of Reiki" (vanderVaart et al.), 191
Systemic lupus erythematosus (SLE),
    111–112
Systolic blood pressure, 54, 82

T

Tacrine, 122
Taglieri, Nevio, 81
Tay, Warren, 76–77
Tay-Sachs disease (TSD), 76–77
TB. See Tuberculosis
TCM (traditional Chinese medicine), 185
Teenagers. See Adolescents
TeenScreen National Center for Mental
    Health Checkups, 46
TeenScreen program, Columbia University,
    45–46, 46(t2.7)
Temperature, 54
"Tenofovir DF, Emtricitabine, and
    Efavirenz vs. Zidovudine, Lamivudine,
    and Efavirenz for HIV" (Gallant et al.),
    145
"Ten-Year Risk of First Recurrent Stroke
    and Disability after First-Ever Stroke in
    the Perth Community Stroke Study"
    (Hardie), 88
Terminally ill, suicide among, 173–174
Terrorism, biological, 148–149
Tertiary prevention
    definition of, 35
    of diabetes, 43–44
Testing
    children for adult-onset disorders, 70–71
    DNA-based gene tests, 66t
    genetic, ethical considerations, 71–72
    genetic, overview of, 65–66, 68
    prenatal genetic, 68–69
    symptomatic genetic, 70
    See also Diagnostic testing; Screening
Tetanus, 134

"Tetrabenazine as Anti-chorea Therapy in
    Huntington Disease: An Open-Label
    Continuation Study" (Frank), 74
Texas, Vioxx case in, 114
Thornton, Timothy N., 37–38
"3-Year Followup of the NIMH MTA
    Study" (Jensen), 164
Throat culture test, 58
Thun, Michael J., 91
Thyroid stimulating hormone (TSH), 57
Ticks, 146
Tobacco
    asthma and, 102
    chronic bronchitis from, 104
    cigarette smoking among men, women,
        high school students, and mothers
        during pregnancy, 82f
    as heart disease risk factor, 82
    as risk factor for cancer, 91, 93
Tolomio, S., 116
Traditional Chinese medicine (TCM), 185
Traditional medical settings
    CAM use in, 181–182
    Reiki in, 191
Traits, genetic. See Inheritance, genetic
Transcendental meditation, 186
Transmission
    of HIV/AIDS, 142–143
    of tuberculosis, 138–139
Transplants, heart, 81–82
Trastuzumab, 101
Treatment
    of AIDS, 143–145
    of Alzheimer's disease, 121–122
    of arthritis, 112–114
    of breast cancer, 100, 101
    of colorectal cancer, 94
    for heart attack, 79–80
    of heart disease, 80–81
    of hypertension, 90
    of mental disorders, numbers seeking,
        154–155
    of mental illness, 60
    of multiple sclerosis, 117
    of osteoporosis, 115–116, 116f
    of Parkinson's disease, 118–119
    of prostate cancer, 102
    of SLE, 112
    tertiary prevention of diabetes, 43–44
"The Treatment for Adolescents with
    Depression Study (TADS): Long-Term
    Effectiveness and Safety Outcomes"
    (March et al.), 158
Treatment of Children with Mental Illness
    (NIMH), 167
"Treatment Preferences for CAM in
    Children with Chronic Pain" (Tsao et
    al.), 186
"Trends in Antipsychotic Drug Use by Very
    Young, Privately Insured Children"
    (Olfsen et al.), 160

*Trends in Spina Bifida and Anencephalus in
    the United States, 1991–2006*
    (Mathews), 16
Tricyclic antidepressants, 158
Triglycerides, 44
Triple-marker screen, 68–69
Tripterygium wilfordii Hook F (Chinese
    Thunder God vine), 185
Tsao, Jennie C., 186
TSD (Tay-Sachs disease), 76–77
TSH (thyroid stimulating hormone), 57
Tuberculosis (TB)
    cases, reported, 139f
    cases in foreign-born persons, 140(f7.7)
    cases in U.S.-born vs. foreign-born
        people, 140(f7.8)
    comeback of, 139–141
    description of, 138–139
    latent TB infection/TB disease, 139t
    multidrug-resistant, in persons with no
        previous TB, by origin of birth, 141t
    multidrug-resistant, in persons with
        previous history of TB, by origin of
        birth, 142t
    number of cases of, 126
Tumors
    benign/malignant, 90
    breast cancer treatment, 100
"Twelve-Month Use of Mental Health
    Services in the United States: Results
    from the National Comorbidity Survey
    Replication" (Wang), 154–155
*2009 Alzheimer's Disease Facts and
    Figures* (Alzheimer's Association), 119
Type 1 diabetes mellitus
    causes of, 105–106
    double diabetes, 107–108
    prevention of, 43
    symptoms of, 104
Type 2 diabetes mellitus
    causes of, 105–106
    description of, prevention of, 43
    double diabetes, 107–108
    symptoms of, 104

U

Ultrasound, 57, 58
"Understanding the Relation between
    Anorexia Nervosa and Bulimia Nervosa
    in a Swedish National Twin Sample"
    (Bulik), 166
United Network for Organ Sharing, 194
United States
    flu activity by state, week ending
        January 2, 2010, 138f
    flu activity by state, week ending
        October 17, 2009, 137f
    H1N1 flu in, 136–138
    health in, 2
    HIV/AIDS in, 141–142

infectious diseases and, 125

mental health in, 151–155

TB, multidrug-resistant, in persons with no previous TB, by origin of birth, 141*t*

TB in, 139–141

TB cases in U.S.-born vs. foreign-born people, 140(*f*7.8)

West Nile virus activity, geographic distribution of, 148*f*

"Universal, selective, and indicated prevention model," 45

Universal programs, for mental health prevention, 45

"An Update on Community-Associated MRSA Virulence" (Kobayashi & DeLeo), 129

Urinalysis, 58

Urine culture test, 58

U.S. Air Force, 48–49

U.S. Department of Health and Human Services (HHS)

action plan to achieve goals of, 51*f*

avian influenza and, 135–136

on childhood depression, 159

on children with OCD, 163

Healthy People 2020, 50–51

on mental health, 151

on physical activity, 83

U.S. Department of Veterans Affairs (VA)

on identification of troops/veterans at risk for suicide, 47

suicide prevention program of, 48

U.S. Food and Drug Administration (FDA)

on antidepressants, 158

arthritis drug treatment and, 113–114

on aztreonam, 73

dietary supplements and, 188, 189

H5N1 vaccine, 135

on prescribing psychoactive drugs to children, 167–168

U.S. Library of Medicine, 64

U.S. military

suicide, active military/veterans at risk for, 47–49

suicide risk, warning signs for, 48*t*

use of CAM, 179–180

U.S. Preventive Services Task Force (USPSTF)

mammogram guidelines of, 92

recommended preventive services, 39, 39*t*

screening guidelines for heart disease, depression, breast cancer, 40

"Using Nontraditional Risk Factors in Coronary Heart Disease Risk Assessment" (USPSTF), 40

"Using Serial Registered Brain Magnetic Resonance Imaging to Measure Disease Progression in Alzheimer Disease" (Fox et al.), 121

USPSTF. *See* U.S. Preventive Services Task Force

"USPSTF Mammography Recommendations Will Result in Countless Unnecessary Breast Cancer Deaths Each Year" (Lee), 40

Usui, Mikao, 190

Uterine cancer, 90–91

"Utilization of Ayurveda in Health Care: An Approach for Prevention, Health Promotion, and Treatment of Disease. Part 1—Ayurveda, the Science of Life" (Sharma et al.), 185

V

VA. *See* U.S. Department of Veterans Affairs

Vaccine

for avian influenza, 135

for biodefense, 149

for H1N1 flu, 136–137

for HPV, 42

immunization for prevention, 132–134

immunization schedule, recommended for adults, by vaccine, age group, 132*f*

for influenza, 134

for Lyme disease, 145–146

vaccines recommended for some adults based on medical/other indications, 133*f*

"Vaccines for Preventing Anthrax" (Donegan, Bellamy, & Gamble), 149

Valdecoxib, 113

Validity, of diagnostic testing, 56–57

VanderVaart, Sondra, 191

Varicella (chicken pox), 125, 134

Vector-borne disease, 145

Venereal Disease Research Laboratory, 57

Very low birth weight (VLBW). *See* Low birth weight

Veterans

suicide, active military/veterans at risk for, 47–49

suicide risk, warning signs for, 48*t*

Vioxx, 113–114

"Vioxx Trial Loss Raises Merck Strategy Questions" (Associated Press), 114

Virus, 134

Vital health statistics, 2

Vital signs, 54

Vitamin D, 115

Vitamin E, 122, 188

"Vitamin E Use Is Associated with Improved Survival in an Alzheimer's Disease Cohort" (Pavlik et al.), 122

VLBW (very low birth weight). *See* Low birth weight

W

Waite, Linda J., 50

Walker, Sydney, III, 53

Wang, Philip S., 154–155

Wardley, Andrew, 101

Warfarin, 88

"Warning on Body Building Products Marketed as Containing Steroids or Steroid-Like Substances" (FDA), 189

Warning signs

of cancer, 92

of diabetes, 104

of heart attack, 79

of Parkinson's disease, 118

Washington State, physician-assisted suicide in, 174

Wechsler, Michael E., 103

Weight

mortality rates and, 19

mother's, effect on LBW, 15

See also Low birth weight; Obesity

Weight Gain during Pregnancy: Reexamining the Guidelines (Rasmussen), 15

Wellness, 1–2

See also Health/wellness

Wender, Paul H., 164

West Nile virus, 146, 148*f*

"West Nile Virus: Statistics, Surveillance, and Control" (CDC), 146

Weyand, Cornelia M., 113

"What Causes ADHD?" (NIMH), 163

"What Causes MS?" (National Multiple Sclerosis Society), 117

"What Is CAM?" (NCCAM), 185

"What Is Sickle Cell Anemia?" (National Heart Lung and Blood Institute), 75

"What Is TB?" (CDC), 139

"Which Groups Have Special Needs When Taking Psychiatric Medications?" (NIMH), 168

Whites, hypertension and, 90

WHO. *See* World Health Organization

"Who Gets MS" (National Multiple Sclerosis Society), 116–117

Wiesner, Georgia L., 71

Wilson, G. Terrence, 165

"Window on the Brain" (Mazziotta), 121

Witt, Claudia M., 183

Wolen, Aaron R., 50

Wolfe, David A., 38

Women. *See* Females

"Women and Cardiovascular Diseases— Statistics 2010" (American Heart Association), 84, 88

"Women's Decisions Regarding Tamoxifen for Breast Cancer Prevention: Responses to a Tailored Decision Aid" (Fagerlin), 70

Work, 49

World Health Organization (WHO)

on avian influenza, 135

definition of health, 1

on H1N1 flu, 136, 138
on infectious diseases, 125
mental illness diagnosis guidelines, 59
on monogenic diseases, 75
Worldwide, HIV/AIDS, 141
Wu, Joanne, 182
Wyatt, Gwen, 178

X

X-linked recessive inheritance, 65*f*
X-rays, 57–58
Xu, Xiaohui, 11, 14

Y

Years of potential life lost (YPLL)
before age 75 by sex/race, 24*t*–28*t*
age and, 23, 29–30
overview of, 20–23
race/gender and, 23
Young, Saundra, 42
"Youth Risk Behavior Surveillance—
United States, 2007" (CDC), 37
Youth violence prevention
goal/objectives of goal, 38(*t*2.3)
mentoring activities, 38(*t*2.4)
possible settings for interventions, 38(*t*2.2)

potential participant groups for
interventions, 37*t*
primary prevention, 37–38
YPLL. *See* Years of potential life lost
Yu, Junying, 119

Z

Zanamivir, 138
Zaslavsky, Alan M., 56
Zbierajewski-Eischeid, Samantha J., 86
ZDV (zidovudine), 143
Zhanel, George G., 127–128
Zidovudine (ZDV), 143